# Pediatric Imaging

## CASE REVIEW

### Third Edition

**Aylin Tekes-Brady, MD**
Associate Professor of Radiology
Deputy Director, Division of Pediatric Radiology and
    Pediatric Neuroradiology
Director, Pediatric Radiology Fellowship Program and
    Education
Johns Hopkins Hospital
Baltimore, Maryland

**Daniel P. Seeburg, MD, PhD**
Practicing Radiologist
Charlotte Radiology
Charlotte, North Carolina

**Thierry A.G.M. Huisman, MD, EDiNR, EDiPNR**
Professor of Radiology, Pediatrics, Neurology and
    Neurosurgery
Chairman, Department of Imaging and Imaging Science,
    JHBMC
Director, Pediatric Radiology and Pediatric Neuroradiology,
    JHH
Co-Director, Neurosciences Intensive Care Nursery, JHH
Co-Director, Children's Center Fetal Program, JHH
Co-Director, Center for Translational and Molecular
    Imaging, JHBMC
Johns Hopkins Medicine
Baltimore, Maryland

**ELSEVIER**

# ELSEVIER

1600 John F. Kennedy Blvd.
Ste 1800
Philadelphia, PA 19103-2899

PEDIATRIC IMAGING: CASE REVIEW, 3rd edition       ISBN: 978-0-323-44728-7

---

### Notices

Knowledge and best practice in this field are constantly changing. As new research and experience broaden our understanding, changes in research methods, professional practices, or medical treatment may become necessary.

Practitioners and researchers must always rely on their own experience and knowledge in evaluating and using any information, methods, compounds, or experiments described herein. In using such information or methods they should be mindful of their own safety and the safety of others, including parties for whom they have a professional responsibility.

With respect to any drug or pharmaceutical products identified, readers are advised to check the most current information provided (i) on procedures featured or (ii) by the manufacturer of each product to be administered, to verify the recommended dose or formula, the method and duration of administration, and contraindications. It is the responsibility of practitioners, relying on their own experience and knowledge of their patients, to make diagnoses, to determine dosages and the best treatment for each individual patient, and to take all appropriate safety precautions.

To the fullest extent of the law, neither the Publisher nor the authors, contributors, or editors, assume any liability for any injury and/or damage to persons or property as a matter of products liability, negligence or otherwise, or from any use or operation of any methods, products, instructions, or ideas contained in the material herein.

---

**Library of Congress Cataloging-in-Publication Data**

Names: Tekes-Brady, Aylin, author. | Seeburg, Daniel P., author. | Huisman, Thierry A. G. M., author.
Title: Pediatric imaging : case review / Aylin Tekes-Brady, Daniel P. Seeburg, Thierry A.G.M. Huisman.
Other titles: Case review series.
Description: Third edition. | Philadelphia, PA : Elsevier, Inc., [2018] | Series: Case review series | Preceded by: Case review: pediatric imaging / Thierry A.G.M. Huisman ... [et al.]. 2nd ed. c2011. | Includes bibliographical references and index.
Identifiers: LCCN 2017001880 | ISBN 9780323447287 (pbk. : alk. paper)
Subjects: | MESH: Diagnostic Imaging–methods | Child | Infant | Pediatrics–methods | Case Reports | Problems and Exercises
Classification: LCC RJ51.R3 | NLM WN 18.2 | DDC 618.92/007575–dc23 LC record available at https://lccn.loc.gov/2017001880

*Content Strategist:* Robin Carter
*Content Development Specialist:* Meghan Andress
*Publishing Services Manager:* Patricia Tannian
*Project Manager:* Ted Rodgers
*Design Direction:* Renee Duenow

Printed in the United States of America

Last digit is the print number:   9   8   7   6   5   4   3   2   1

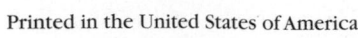

Working together
to grow libraries in
developing countries

www.elsevier.com • www.bookaid.org

# Pediatric Imaging

## CASE REVIEW

### Third Edition

Series Editor

**David M. Yousem, MD, MBA**
Professor of Radiology
Director of Neuroradiology
Russell H. Morgan Department of Radiology and Radiological Science
The Johns Hopkins Medical Institutions
Baltimore, Maryland

**Other Volumes in the CASE REVIEW Series**

I have been very gratified by the popularity and positive feedback that the authors of the Case Review series have received on the publication of the editions of their volumes. Reviews in journals and online sites as well as word-of-mouth comments have been uniformly favorable. The authors have done an outstanding job in filling the niche of an affordable, easy-to-access, case-based learning tool that supplements the material in The Requisites series. I have been told by residents, fellows, and practicing radiologists that the Case Review series books are the ideal means for studying for oral board examinations and subspecialty certification tests.

Although some students learn best in a non-interactive study book mode, others need the anxiety or excitement of being quizzed. The selected format for the Case Review series (which consists of showing a few images needed to construct a differential diagnosis and then asking a few clinical and imaging questions) was designed to simulate the board examination experience. The only difference is that the Case Review books provide the correct answer and immediate feedback. The limit and range of the reader's knowledge are tested through scaled cases ranging from relatively easy to very hard. The Case Review series also offers feedback on the answers, a brief discussion of each case, a link back to the pertinent The Requisites volume, and up-to-date references from the literature. In addition, we have recently included labeled figures, figure legends, and supplemental figures in a new section at the end of the book, which provide the reader more information about the case and diagnosis.

Because of the popularity of online learning, we have been rolling out new editions on the web. We also have adjusted to the new Boards format, which will be electronic and largely case-based. We are ready for the new boards! The Case Reviews are now hosted online at www.expertconsult.com, powered by Inkling. The interactive test-taking format allows users to get real-time feedback, "pinch-and-zoom" figures for easier viewing, and link to supplemental figures and online references. Personally, I am very excited about the future. Join us.

**David M. Yousem, MD, MBA**

Over the years I have come to appreciate that pediatric radiology is not at all the imaging of adult diseases in children. The entities that people in this specialty must address are very often unique and cannot be compared to the adult world. It is no surprise then that this specialty has its own ACGME-approved fellowship, societies, guidelines, and identity. To learn pediatric radiology, you must read pediatrics-specific books. At the Case Review Series, we got you covered.

The third edition *of Pediatric Imaging: Case Review* by my friends and colleagues, Drs. Aylin Tekes-Brady, Daniel P. Seeburg, and Thierry A.G.M. Huisman, builds on the success of the second edition. It includes question-and-answer cases that emphasize fetal, neonatal, infant, and childhood diseases. In addition, this version is unique in its inclusion of material from the non-interpretive skills arena, physics, and radiation safety policies. As always you will find the popular format of the Case Review Series: excellent quality images, multiple choice boards-style questions, accurate answers, graphic explanations, and up-to-date references and links back to the Requisites series textbook.

Congratulations to Drs. Tekes-Brady, Seeburg, and Huisman for bringing us the new and improved *Pediatric Imaging: Case Review*, 3rd edition.

**David M. Yousem, MD, MBA**

The 3rd edition of *Pediatric Imaging: Case Review* is fully revised, taking into account the most up-to-date advances in pediatric imaging. High-yield exemplary cases of common, rare but classic, or do not miss/do not overcall cases of childhood diseases from fetus to young adults are presented. Utility of imaging modalities, common and variant imaging findings, and imaging information relevant to management morbidity/mortality are presented with questions and multiple choices and followed by brief text to match the format of the ABR core and certifying examinations.

The contributing authors have been carefully selected. In addition to a high level of overall expertise, we aimed to include experts with many levels of professional experience. Dr. Daniel P. Seeburg graduated from the Johns Hopkins radiology residency program after he had served as chief resident. His contributions guarantee that the selected cases are in tune with the needs of a trainee. Dr. Aylin Tekes-Brady provides 10-plus years of experience in academic pediatric radiology and pediatric neuroradiology, while Dr. Thierry A.G.M. Huisman contributes the most senior member of the editorial board with national and international recognition in pediatric radiology and pediatric neuroradiology. Our case review book can serve as a launching point to familiarize yourself with pediatric radiology or an invitation to deepen your knowledge. Another way to use this book is to test your knowledge acquired in lectures, textbooks, and daily practice.

We sincerely thank our resident-fellow of 2016, Dr. Elizabeth Snyder, for contributing with the questions on QI/QA, and our physicist Dr. Mahadevappa Mahesh for contributions related to radiology physics.

**Aylin Tekes-Brady**
**Daniel P. Seeburg**
**Thierry A.G.M. Huisman**

*To my mother, Nurten Tekes, and to all women who have advanced
the education and knowledge of their fellow men and women in the journey
through life.*

**AYLIN TEKES-BRADY**

*To the loving memory of my father, who taught me to always question preconceived
ideas.*

**DANIEL SEEBURG**

*To all those parents who trust their most precious children in our hands.
It is always a privilege to become part of their life, either by an encounter during
an imaging study or a cheerful moment after a completed treatment.
But foremost by helping them to get healthy and happy.*

**THIERRY A.G.M. HUISMAN**

# TABLE OF CONTENTS

# Opening Round

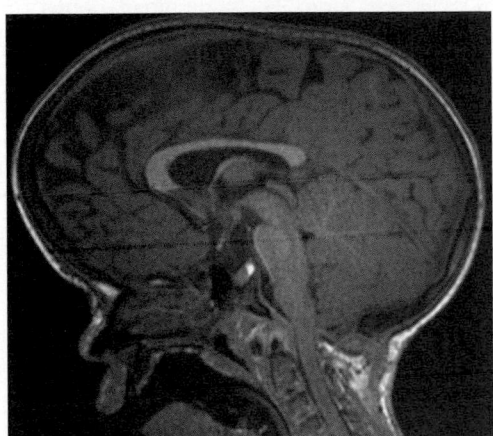

Fig. 1.1

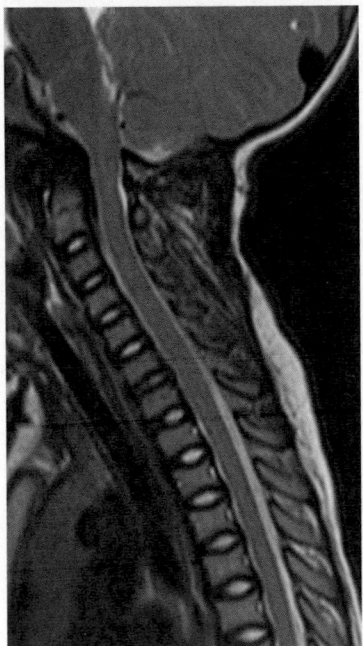

Fig. 1.2

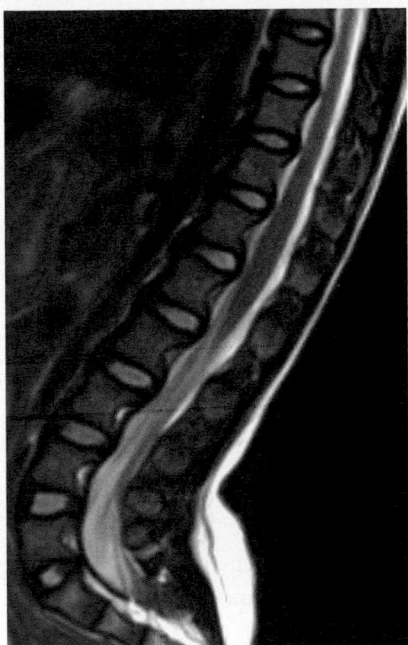

Fig. 1.3

1. What is the most common nonlethal skeletal dysplasia?
   A. Osteogenesis imperfecta
   B. Achondroplasia
   C. Thanatophoric dysplasia
   D. Hypochondroplasia

2. Which option represents classic imaging findings of achondroplasia?
   A. Occipital bossing
   B. Widening of the foramen magnum
   C. Flattening of the posterior vertebral bodies
   D. Reduced interpediculate distance

3. Which option is accurate for the achondroplasia phenotype?
   A. Rhizomelic shortening
   B. Frontal bossing, midface hypoplasia, saddle nose
   C. Exaggerated lumbar lordosis
   D. All of the above

4. Which option represents the most common mode of inheritance?
   A. Autosomal dominant
   B. X-linked
   C. Autosomal recessive
   D. New (de novo) mutations

## CASE 1

### Achondroplasia

1. B
2. D
3. D
4. D

### Comment

Achondroplasia is the most common nonlethal skeletal dysplasia and is caused by gain-of-function mutations of the fibroblast growth factor receptor 3 (FGR3) gene. The most common mode of inheritance is de novo mutations (80%), followed by autosomal dominant inheritance. Impaired endochondral growth results in stenosis of the foramen magnum and vertebral canal. The head is usually large with frontal bossing. Midface hypoplasia and relative tonsillar hypertrophy contribute to sleep apnea in these patients. Disproportionately short stature with rhizomelic shortening of the extremities is seen as a result of defective endochondral bone formation. Midface hypoplasia and saddle nose (flat nasal bridge) are typical facial features. In addition to foramen magnum stenosis, basilar impression can be seen. Decreased interpediculate distances are seen in the anteroposterior (AP) view of the spine, which become progressively smaller lower in the lumbar spine (opposite of normal). Vertebral bodies are short, flat, and bullet shaped in early life with a concave posterior surface (scalloping); there is also decreased height, which makes disc spaces look relatively large. Thoracolumbar gibbus or kyphosis in infancy normalizes after 4 to 6 years of age. The iliac wings are squared and hands have a trident look. There is increased lumbar lordosis as the child's ambulation increases. Cervical instability is a clinical concern. Foramen magnum stenosis leads to venous hypertension resulting in ventriculomegaly. Distal femoral epiphysis is chevron shaped. Genu varum and bowing of the legs are seen.

### Reference

Shirley ED, Ain MC. Achondroplasia: manifestations and treatment. *J Am Acad Orthop Surg*. 2009;17(4):231–241.

### Cross-reference

Walters MM, Robertson RL. *Pediatric Radiology: The Requisites*. 4th ed. Philadelphia: Elsevier. 2017:203–204.

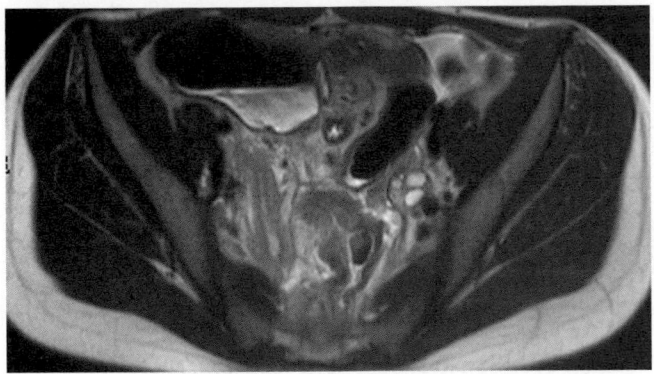

Fig. 2.1

1. What is the diagnosis?
   A. Ruptured right ovarian cyst
   B. Crohn disease
   C. Ruptured appendicitis with abscess
   D. Appendicitis

2. What are the pertinent imaging findings?
   A. Thickening wall of appendix in the right lower quadrant/pelvis with free fluid
   B. Thickened wall of the terminal ileum
   C. Enlarged ovarian cyst
   D. Enlarged salpinx with wall thickening

3. True or false?
   A. Appendicolith can be seen with plain film and computed tomography (CT) but not with ultrasonography (US).
   B. Presence of appendicolith requires surgical intervention.

4. True or false?
   A. ≥6-mm tubular blind-ending structure in the right lower quadrant is highly suggestive of appendicitis in a child presenting with right lower quadrant pain.

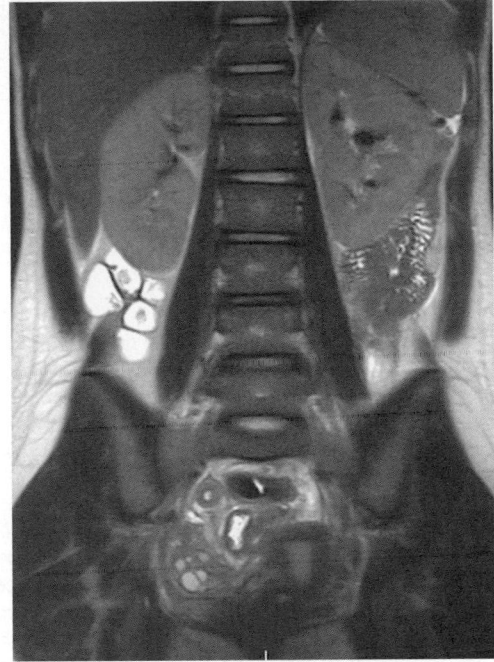

Fig. 2.2

   B. Thickened appendix wall with lumen diameter measuring 5 mm (from serosa to serosa) in a child with additional descending colon and rectal wall thickening is most suggestive of inflammatory bowel disease–related changes.

## CASE 2

### Appendicitis

1. D

2. A

3. A) False, B) False

4. A) True, B) True

### *Comment*

Acute appendicitis is the most common condition requiring emergent abdominal surgery in childhood. The clinical diagnosis of acute appendicitis may be challenging in cases presenting with atypical clinical findings. There has been a great deal of variability in the use of imaging modalities in children with this suspected diagnosis. The principal advantages of ultrasonography (US) are its lower cost, lack of ionizing radiation, and its ability to assess vascularity through color Doppler techniques and provide dynamic information through graded compression. The principal advantages of computed tomography (CT) include less operator dependency than US, as reflected by higher diagnostic accuracy in some studies, and enhanced delineation of disease extent in a perforated appendix. With the advent and use of quick T2-weighted imaging and its clinical applications, magnetic resonance imaging (MRI) has gained popularity in pediatric emergencies since the late 1990s. Cross-sectional imaging capability, lack of ionizing radiation exposure, and superior soft tissue contrast make MRI desirable not only for diagnosis, but also for safely ruling out the suspected differential diagnosis. Regarding technique, half-acquisition single-shot fast spin-echo (SSFSE) pulse sequences are crucial. Although gadolinium-enhanced T1-weighted pulse sequences might be helpful, any benefit beyond noncontrast MRI has not been confirmed. This protocol is successfully implemented in children 5 years and older without sedation or anesthesia, and has the advantage of short acquisition times and relative insensitivity of the SSFSE sequence to motion. Use of this protocol in children younger than 5 years of age is a case-by-case decision, and reasonable success rates can be obtained especially with the support of child life specialists.

In our institution, right lower quadrant and/or pelvic ultrasonography is the first line of imaging. In cases where the appendix cannot be seen, we proceed with MRI with the above-mentioned protocol. Each hospital or children's center should work on an imaging algorithm in pediatric appendicitis with a multidisciplinary approach that includes the emergency physicians, surgeons, and radiologists.

### References

Incesu L, Coskun A, Selcuk MB, Akan H, Sozubir S, Bernay F. Acute appendicitis: MR imaging and sonographic correlation. *Am J Roentgenol.* 1997;168(3):669–674.

Moore MM, Kulaylat AN, Hollenbeak CS, Engbrecht BW, Dillman JR, Methratta ST. Magnetic resonance imaging in pediatric appendicitis: a systematic review. *Pediatr Radiol.* 2016;46(6):928–939.

### Cross-reference

Walters MM, Robertson RL. *Pediatric Radiology: The Requisites.* 4th ed. Philadelphia: Elsevier; 2017:116.

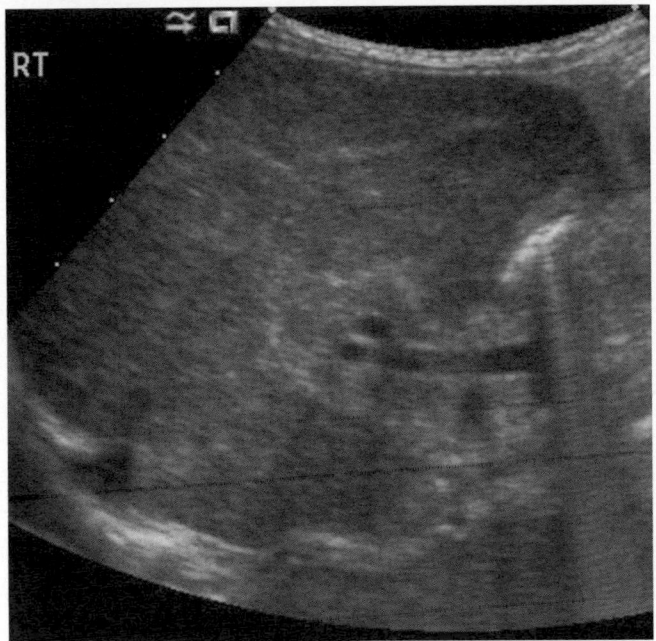

Fig. 3.1

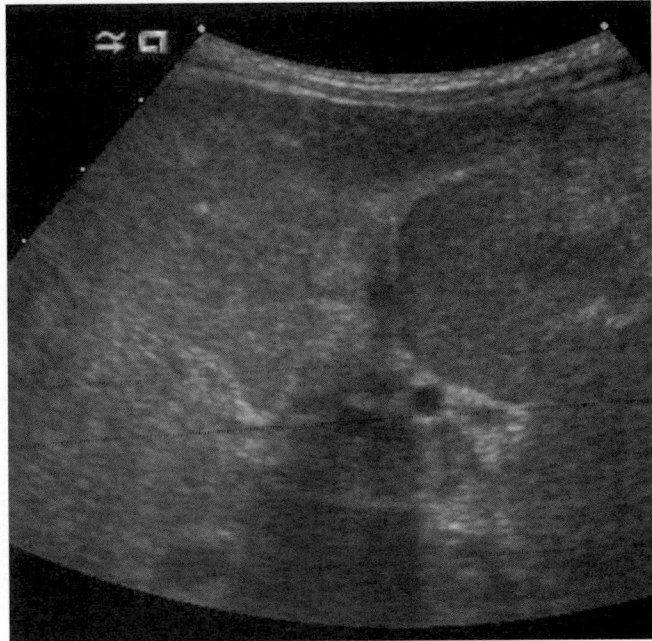

Fig. 3.2

**HISTORY:** Full term male neonate with jaundice

1. Which option is less likely in a neonate presenting with cholestasis?
   A. Biliary atresia
   B. Neonatal hepatitis
   C. Alagille syndrome
   D. All of the above are equally likely.

2. What is the most likely diagnosis in this patient?
   A. Biliary atresia
   B. Neonatal hepatitis
   C. Choledochal cyst
   D. Cystic fibrosis

3. True or false?
   A. Presence of gallbladder in liver ultrasound excludes biliary atresia.
   B. Best time to do ultrasound is 1 hour after feeding.

4. What is the best time to perform the Kasai procedure?
   A. First 8 days of life
   B. First 8 weeks of life
   C. Before kindergarten age
   D. Kindergarten age

## CASE 3

### Biliary Atresia

1. C

2. A

3. A) False, B) False

4. B

### Comment

Biliary atresia (BA) presents as an obliterative cholangiopathy with neonatal jaundice and pale stools. Although the exact cause is not known, viral infections, immune dysregulation, gene polymorphism, and toxins have been speculated. BA is a rare disorder (1 in 10,000 to 19,000 in Europe and North America), but it is one of the most common reasons for neonatal jaundice. Early diagnosis is critical because prognosis is highly related to timely surgical correction (ideally within 30 days); however, in most cases the average age at diagnosis is 60 days. The blockage of bile flow leads to hepatocyte injury, fibrosis, and cirrhosis. Bile duct absence can occur at any level; surgically approachable disease is confined to abnormality at the level of the right and left hepatic ducts and below.

Ultrasound can detect abnormalities that are highly associated with BA, although no sign is absolutely specific. At the organ level, heterotaxy (transverse liver, polysplenia, or asplenia) should raise suspicion that BA is also present. A gallbladder should be carefully searched for (but only after the infant has received nothing by mouth for 3 to 4 hours to maximize gallbladder distention). The presence of a gallbladder does not exclude BA; if it appears small and irregular, or if a thick, echogenic cord is found in the gallbladder bed, then BA may well be present. A gallbladder that does not contract after a milk feeding suggests obstruction by BA. Another echogenic cord paralleling the portal vein (triangular in cross-section) is thought to represent the fibrosed common duct. No proximal duct dilation occurs within the liver, although irregular bile lakes adjacent to portal triads may be seen.

Lack of isotope excretion into the bowel over 24 hours on nuclear medicine (technetium-99m iminodiacetic acid [99mTc-IDA]) scan can be helpful (as shown in this case) and is a classic finding. Ultrasound failed to show a gallbladder. Biopsy looks for bile duct proliferation, periportal fibrosis, and giant cell proliferation, but these findings also overlap findings for neonatal hepatitis.

In the Kasai procedure, the surgeon cuts back through the porta hepatis to expose patent bile ducts. A small bowel loop is then brought up to this hepatic plate to funnel the bile into the gastrointestinal tract. This procedure has its best chance of success if it is performed before the infant is 8 weeks old.

Reference

Verkade HJ, Bezerra JA, Davenport M, et al. Biliary atresia and other cholestatic childhood diseases: advances and future challenges. *J Hepatol*. 2016;65(3):631–642.

Cross-reference

Walters MM, Robertson RL. *Pediatric Radiology: The Requisites*. 4th ed. Philadelphia: Elsevier; 2017:118–120.

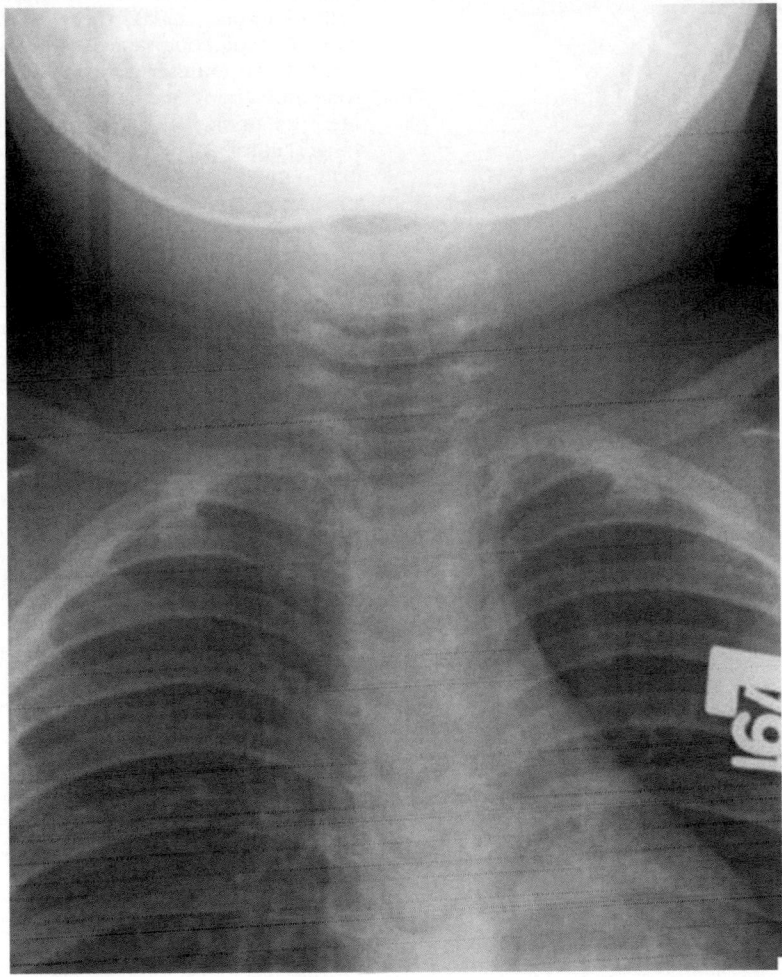

**Fig. 4.1**

**HISTORY:** Two-year-old child presenting with cough

1. Given the images presented, what is the best diagnosis?
   A. Epiglottitis
   B. Croup
   C. Exudative tracheitis
   D. Retropharyngeal abscess

2. What is the most common organism associated with croup?
   A. *Haemophilus influenzae* type B
   B. Group A beta-hemolytic *Streptococcus pneumonia*
   C. Parainfluenza virus
   D. *Moraxella catarrhalis*

3. What is the primary role of imaging in croup?
   A. To confirm the diagnosis
   B. To rule out other, more serious causes of upper airway obstruction
   C. To help plan treatment
   D. To look for complications

4. What causes the imaging appearance of the "steeple" sign?
   A. Inflammation and thickening of the aryepiglottic folds
   B. Inflammation and effacement of the pyriform sinus
   C. Inflammation and effacement of the subglottic arch
   D. Inflammation and obstruction of the laryngeal ventricle

## Croup

1. B
2. C
3. B
4. C

## Comment

Croup, or laryngotracheobronchiolitis, is the most common cause of acute upper airway obstruction in young children. Its peak incidence is between 3 months and 3 years. The most common causative organism is type I parainfluenza virus, and treatment is typically supportive. The diagnosis is normally made on clinical grounds. Initially the child may have mild cold symptoms, and as the airways become more inflamed a harsh barking cough may occur. Imaging is not routinely indicated because the diagnosis is often made clinically. Imaging is sometimes performed to rule out other, more serious causes of upper airway obstruction, including epiglottitis or retropharyngeal abscess. The "steeple" sign on the anteroposterior (AP) plain radiograph of the neck is due to mucosal edema of the subglottic larynx, which results in effacement of the normally rounded (inward concave) subglottic arch.

### Reference

Darras KE, Roston AT, Yewchuk LK. Imaging acute airway obstruction in infants and children. *Radiographics.* 2015;35(7):2064–2079.

### Cross-reference

Walters MM, Robertson RL. *Pediatric Radiology: The Requisites.* 4th ed. Philadelphia: Elsevier; 2017:16–17.

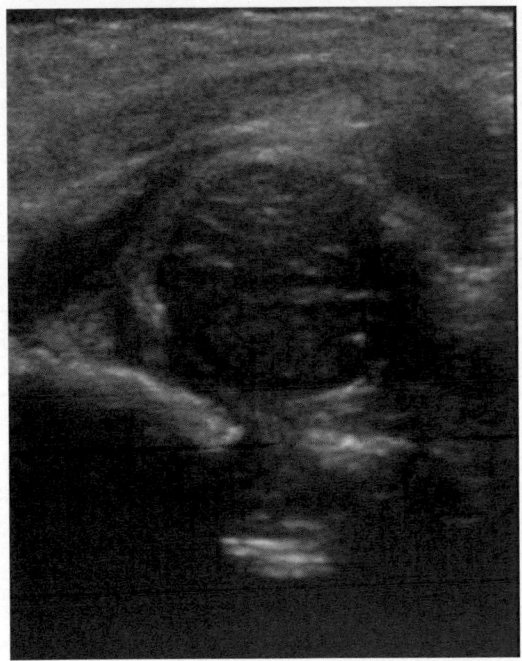

Fig. 5.1

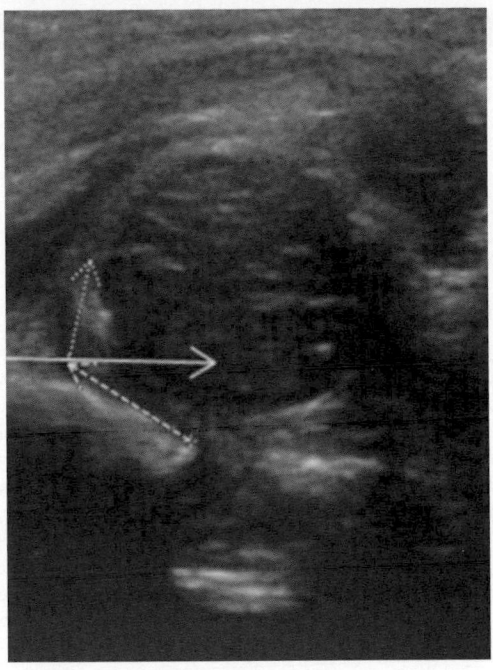

Fig. 5.2

**HISTORY:** Three-week old infant presenting with clicking sound in the hips

1. When is the best time to screen infants for this abnormality?
   A. Within the first 1 week after birth
   B. After about 2 to 4 weeks of age
   C. After 3 months
   D. After 6 months

2. All of the following are risk factors for developing developmental dysplasia of the hip (DDH), except:
   A. Male gender
   B. Multiple gestation
   C. Breech presentation
   D. Caucasian race

3. The normal alpha angle in an infant 6 weeks of age should be at least:
   A. 45 degrees
   B. 50 degrees
   C. 55 degrees
   D. 60 degrees

4. Which of the following is (are) the correct relationship(s) between the Perkin (perpendicular) line and the proximal femur? (Choose all that apply.)
   A. Intersects the femoral epiphysis
   B. Intersects the femoral metaphysis
   C. Lies lateral to the femoral epiphysis
   D. Lies lateral to the femoral metaphysis

## CASE 5

### Developmental Dysplasia of the Hip

1. B
2. A
3. B
4. B and C

## Comment

Developmental dysplasia of the hip (DDH) refers to a spectrum of abnormalities including abnormal development and configuration of the acetabulum, increased laxity of the ligaments around the hip, and femoral head malpositioning. Risk factors include female gender (F/M: 8/1), multiple gestation, breech presentation, positive family history, Caucasian race, and oligohydramnios. Imaging should be delayed in infants until 2 to 4 weeks after birth because maternal hormones linger and contribute to joint laxity. After 4 to 5 months, the femoral epiphyses begin to ossify, precluding good visualization with ultrasound and necessitating plain radiographs for optimum evaluation. In the immature hip on ultrasound (<3 months of age), alpha angles of more than 50 degrees are considered normal, with at least 45% coverage and no instability with stress maneuvers. After 3 months of age, the alpha angle should be more than 60 degrees, and there should be more than 50% coverage. On plain radiographs, the femoral epiphysis should be located in the lower inner quadrant, delineated by the crossing of the Hilgenreiner line (horizontal line through triradiate cartilages) and the Perkin line (vertical line through the upper outer margin of the acetabulum). The Perkin line should intersect the proximal femoral metaphysis, and the Shenton arch should be a continuous arc from the upper margin of the obturator foramen to the medial femoral metaphysis. The acetabular angle (angle between the acetabular roof and the Hilgenreiner line) should be less than 30 degrees. Magnetic resonance imaging is increasingly used for treatment planning and is now widely used in the postoperative period.

### Reference

Starr V, Ha BY. Imaging update on developmental dysplasia of the hip with the role of MRI. *AJR Am J Roentgenol*. 2014;203(6):1324-1335.

### Cross-reference

Walters MM, Robertson RL. *Pediatric Radiology: The Requisites*. 4th ed. Philadelphia: Elsevier; 2017:217-218.

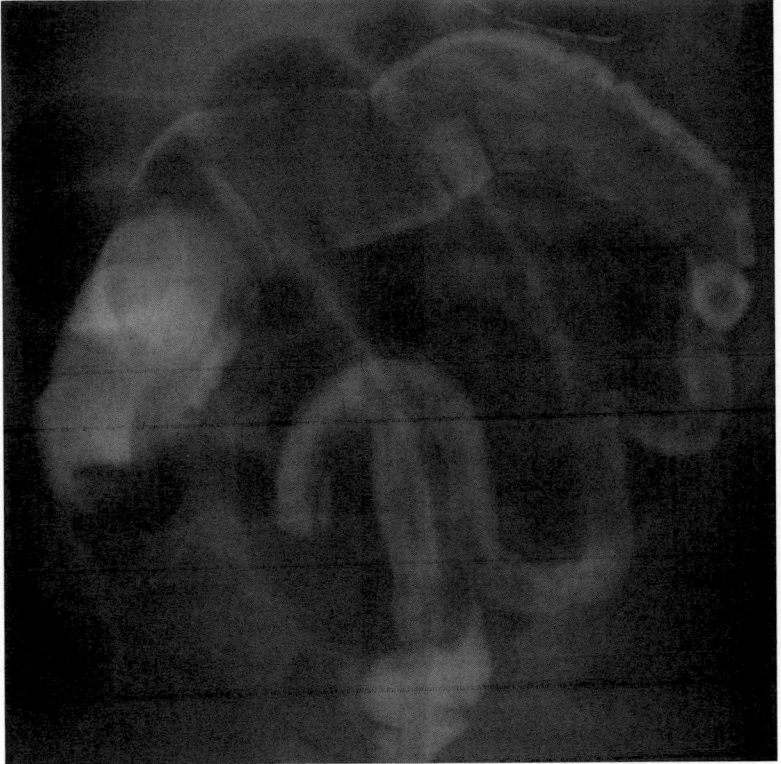

Fig. 6.1

1. What is your diagnosis?
   A. Small left colon syndrome
   B. Hirschsprung disease
   C. Crohn disease
   D. Meconium ileus

2. Which of the following are synonyms for this entity?
   A. Small left colon syndrome
   B. Meconium plug syndrome
   C. Functional immaturity of the colon
   D. A, B, and C

3. Which of the following imaging features is not part of meconium plug syndrome?
   A. Small-caliber sigmoid and descending colon to the level of the splenic flexure
   B. Multiple filling defects in the distal colon
   C. Multiple dilated bowel loops
   D. All of the above.

4. Which option best describes the most appropriate counseling for parents with children diagnosed with functional immaturity of the colon?
   A. This is a temporary state that usually resolves within a few days.
   B. An enema is not therapeutic; surgery is needed in almost 45% of cases.
   C. A rectal biopsy should be performed.
   D. None of the above.

## CASE 6

### Meconium Plug Syndrome

1. A
2. D
3. D
4. A

### Comment

Meconium plug syndrome (MPS) is a transient functional colonic obstruction of the newborn. Neonates typically present with abdominal distention, delayed passage of meconium, and sometimes bilious emesis. Increased incidence of meconium plug is seen in infants of diabetic mothers or mothers who received magnesium sulfate. MPS is an example of low intestinal obstruction in a neonate. Differential diagnosis include, Hirchsprung disease Colonic atresia, Meconium ileus, Ileal atresia Anorectal malformations. Plain abdominal radiography shows multiple dilated bowel loops as in neonatal distal bowel obstruction, and therefore an enema is the next diagnostic step. Remember that dilated large versus small bowel loops cannot be reliably differentiated in neonates by morphology or size!

A water-soluble low osmolality contrast enema is recommended because barium may hinder passage of meconium. The enema shows a small-caliber left colon to the level of the splenic flexure, with an abrupt transition to normal or mildly dilated proximal colon. The rectosigmoid ratio is typically >1. An enema is usually diagnostic and therapeutic. Meconium plugs in the left colon are not the cause, but are secondary to functional obstruction. MPS has excellent outcomes regardless of gestational age at the time of presentation. Although some association with Hirschsprung disease has been reported, there are other reports suggesting otherwise. Suction rectal biopsy is only recommended in neonates that have persisting symptoms after a typical enema and clinical findings of MPS.

### References

Cuenca AG, Ali AS, Kays DW, Islam S. "Pulling the plug"—management of meconium plug syndrome in neonates. *J Surg Res.* 2012;175(2): e43–e46.

Keckler SJ, St Peter SD, Spilde TL, et al. Current significance of meconium plug syndrome. *J Pediatr Surg.* 2008;43(5):896–898.

### Cross-reference

Walters MM, Robertson RL. *Pediatric Radiology: The Requisites.* 4th ed. Philadelphia: Elsevier; 2017:95–97.

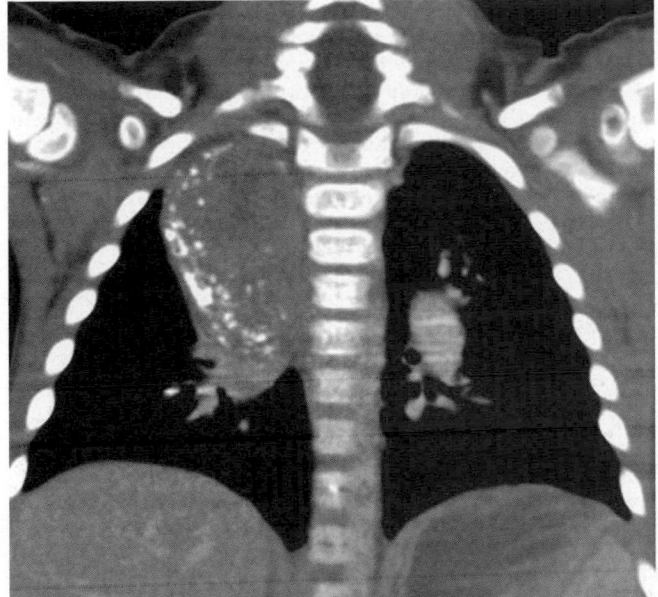

Fig. 7.1

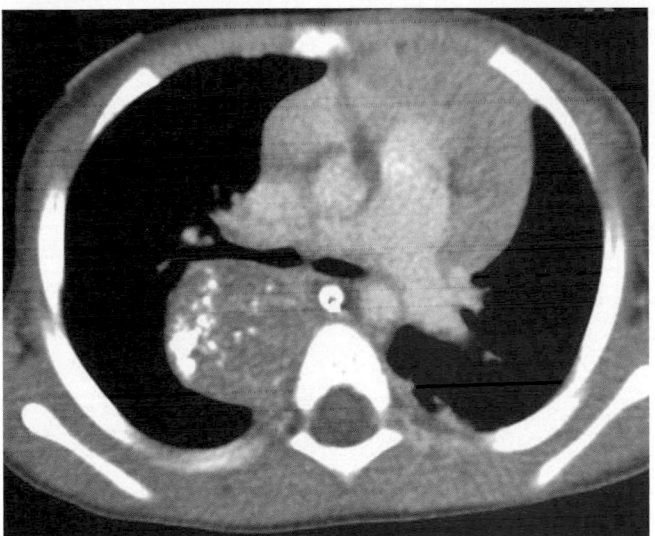

Fig. 7.2

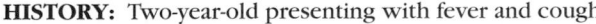

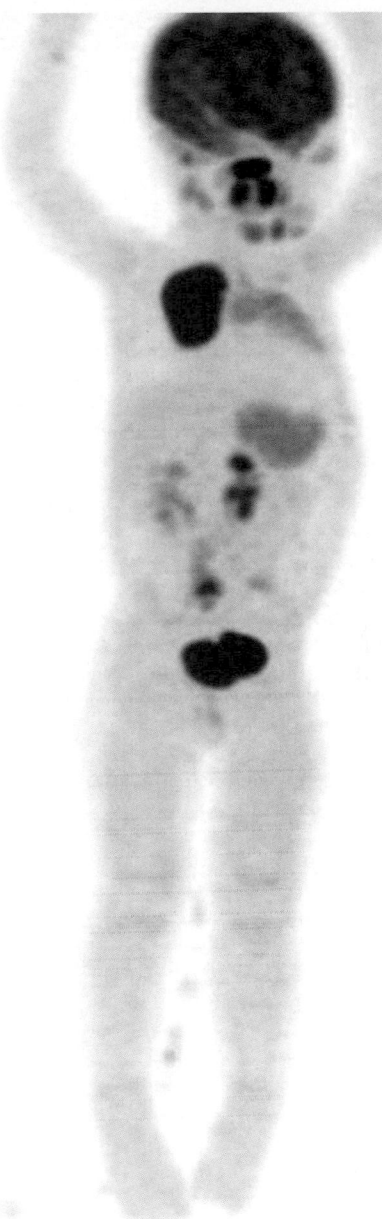

Fig. 7.3

**HISTORY:** Two-year-old presenting with fever and cough

1. What is the most likely diagnosis?
   A. Teratoma
   B. Neuroblastoma
   C. Thymoma
   D. Chronic pneumonia

2. Which option indicates a better prognosis in neuroblastoma (NB)?
   A. Increased copies of n-myc proto-oncogene
   B. Increased CD44 glycoprotein on the surface
   C. Patient is older than 1 year at diagnosis
   D. Anatomical stage 3S

3. Which option is a common imaging feature of NB?
   A. Invasion into the neural foramina
   B. Surrounds and engulfs the vessels
   C. Invasion into the renal vein and inferior vena cava
   D. A and B

4. True or false?
   A. Approximately 3/4 of NB cases demonstrate calcification on computed tomography (CT)
   B. Metastasis to the lung rather than liver and bone

## CASE 7

### Thoracic Neuroblastoma

1. B
2. B
3. D
4. A) True, B) False

### *Comment*

Neuroblastoma (NB) is a malignant tumor of primitive neural crest cells that most commonly arises from the adrenal gland, but can be seen anywhere along the sympathetic chain. NB can present in the adrenal glands (35%), extraadrenal retroperitoneum (30% to 35%), posterior mediastinum (20%), pelvis (2% to 3%), and neck (1%). NB is the third most common malignant tumor in children following leukemia/lymphoma and brain tumors. The International Neuroblastoma Staging System (INSS) is commonly used and takes into account surgical results (see the NB stage 4S case in this book). A risk-group staging model, the International Neuroblastoma Risk Group Staging System (INRGSS), has gained popularity in recent years. It is similar to the INSS, but it does not use the results of surgery to help define the stage. Instead, the INRGSS bases its staging on imaging results to guide resectability evaluation of the tumor. The INRGSS uses image-defined risk factors (IDRFs), which are factors seen on imaging tests that might mean the tumor will be harder to remove. The INRGSS divides NBs into four stages: L1: A tumor that has not spread from the origin and is confined to one body compartment, such as the neck, chest, or abdomen. L2: A tumor that has not spread far from its origin (e.g., it may have grown from the left side of the abdomen into the left side of the chest), but has at least one IDRF. M: A tumor that has spread (metastasized) to a distant part of the body (except tumors that are stage MS). MS: Metastatic disease in children younger than 18 months with cancer spread only to skin, liver, and/or bone marrow. No more than 10% of marrow cells are cancerous, and an metaiodobenzylguanidine (MIBG) scan does not show spread to the bones and/or the bone marrow.

Children younger than 12 to 18 months are more likely to be cured than older children. In infants, hyperdiploid cells tend to be associated with earlier stages of disease, respond better to chemotherapy, and usually predict a more favorable prognosis (outcome) than diploid cells. Ploidy is not as useful a factor in older children. MYCN is an oncogene, a gene that helps regulate cell growth. NBs with increased amplification of the MYCN oncogene tend to grow quickly and have a worse prognosis. Chromosome 1p deletions or 11q deletions may predict a less favorable prognosis. Having an extra part of chromosome 17 (17q gain) is also linked with a worse prognosis. NB cells release ferritin, a chemical that is an important part of the body's normal iron metabolism, into the blood. Patients with high ferritin levels tend to have a worse prognosis.

Ninety-five percent of patients have elevated levels of catecholamines and increased vanillylmandelic acid (VMA) in their urine.

http://www.cancer.org/cancer/neuroblastoma/detailedguide/neuroblastoma-staging

### References

Elsayes KM, Mukundan G, Narra VR, et al. Adrenal masses: MR imaging features with pathologic correlation. *Radiographics*. 2004;24(Suppl 1): S73–S86.

Pinto NR, Applebaum MA, Volchenboum SL, et al. Advances in risk classification and treatment strategies for neuroblastoma. *J Clin Oncol*. 2015;33(27):3008–3017.

### Cross-reference

Walters MM, Robertson RL. *Pediatric Radiology: The Requisites*. 4th ed. Philadelphia: Elsevier; 2017:172–173.

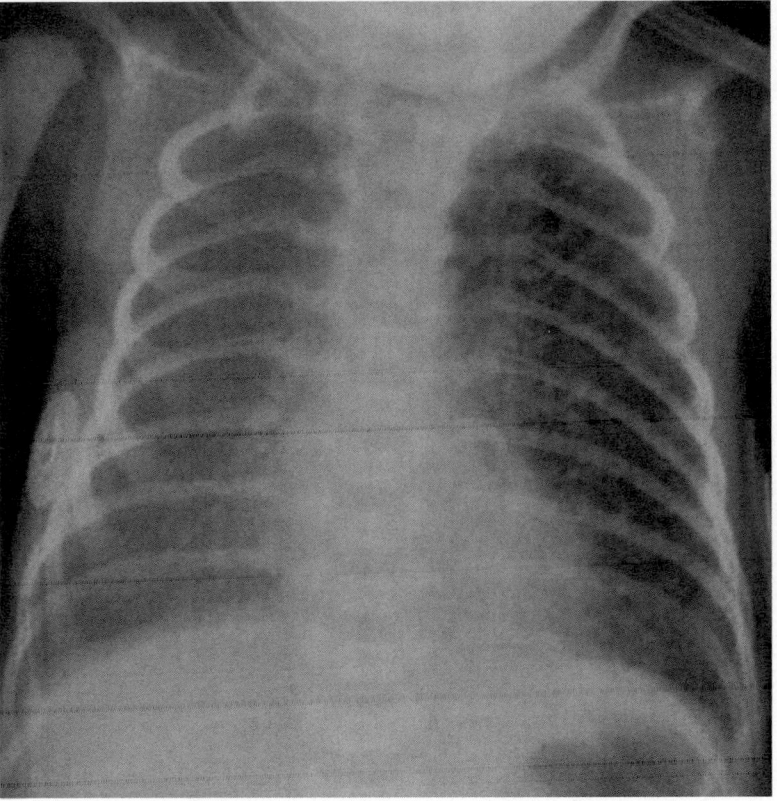

**Fig. 8.1**

**HISTORY:** Four-day-old premature infant with increased oxygen requirement

1. What is the most likely diagnosis?
   A. Meconium aspiration
   B. Pulmonary interstitial edema
   C. Chronic lung disease of prematurity
   D. Pulmonary interstitial emphysema

2. What is the most likely cause?
   A. Iatrogenic
   B. Postsurgical change
   C. Aspiration
   D. Congenital

3. Which option is true regarding this entity?
   A. It is a transient disease that typically resolves within 48 hours after birth.
   B. There is decreased risk of reactive airway disease compared to controls.
   C. It typically occurs in infants who are more than 34 gestational weeks.
   D. Preterm infants requiring ventilation support are the most common patient population.

## CASE 8

### Pulmonary Interstitial Emphysema

1. D
2. A
3. D

### *Comment*

Pulmonary interstitial emphysema (PIE) is one of the presentations of air leak syndrome in a neonate. Other manifestations of air leak include pneumothorax, pneumatocele, pneumomediastinum, pneumopericardium, pneumoperitoneum, subcutaneous emphysema, and systemic air embolism. The incidence of air leak is inversely related to birth weight, especially in very-low–birth weight preterm infants. Often, the cause is barotrauma, that is, inadequate mechanical ventilation of the immature lungs. High-frequency ventilation, maneuvers to decrease ventilation in the affected lung such as positioning the baby on the ipsilateral side, and, less frequently, selective ventilation of the unaffected lung are some of the nonsurgical interventions for treatment of PIE. Large air leaks collecting in a space are usually treated with drainage. PIE may affect one lobe of the lung, an entire single lung (as shown in this case), or both lungs (rare). Diagnosis is established with plain radiography, with uniform small focal lucencies of similar size extending from a hilum toward the periphery of the lung in a linear fashion. PIE most commonly presents within the first week of life in premature infants with surfactant deficiency disease, although the imaging appearance may mimic that of chronic lung disease of prematurity. The young age of the infant (<1 week old) and the involvement of a single lung or one or two lobes of a lung help differentiate PIE from chronic lung disease of prematurity.

### Reference

Joseph LJ, Bromiker R, Toker O, Schimmel MS, Goldberg S, Picard E. Unilateral lung intubation for pulmonary air leak syndrome in neonates: a case series and a review of the literature. *Am J Perinatol.* 2011;28(2):151–156.

### Cross-reference

Walters MM, Robertson RL. *Pediatric Radiology: The Requisites.* 4th ed. Philadelphia: Elsevier; 2017:53.

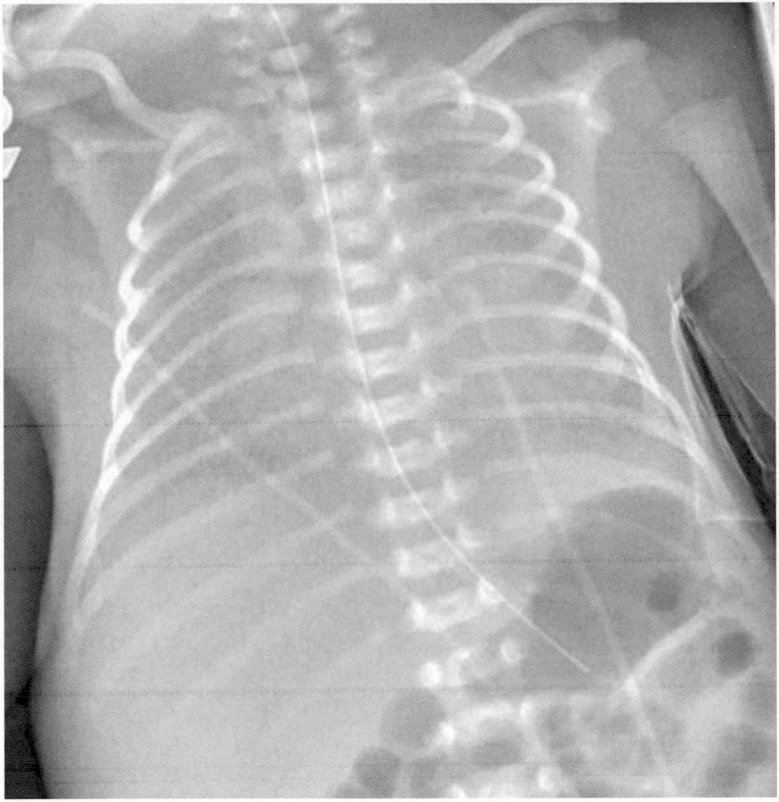

**Fig. 9.1**

**HISTORY:** Newborn infant at day of life 0, presenting with respiratory distress.

1. Name the disease shown in the image.
   A. Infant respiratory distress syndrome
   B. Surfactant deficiency disease
   C. Hyaline membrane disease
   D. All of the above

2. Which option represents the least likely clinical scenario?
   A. Male infant born at 27 gestational weeks
   B. Female infant born at 26 gestational weeks
   C. Male infant born at 38 gestational weeks
   D. Female infant less than 1500 g

3. Which condition could be considered in the differential diagnosis in this 27-gestational-week preterm infant?
   A. Meconium aspiration
   B. Group B streptococcal pneumonia
   C. Transient tachypnea of the newborn
   D. Pulmonary interstitial emphysema

4. Which option describes acute complications?
   A. Necrotizing enterocolitis, bronchopulmonary dysplasia
   B. Pulmonary interstitial emphysema, pulmonary hemorrhage
   C. Pneumothorax, retinopathy of prematurity
   D. Neurologic impairment, patent ductus arteriosus

## CASE 9

### Surfactant Deficiency Disease

1. D
2. C
3. B
4. B

### Comment

Surfactant deficiency disease is the preferred terminology, although multiple different names have been used to refer to this disease, such as hyaline membrane disease. Surfactant deficiency disease is the most common lung disease in premature infants due to lack of surfactant. Immature type II pneumocytes cannot produce surfactant in the preterm infant. Rarely, secondary surfactant deficiency can be seen due to meconium aspiration and pneumonia causing deactivation of surfactant. Even more rarely, primary surfactant deficiency can be seen due to genetic mutations affecting surfactant production in term infants. Males are more commonly affected than females. Maternal diabetes is a risk factor as well. Radiographic findings change depending on the stage of the disease; however, low lung volumes with diffuse reticular granular homogeneous densities are the classic radiographic findings prior to treatment. Areas of atelectasis and heterogeneous densities can be observed during the course of the disease, which may result from uneven distribution of intratracheal surfactant administration and be secondary to intubation/ventilator support. Patent ductus arteriosus may result in superimposed edema, typically presenting around the fifth day of life. It is important to know the gestational age at birth, because meconium aspiration and transient tachypnea of the newborn are typically seen in full-term infants. Group B streptococcal pneumonia is the most common pneumonia in neonates, with higher incidence in preterm infants. Although the radiographic findings are quite similar, the presence of pleural effusion in group B streptococcal pneumonia helps differential diagnosis. Chronic lung disease of prematurity may develop in up to half of the cases.

### Reference

Lopez E, Gascoin G, Flamant C, et al. Exogenous surfactant therapy in 2013: what is next? Who, when and how should we treat newborn infants in the future? *BMC Pediatr*. 2013;13:165.

### Cross-reference

Walters MM, Robertson RL. *Pediatric Radiology: The Requisites*. 4th ed. Philadelphia: Elsevier; 2017:52–55.

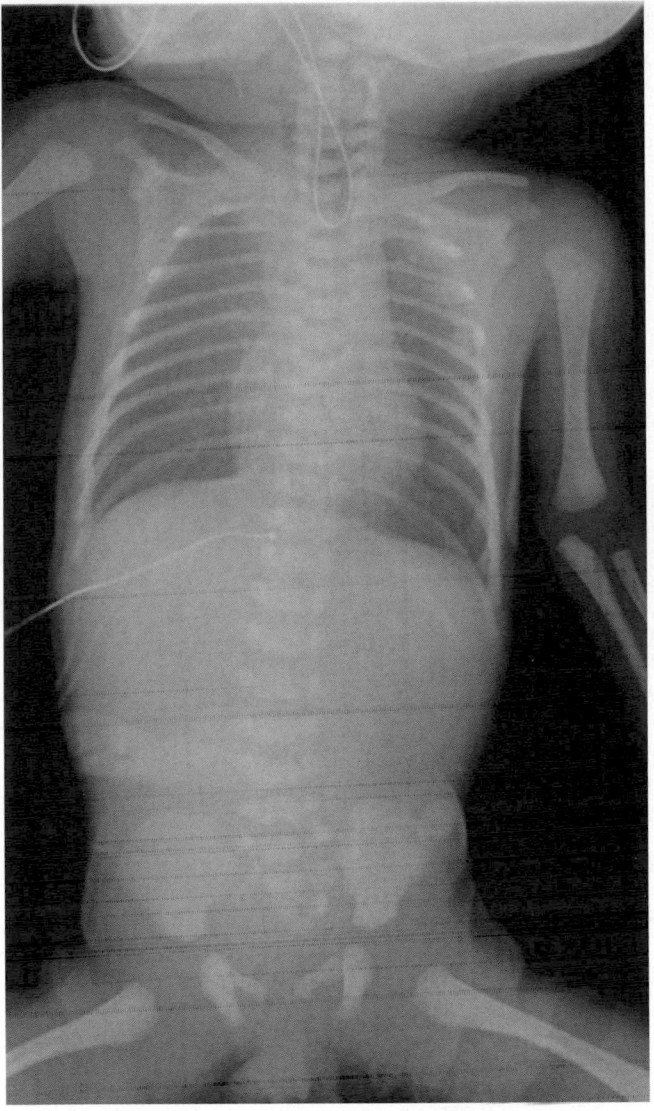

Fig. 10.1

**HISTORY:** Neonatal radiography at 1 day of life

1. Which principal finding is seen on the neonatal radiography?
   A. Air distended proximal esophagus
   B. Air distended distal esophagus
   C. Air within the mediastinum
   D. Air within the pleural space

2. What is the most likely diagnosis?
   A. Traumatic esophageal perforation
   B. Esophageal duplication cyst
   C. Esophageal atresia
   D. Bronchogenic cyst

3. Esophageal atresia is most frequently combined with which of the following?
   A. A distal tracheoesophageal fistula
   B. A proximal and distal tracheoesophageal fistula
   C. An isolated H-type tracheoesophageal fistula
   D. A proximal tracheoesophageal fistula

4. Which statement is correct?
   A. In the VACTERL association, the T and E refer to the thorax and esophagus.
   B. Esophageal atresia may be related to oligohydramnios.
   C. Esophageal atresia may be related to polyhydramnios.
   D. In the VACTERL association, the V and A refer to the veins and arteries.

## CASE 10

### Esophageal Atresia

1. A
2. C
3. A
4. C

## Comment

Esophageal atresia is a congenital defect in which the continuity of the esophagus is interrupted. The esophagus may be blind, ending in a pouch, or a complex fistulous connection between the esophagus and trachea may exist. Typically, esophageal atresia is classified in five types depending on the level and complexity of the coexisting tracheoesophageal fistula. The most frequent type is characterized by a blind-ending upper esophageal pouch, a large esophageal gap, and a connection between the distal esophageal pouch and the trachea (86%). The next most frequent type is characterized by the presence of a large gap between the two blind-ending esophageal pouches without any anomalous connection to the trachea (9%). The third most frequent esophageal malformation is known as the H-type malformation in which the continuity of the esophagus is preserved; however, an abnormal focal connection/fistula is present between the esophagus and trachea (6%). The remaining types are very infrequently encountered and are characterized by a true esophageal gap in which the proximal and distal esophagus connect to the trachea (2%) or the proximal esophagus connects to the adjacent trachea while the distal esophagus does not connect to the trachea (1%).

On plain radiography of the neonatal chest, an air-filled distended pharyngeal pouch or dilated proximal esophagus is typically noted. Depending on the presence of a coexisting tracheoesophageal fistula, air may be noted in the stomach and bowel loops. In addition, enteric feeding tubes may terminate or coil in the proximal esophageal pouch.

Esophageal atresia, with or without tracheoesophageal fistula, may be seen in association with multiple other congenital findings. The VACTERL association is the best known and refers to various combinations of anomalies involving the Vertebral column and the Anorectal canal, as well as Cardiac, Tracheal, Esophageal, Renal, and Limb abnormalities. Esophageal atresia typically presents with polyhydramnios in the third trimester of pregnancy. Digestive, motility, and nutritional issues are not uncommon after repair.

### Reference

Berrocal T, Torres I, Gutierrez J, Prieto C, del Hoyo ML, Lamas M. Congenital anomalies of the upper gastrointestinal tract. *Radiographics*. 1999;19:855–872.

### Cross-reference

Walters MM, Robertson RL. *Pediatric Radiology: The Requisites*. 4th ed. Philadelphia: Elsevier; 2017:102–104.

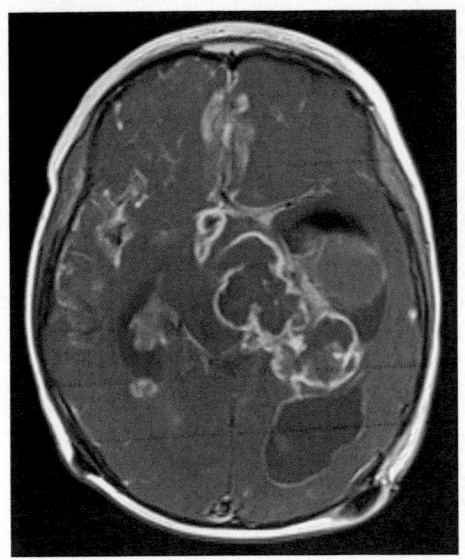

Fig. 11.1

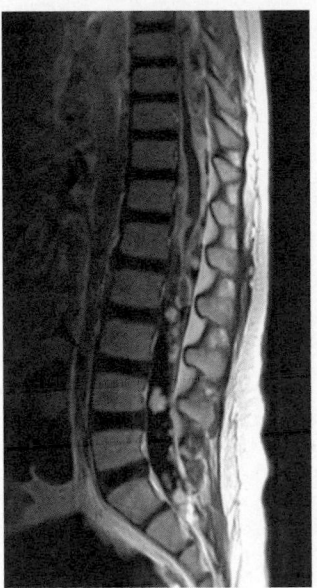

Fig. 11.2

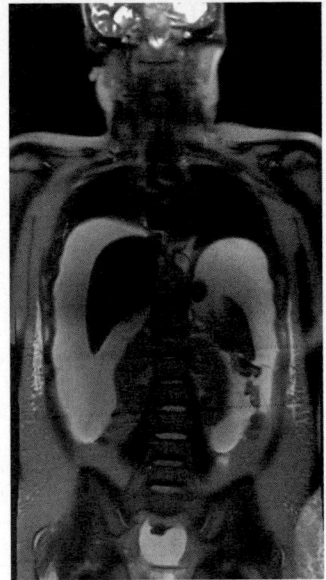

Fig. 11.3

**HISTORY:** Multiplanar magnetic resonance imaging (MRI) of a young child with a high-grade astrocytoma

1. Which complication is seen on the brain and spinal cord MRI?
   A. Tumor seeding into the ventricular system
   B. Tumor seeding along the spinal canal
   C. Tumor seeding into the peritoneal cavity
   D. All of the above

2. How can intraperitoneal tumor seeding be explained?
   A. Direct infiltration from the dural sac
   B. Hematogenous spread from the primary brain tumor
   C. Lymphogenic spread from the primary brain tumor
   D. Intraperitoneal seeding via the ventriculoperitoneal (VP) shunt

3. Which of the following primary brain tumors may present with drop metastases?
   A. Pilocytic astrocytoma
   B. Pilocystic astrocytoma
   C. Anaplastic astrocytoma
   D. Multicystic astrocytoma

4. Which statement is incorrect?
   A. A small amount of "ascitis" without peritoneal contrast enhancement is a common finding in shunted hydrocephalus.
   B. Migration of the shunt tip within the peritoneal cavity suggests shunt disconnection.
   C. In case of a ruptured appendix, ventriculitis may occur via a VP shunt.
   D. A VP shunt status should cover the entirety of the shunt course.

## CASE 11

### Ventriculoperitoneal Shunt Complication

1. D
2. D
3. C
4. B

### *Comment*

Ventriculoperitoneal (VP) shunts divert excess cerebrospinal fluid from dilated or obstructed ventricles to the peritoneal cavity, pleural space, or right atrium. The etiology can be related to intracranial hemorrhage primarily affecting the ventricular system, or to trauma, infection, or intracranial neoplasms, to name a few possibilities. In metastatic brain tumors, this may occasionally result in a tumor seeding via the VP shunt as shown in this case. In these rare instances, large tumor masses may be seen within the dependent or lower parts of the peritoneal cavity. The tumor may appear like a second focal tumor, possibly complicated by excessive amounts of free fluid (ascites) within the abdomen. Contrast-enhanced magnetic resonance imaging (MRI) may show enhanced masses, partially outlining the abdominal organs. Usually, the metastatic mass exhibits a contrast pattern similar to metastatic lesions within the spinal canal. In most cases, the prognosis is dismal.

In the diagnostic workup of high-grade primary brain tumors, which are at risk for metastatic lesions, the presence of a VP shunt should alert the radiologist to actively exclude metastatic lesions outside of the cranial vault or spinal canal. In most reported cases, VP shunt–mediated metastatic disease is seen in close proximity to the tip of the VP shunt. An increased enhancement of the peritoneal lining may be seen as a complication of intraperitoneal tumor seeding, however peritonitis secondary to, e.g., an appendicitis, may result in ventriculitis or meningitis from retrograde spread of infection via an existing VP shunt.

About 40% of shunts eventually fail because of infection or mechanical dysfunction. The imaging algorithm should consider the detrimental effects of cumulative radiation in children with hydrocephalus. Fast/limited MRI is preferred over computed tomography (CT). Shunt series are recommended only after cross-sectional imaging of the ventricular system.

### Reference

Narayan A, Jallo G, Huisman TA. Extra-cranial, peritoneal seeding of primary malignant brain tumors through ventriculo-peritoneal shunts in children. Case report and review of the literature. *Neuroradiol J.* 2015;28(5):536–539.

### Cross-reference

Walters MM, Robertson RL. *Pediatric Radiology: The Requisites.* 4th ed. Philadelphia: Elsevier; 2017:286–287.

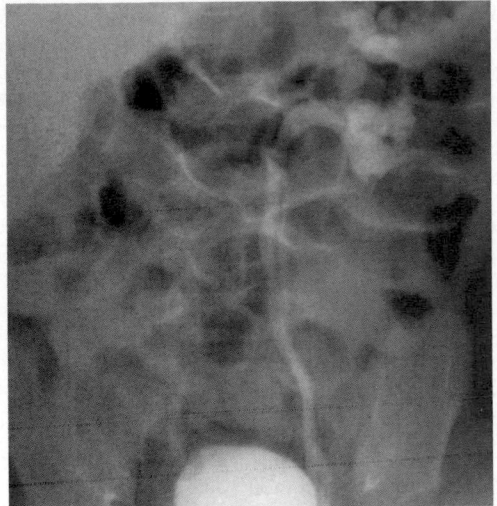

Fig. 12.1

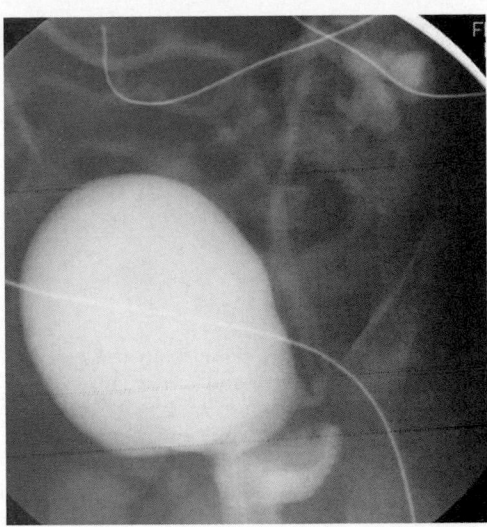

Fig. 12.2

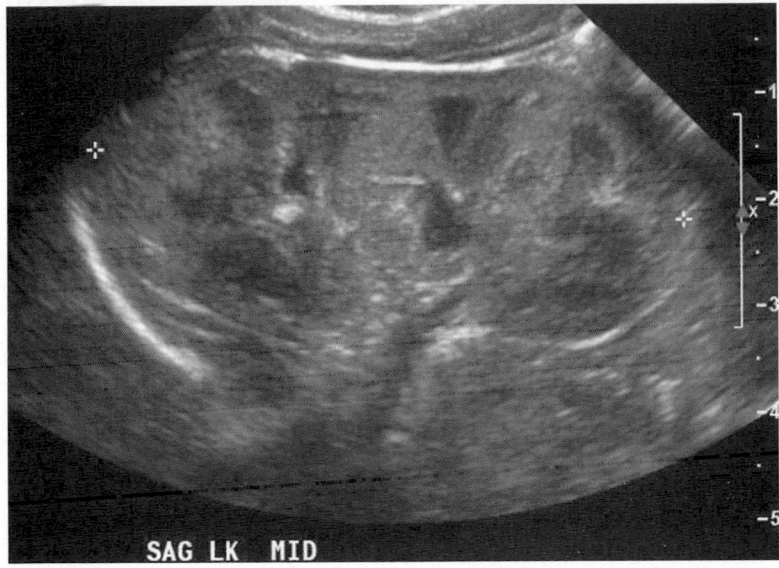

Fig. 12.3

**HISTORY:** Urinary tract infection

1. Which option is the best diagnosis?
   A. Vesicoureteral fistula
   B. Vesicureteral reflux
   C. Vesicoureteral remnant
   D. Vesicoureteral duplication without reflux

2. Which of the following best describes the name of the test presented in this entity?
   A. Voiding cystourethrogram
   B. Retrograde cystogram
   C. Nuclear cystogram
   D. All of the above

3. True or false?
   A. Females are more commonly affected than males.
   B. Shortened or abnormally angulated insertion of the ureter into the bladder is theorized to result in vesicoureteral reflux (VUR).

4. Which committee's grading system is most commonly used in vesicoureteral reflux (VUR)?
   A. International Reflux Study Committee
   B. International Study for the Grading of Renal Abnormalities
   C. Committee of Renal Diseases, Radiological Society of North America
   D. Committee of Renal Diseases, Society for Pediatric Radiology

## CASE 12

### Vesicoureteral Reflux

1. B

2. A

3. A) True, B) True

4. A

## Comment

Abnormal retrograde flow of urine from the bladder toward the kidney is called vesicoureteral reflux (VUR). The International Reflux Study Committee's grading system is accepted worldwide: grade 1 includes reflux into the ureter only, grade 2 includes reflux that reaches the renal pelvis but no calyceal blunting, grade 3 includes mild calyceal blunting, grade 4 includes progressive calyceal and ureteral dilation, and grade 5 includes a very dilated and tortuous collecting system and intrarenal reflux. VUR is an intermittent phenomenon that most commonly occurs in a full bladder and during voiding. Diagnosis is established with a voiding cystourethrogram, which is performed under fluoroscopy after catheterization of the bladder. Water-soluble contrast is administered under gravity.

Females are more commonly affected than males. White Caucasian children are more commonly affected than are other races. Approximately 80% of children grow out of VUR by puberty. Older age at the time of diagnosis, associated renal anomalies (duplication, ureteropelvic junction obstruction), or associated ureteral anomalies (ectopic insertion, ureterocele) decrease the likelihood of spontaneous resolution.

Prophylactic antibiotic therapy is common to decrease/eliminate breakthrough infections and pyelonephritis. Ureteral reimplantation surgery or endoscopic periureteral injections (such as Deflux) are other treatment options. Deflux injections may appear as focal hyperechogenicity at the vesicoureteral junctions, not to be confused with bladder wall lesions.

### Reference

Berrocal T, López-Pereira P, Arjonilla A, Gutiérrez J. Anomalies of the distal ureter, bladder, and urethra in children: embryologic, radiologic, and pathologic features. *Radiographics*. 2002;22(5):1139–1164.

### Cross-reference

Walters MM, Robertson RL. *Pediatric Radiology: The Requisites*. 4th ed. Philadelphia: Elsevier. 2017:145, 151.

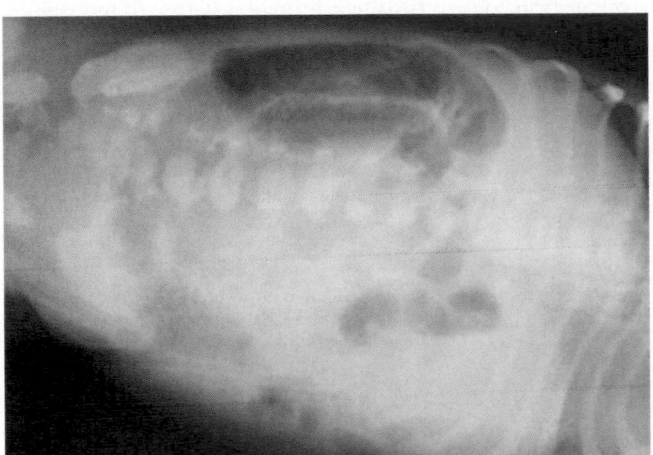

Fig. 13.1

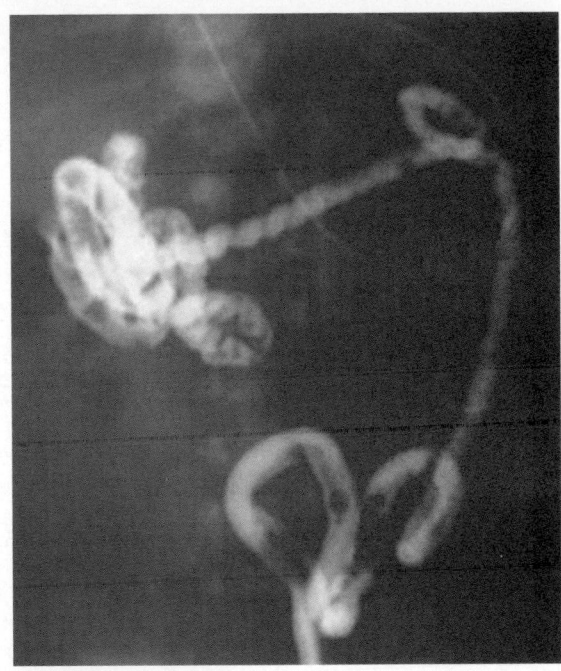

Fig. 13.2

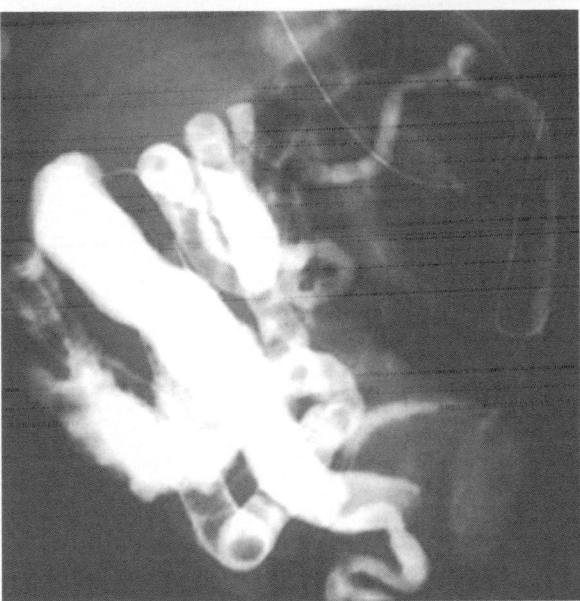

Fig. 13.3

**HISTORY:** Full term infant with no passage of meconium at day of life 2.

1. What is your diagnosis?
   A. Meconium ileus
   B. Meconium plug
   C. Ileal atresia
   D. Megacystic microcolon intestinal hypoperistalsis syndrome

2. Which option provides the best description of the entity shown?
   A. Functional obstruction of the colon due to intrinsic ganglion cells
   B. Transient functional obstruction of the colon due to meconium plugs
   C. Neonatal obstruction of the distal ileum due to thick, tenacious meconium
   D. Chemical peritonitis from in utero bowel perforation and leakage of meconium

3. Which statement is accurate for meconium ileus?
   A. Meconium ileus is more prevalent in infants of diabetic mothers and mothers treated with magnesium sulfate.
   B. Almost all patients with meconium ileus have cystic fibrosis.
   C. Most infants with meconium ileus syndrome have associated central nervous system (CNS) anomalies.
   D. Most infants who fail to pass meconium have meconium ileus.

4. Choose the best answer for classic imaging findings of meconium ileus.
   A. Very small microcolon with normal morphology
   B. Small left colon to the level of the splenic flexura
   C. Rectum smaller than sigmoid (R/S ration <1)
   D. Normal-caliber colon

## CASE 13

### Meconium Ileus

1. A
2. C
3. B
4. A

### *Comment*

Meconium ileus (MI) is the earliest manifestation of cystic fibrosis (CF) and presents with obstruction of the distal ileum due to thick tenacious meconium. MI occurs in 10% to 20% of CF patients, and approximately 90% of patients who have MI are diagnosed with CF. MI is most commonly seen in white Caucasians and exhibits no gender preference. MI is primarily associated with CF transmembrane (conductance) regulator mutations in chromosome 7. Imaging diagnosis can be established during fetal life with the presence of hyperechoic masses and dilated bowels in an ultrasound exam of the high-risk neonate. MI can be simple (50%) or complicated (50%). The simple form is basically obstruction in the mid/distal ileum and dilation in the proximal bowel segments. In complicated MI, the obstruction may lead to segmental volvulus, atresia, necrosis, perforation, meconium peritonitis (generalized), or meconium pseudocyst formation. Initial plain radiography shows multiple dilated bowel loops typical of neonatal distal bowel obstruction. Due to air mixture in the meconium, there may be bubbly lucencies in the right lower quadrant. Air-fluid levels are rare, due to the thick/tenacious nature of meconium. A water-soluble hyperosmotic enema is the diagnostic imaging modality; it is also the first choice of treatment in simple MI and can be repeated for therapeutic purposes if necessary. Contrast medium that is refluxed into the terminal ileum may outline obstructing meconium pellets. However, obstruction may not allow contrast passage in some instances, in which case the imaging findings mimic that of ileal atresia. Complicated MI requires surgery.

### Reference

Caryyle BE, Borowotz DS, Glick PL. A review of pathophysiology and management of fetuses and neonates with meconium ileus for the pediatric surgeon. *J Pediatric Surg*. 2012;47(4):772–781.

### Cross-reference

Walters MM, Robertson RL. *Pediatric Radiology: The Requisites*. 4th ed. Philadelphia: Elsevier; 2017:97–98.

# CASE 14

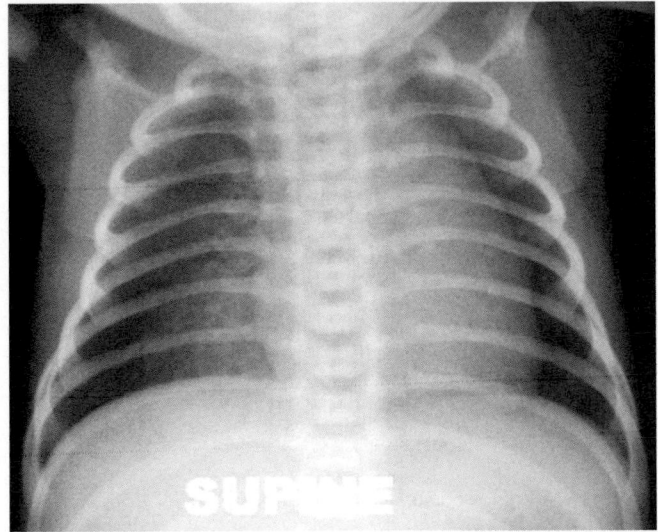

Fig. 14.1

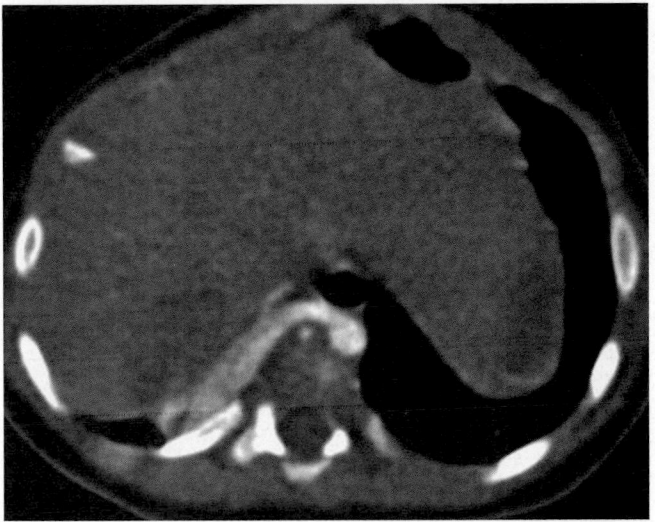

Fig. 14.2

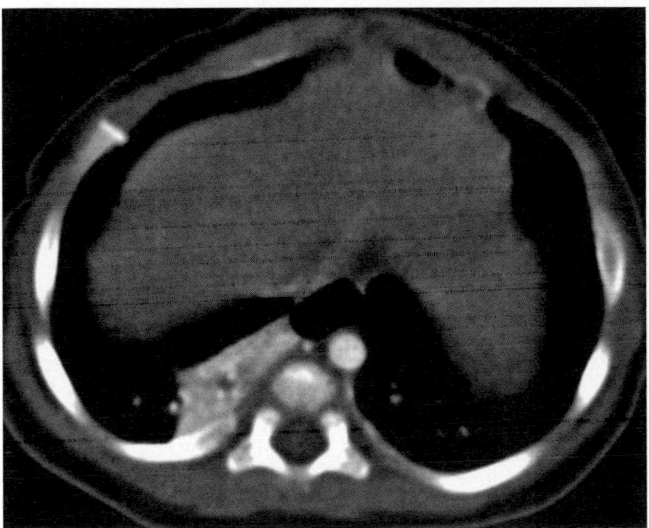

Fig. 14.3

**HISTORY:** Prenatally diagnosed lung mass

1. Based on the imaging appearance on the plain radiograph, which of the following should be included in the differential diagnosis for this lesion? (Choose all that apply.)
   A. Cystic pulmonary adenomatoid malformation
   B. Foregut duplication cyst
   C. Pulmonary sequestration
   D. Pleuropulmonary blastoma

2. What is the most common location of pulmonary sequestration?
   A. Right upper lobe
   B. Right lower lobe
   C. Left upper lobe
   D. Left lower lobe

3. All of the following statements about pulmonary sequestration are true, *except*:
   A. Typically, a cystic or solid mass without connection with the bronchial tree.
   B. Extralobar sequestration can sometimes occur below the diaphragm.
   C. Intralobar sequestration has its own pleural investment.
   D. Both intralobar and extralobar sequestration have a systemic arterial supply.

4. Which statement about pulmonary sequestration is *true*?
   A. Pulmonary sequestration can sometimes occur as a hybrid lesion with cystic pulmonary airway malformation (CPAM).
   B. Intralobar sequestration typically presents at birth.
   C. Intralobar sequestration is commonly associated with other congenital anomalies.
   D. Extralobar sequestration usually has pulmonary venous drainage.

## CASE 14

### Pulmonary Sequestration

1. A, B, C, D
2. D
3. C
4. A

### Comment

Pulmonary sequestration refers to dysplastic nonfunctional lung tissue that does not connect to the bronchial tree. It is almost always in the lower lobes, and more commonly on the left. It can sometimes be seen as a hybrid lesion with cystic pulmonary airway malformation (CPAM), in which case it may appear cystic. The key to this diagnosis and to differentiate it from other masses that may otherwise present similarly is detecting the presence of a systemic arterial supply. This is also important for surgical planning. There are two main types, extralobar and intralobar. Extralobar sequestration has its own pleural investment, typically presents in the pre- or perinatal period, may be asymptomatic, and usually has systemic venous drainage. It is commonly associated with other congenital anomalies, including congenital diaphragmatic hernia and cardiac anomalies. Intralobar sequestration shares its pleural investment with the normal lung, typically presents in older children with recurrent pneumonia, and usually has pulmonary venous drainage. It is not associated with other anomalies, and its etiology may be related to chronic postnatal inflammation.

### Reference

Odev K, Guler I, Altinok T, Pekcan S, Batur A, Ozbiner H. Cystic and cavitary lung lesions in children: radiologic findings with pathologic correlation. *J Clin Imaging Sci.* 2013;3:60.

### Cross-reference

Walters MM, Robertson RL. *Pediatric Radiology: The Requisites.* 4th ed. Philadelphia: Elsevier; 2017:29–31.

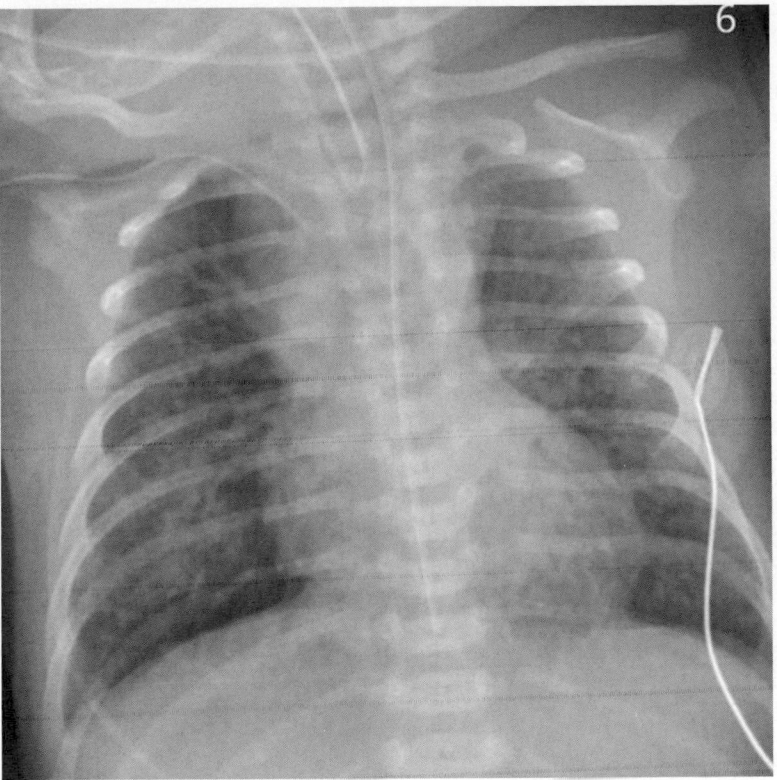

**Fig. 15.1**

**HISTORY:** Full term infant presenting with respiratory distress.

1. Which statement is most accurate regarding this disease?
   A. This is a transient disease that typically resolves within 48 hours after birth.
   B. There is decreased risk of reactive airway disease compared to controls.
   C. This disease typically occurs in infants at 34 or more gestational weeks.
   D. None of the above.

2. Which option is not part of typical radiographic findings of meconium aspiration?
   A. Bilateral diffuse symmetric granular densities
   B. Hyperinflation
   C. Asymmetric focal areas of atelectasis
   D. Pneumothorax, pneumomediastinum

3. Which option is incorrect regarding meconium aspiration syndrome (MAS)?
   A. MAS is a chemical pneumonitis occurring secondary to aspiration of meconium.
   B. Meconium aspiration results in deactivation of surfactant, and thus surfactant administration may be useful during treatment.
   C. MAS occurs in infants who experienced in utero or intrapartum hypoxia.
   D. Extracorporeal membrane oxygenation (ECMO) is not an option for infants with MAS because they may develop pulmonary hypertension.

4. In addition to respiratory distress, which of the following symptoms can be seen?
   A. Metabolic acidosis
   B. Syndrome of inappropriate secretion of antidiuretic hormone (SIADH) or acute renal failure
   C. Anoxic brain injury
   D. All of the above

## CASE 15

### Meconium Aspiration

1. C
2. A
3. D
4. D

### Comment

Meconium aspiration syndrome (MAS) occurs in term or post-term infants who are born through meconium-stained amniotic fluid. Although 10% to 15% of deliveries have meconium-stained amniotic fluid, only 4% to 5% of these infants have MAS. Maternal risk factors include preeclampsia, diabetes, chorioamnionitis, and illicit substance abuse. Infants with MAS develop symptoms within a few hours of birth. In utero meconium passage is a sign of fetal distress that is a result of anal sphincter relaxation. Meconium aspiration results in airway obstruction, surfactant dysfunction, and chemical pneumonitis. Radiographic findings can be variable, but hyperinflation, interstitial thickening, and asymmetric areas of atelectasis are typically observed. Radiographs are helpful in assessing complications like pneumothorax (20% to 40%), pneumomediastinum, or pulmonary interstitial emphysema. Extracorporeal membrane oxygenation (ECMO) may be necessary in cases with severe pulmonary hypertension. Outcomes depend on the severity of the disease; some infants recover within the first 3 days of life and some develop chronic lung disease–like symptoms. The mortality rate is approximately 10%. Perinatal asphyxia may result in hypoxic brain injury. ECMO may further contribute to brain injury.

### Reference

Pramanik AK, Rangaswamy N, Gates T. Neonatal respiratory distress: a practical approach to its diagnosis and management. *Pediatr Clin North Am.* 2015;62(2):453–469.

### Cross-reference

Walters MM, Robertson RL. *Pediatric Radiology: The Requisites.* 4th ed. Philadelphia: Elsevier; 2017:56.

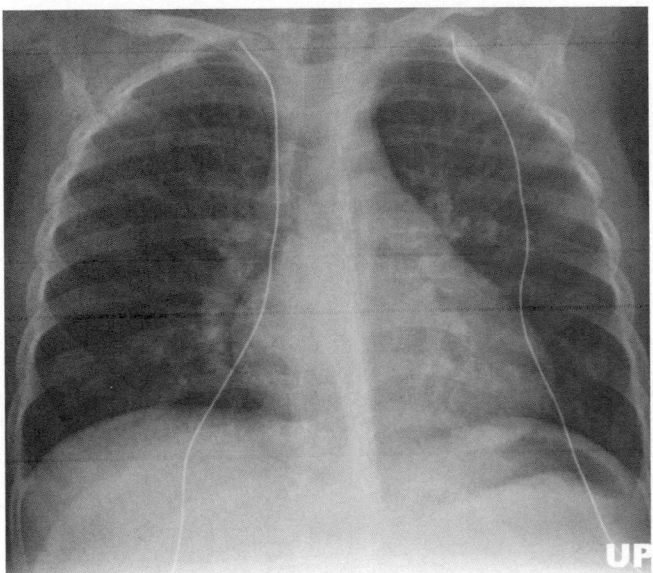

Fig. 16.1

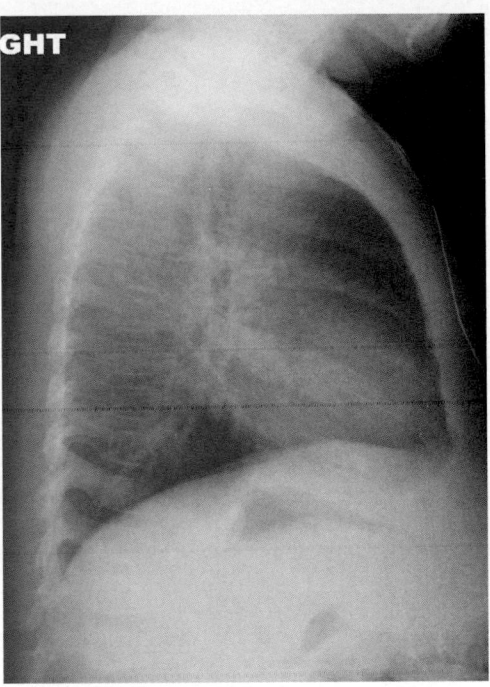

Fig. 16.2

1. What is the most common cause for the illness shown on the radiographs in this 1-year-old child?
   A. Respiratory syncytial virus (RSV)
   B. *Streptococcus pneumoniae*
   C. Herpes virus
   D. *Neisseria gonorrhoeae*

2. Which option describes the best imaging clue(s) for the diagnosis of bronchiolitis?
   A. Hyperinflation
   B. Increased peribronchial markings
   C. Lack of focal consolidation
   D. All of the above

3. Which statement is correct?
   A. Presence of hilar adenopathy in young children is alarming in the setting of viral infection.
   B. Subsegmental atelectasis is a concern for bacterial pneumonia in patients with bronchiolitis.
   C. Symmetric coarse linear markings radiating from the hila resulting in dirty/busy parahilar regions is a classic radiographic finding of bronchiolitis.
   D. None of the above are true.

4. Which of the following entities should be considered in the differential diagnosis?
   A. Cardiac disease with left to right shunts
   B. Bronchial foreign body
   C. Asthma
   D. All of the above

## CASE 16

### Bronchiolitis

1. A
2. D
3. C
4. D

### *Comment*

Respiratory tract infection is the most common cause of illness in children and continues to be a significant cause of morbidity and mortality. Although the reported proportion of hospitalizations for each virus differs by geography, the most common pathogen is respiratory syncytial virus (RSV) followed by rhinovirus. Children younger than 2 years of age suffer from viral infection more commonly than bacterial infection. Most common clinical symptoms are wheezing, cough, and maybe fever. Viral infection affects small airways, resulting in inflammation: narrowing of small airways lumen from edema, necrotic debris and mucus to small airway occlusion, leading to subsegmental atelectasis and air trapping. Classic radiographic findings are therefore hyperinflation of the lungs, peribronchial wall thickening, and subsegmental atelectasis. Clinically, it is important to differentiate viral illness from bacterial infection; chest radiographs have 92% negative predictive value by demonstrating lack of lung consolidation, the hallmark of bacterial infection. Counting ribs is usually not reliable in assessment of hyperinflation in children. For assessment of hyperinflation, evaluate the diaphragm (flattened, or loss of normal convexity) and presence of retrosternal aerated lung tissue in the lateral radiograph. Severe bronchiolitis early in life is associated with increased risk of asthma.

### Reference

Meissner HC. Viral bronchiolitis in children. *N Engl J Med*. 2016;374(1): 62-72.

### Cross-reference

Walters MM, Robertson RL. *Pediatric Radiology: The Requisites*. 4th ed. Philadelphia: Elsevier; 2017:37.

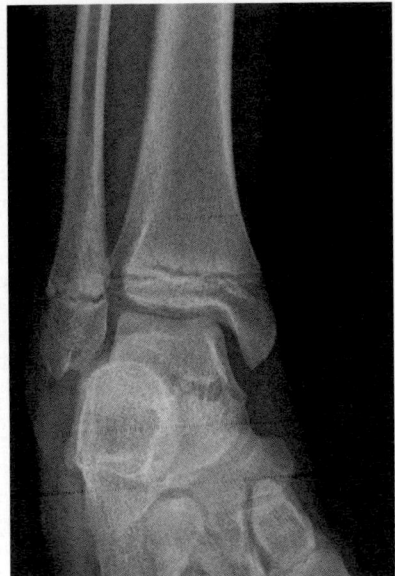

Fig. 17.1

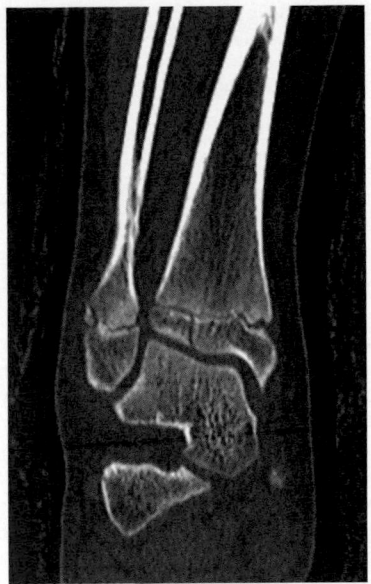

Fig. 17.2

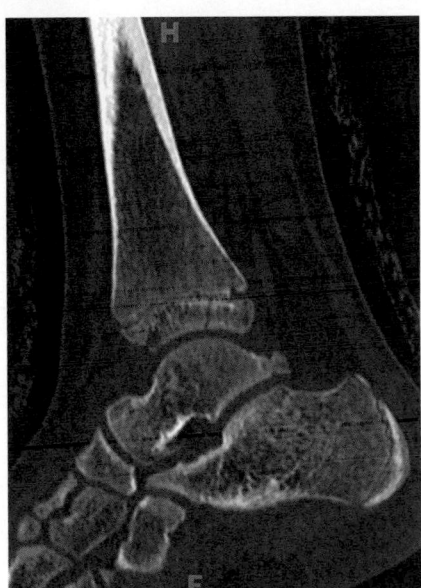

Fig. 17.3

**HISTORY:** Fall.

1. Which part(s) of the bone is/are abnormal?
   A. Physis and epiphysis
   B. Physis and metaphysis
   C. Epiphysis and metaphysis
   D. Hypophysis and epiphysis

2. How do you classify these physeal injuries?
   A. Salter-Morris fractures
   B. Salter-Harris fractures
   C. Halter-Sarris fractures
   D. Malter-Sorris fractures

3. How many types of physeal fractures are frequently described in everyday clinical practice?
   A. 3
   B. 5
   C. 7
   D. 9

4. Which is the most often encountered type of physeal injury?
   A. Type 1
   B. Type 2
   C. Type 3
   D. Type 4

## CASE 17

### Salter-Harris Fracture

1. A
2. B
3. B
4. B

### Comment

Physeal fractures, also known as Salter-Harris fractures, involve the open physis (growth plate) in various ways. Based upon the involvement of the epiphysis, physis, or metaphysis, up to nine different types of Salter-Harris fractures are known. In type I, a transverse fracture runs solely through the physis (6%). Type II fractures are characterized by a fracture extending from the physis into the adjacent metaphysis (75%). The type III fracture extends from the physis into the adjacent epiphysis (8%) (as shown in this case), and simultaneous extension from a physeal fracture into both the meta- and epiphysis is classified as a type IV Salter-Harris fracture (10%). Finally, a crush or compression injury to the physis is known as a type V fracture (1%). The remaining types 6 to 9 are much rarer.

The SALTER mnemonic can be used to remember the five most frequent types of physeal injuries. The "S" refers to *slipped* in type 1, the "A" refers to *above the physis* (i.e., metaphyseal) (type 2), the "L" refers to *lower than the physis* (i.e., epiphyses) (type 3), "TE" refers to *through everything* (type 4), and, finally, the "R" refers to *rammed* or *crushed* (type 5).

Conventional radiography of the physis in two planes usually allows identification of the extent, severity, and consequently the type of physeal injury. A Salter-Harris type 5 fracture occasionally requires a comparison with the contralateral side to evaluate for the compression or loss of width of the physis. A computed tomography (CT) study with multiplanar two-dimensional or three-dimensional reconstruction may be helpful for the evaluation of complex multiplanar fractures involving the physis. Finally, magnetic resonance imaging (MRI) may be considered to determine/evaluate a possible focal premature closure of the physis after a previous trauma.

Growth disturbance is the biggest concern in Salter-Harris fractures. Type II fractures infrequently result in growth disturbance. As the fractures become more severe, especially in the rare type 5, growth interruption becomes more common. The prognosis is worse when the fracture involves the lower extremity, irrespective of the Salter-Harris classification.

### Reference

Rogers LF, Poznanski AK. Imaging of epiphyseal injuries. *Radiology*. 1994;191:297–308.

### Cross-reference

Walters MM, Robertson RL. *Pediatric Radiology: The Requisites*. 4th ed. Philadelphia: Elsevier; 2017:250, 257.

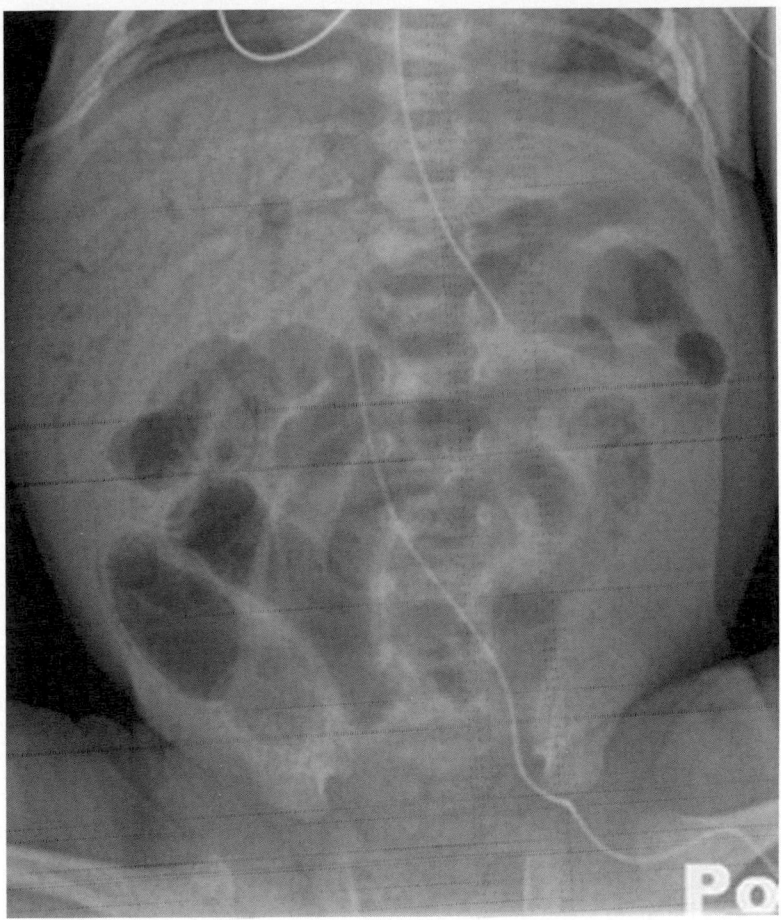

Fig. 18.1

**HISTORY:** Conventional abdominal radiography of a preterm infant.

1. Which signature pathological imaging finding do you see?
   A. Air in the lumen of the small bowel
   B. Air in the lumen of the large bowel
   C. Air in the wall of the small bowel
   D. Air in the wall of the large bowel

2. Where else do you see "abnormal" air bubbles on this abdominal radiograph?
   A. In the biliary tree
   B. In the hepatic veins
   C. In the portal vein
   D. In the hepatic arteries

3. What is the most likely diagnosis?
   A. Necrotizing enterocolitis (NEC)
   B. Necrotizing fasciitis
   C. Necrotizing hepatitis
   D. Necrotizing urosepsis

4. Which of the following is not considered to be a risk factor for this entity?
   A. Prematurity
   B. Congenital heart disease
   C. Cesarean section
   D. Respiratory distress due to surfactant deficiency disease

## CASE 18

### Necrotizing Enterocolitis

1. D

2. C

3. A

4. C

### Comment

Necrotizing enterocolitis (NEC) is a potentially life-threatening entity characterized by a combination of ischemia and infection of the large bowel. The disease typically occurs in preterm neonates, but may occasionally be seen in critically ill term neonates. The large bowel may be segmentally affected; however, in severe cases, the entirety of the colon may be involved. In rare cases, the small bowel is also affected. The etiology is multifactorial. NEC is believed to result from a combination of intestinal ischemia due to systemic hypoperfusion and hypoxia, bacterial overgrowth, bowel immaturity, oral feeding, and overall neonatal prematurity. In many cases, coexisting respiratory insufficiency resulting from surfactant deficiency disease, and systemic hypoperfusion due to, for example, cardiac failure or congenital heart disease, may aggravate the severity of NEC.

NEC becomes clinically apparent by progressive abdominal distention, bloody loose stools, feeding intolerance, bradycardia, hemodynamic instability, sepsis, and lethargy.

NEC is typically diagnosed by conventional abdominal radiography. Various direct and indirect imaging findings may be seen including air bubbles within the bowel wall (pneumatosis), portal venous air, free intraperitoneal air (after perforation). Earliest signs might be progressive air distention of smooth, "featureless" bowel loops, thickened bowel wall, and fixed bowel loops with little propagation of air through the bowel loops on serial imaging. The pearl string of intramural air bubbles are usually particularly well seen along the lateral contour of the descending or ascending colon. Occasionally air will be seen outlining the falciform ligament. Lateral supine views or anterioposterior views in the left lateral decubitus position may facilitate detection of free air. Intestinal ultrasound is another helpful and sensitive imaging tool to detect intramural, hyperechogenic air bubbles. Furthermore, cine studies may show moving air bubbles within the portal venous system, occasionally extending into the periphery of the liver. In later stages of the disease, strictures and adhesions may lead to mechanical ileus.

### Reference

Epelman M, Daneman A, Navarro OM, et al. Necrotizing enterocolitis: review of state-of-the-art imaging findings with pathologic correlation. *Radiographics*. 2007;27:285–305.

### Cross-reference

Walters MM, Robertson RL. *Pediatric Radiology: The Requisites*. 4th ed. Philadelphia: Elsevier; 2017:104–107.

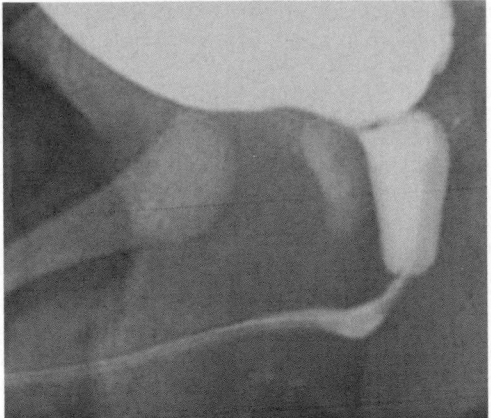

**Fig. 19.1**

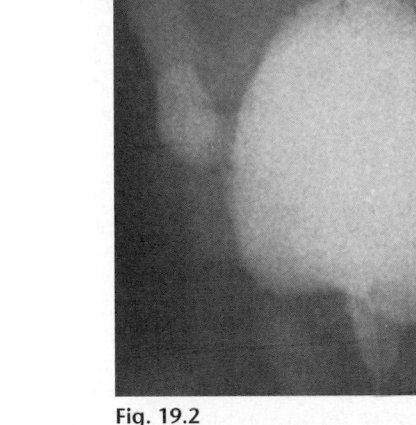

**Fig. 19.2**

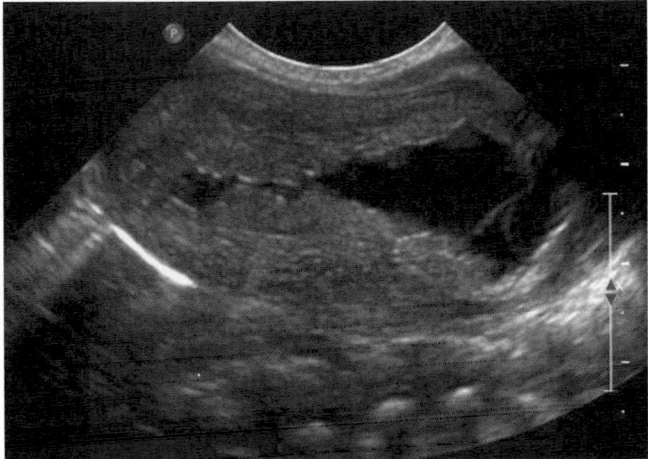

**Fig. 19.3**

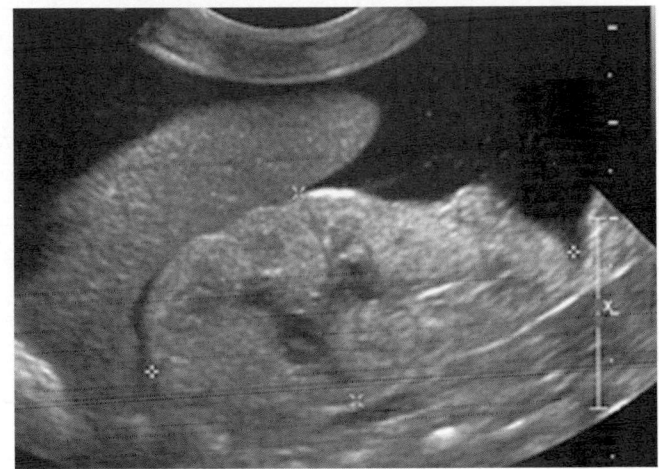

**Fig. 19.4**

**HISTORY:** Neonate with prenatal diagnosis of bilateral hydronephrosis and oligohydramnios

1. Which signature pathological imaging finding do you see on the voiding cystourethrogram?
   A. Dilated posterior urethra
   B. Bilateral high-grade vesicoureteral reflux (VUR)
   C. Trabeculated, deformed urinary bladder
   D. All of the above

2. What are the additional findings on the abdominal ultrasound (US)?
   A. High-grade hydronephrosis, ascites
   B. Nephrocalcinosis and blood in the peritoneal cavity
   C. Renal dysplasia, uroascites, hypertrophic bladder
   D. Renal cysts, patent urachus, and bladder stones

3. What is the most likely diagnosis?
   A. Bilateral ureteropelvic junction obstruction
   B. Primary VUR
   C. Primary obstructive megaureter
   D. Posterior urethral valves (PUVs)

4. Which of the following statements is correct?
   A. PUVs are frequently seen in polycystic recessive kidney disease.
   B. PUVs are associated with polyhydramnios during pregnancy.
   C. PUVs can be seen in association with hydrometrocolpos.
   D. PUVs may be complicated by end-stage renal disease.

## CASE 19

### Posterior Urethral Valves

1. D
2. C
3. D
4. D

## Comment

Posterior urethral valves (PUVs) are among the most frequent reasons for urethral obstruction in boys. These "valves" result from fusion and adhesions of mucosal folds in the urethra just below the verumontanum. Depending on the type and size of the valves, various degrees of pre- and postnatal chronic outlet obstruction of the bladder may be seen. In mild cases, an abnormal voiding pattern with a poor stream, incomplete voiding, and recurrent urinary tract infections are seen. In moderate to severe cases, the chronic obstruction may lead to bladder wall hypertrophy with extensive trabeculation, and progressive renal injury or failure due to chronic obstruction and vesicoureteral reflux (VUR), which is seen in 40% to 60% of children. PUVs that become apparent during fetal life are usually significant and are linked to a cascade of complications including renal dysplasia and oligohydramnios with subsequent pulmonary hypoplasia. Uroascites may result from fetal urine leaking into the peritoneal cavity after forniceal rupture (pop-off).

Prenatal ultrasound (US) or fetal magnetic resonance imaging (MRI) findings include megacystis, bladder wall thickening, dilated posterior urethra, symmetrical or asymmetrical hydroureteronephrosis, uroascites, renal dysplasia, oligohydramnios, and possibly associated pulmonary hypoplasia.

Postnatally, the US and MRI imaging features are similar. PUVs are, however, best seen on a retrograde urethrogram or on a dynamic voiding cystourethrogram (VCUG). VCUG typically demonstrates a significant dilation of the posterior urethra up to the level of the PUV. In addition, VCUG may reveal extensive VUR into dilated, tortuous ureters. Intrarenal reflux is occasionally noted. Catheterization of the urinary bladder may be difficult because the catheter may coil into the enlarged posterior urethra just superior to the valves. The use of a coudé catheter may be helpful. Early diagnosis and prompt, possibly intrauterine treatment are essential in limiting the degree of renal injury or failure.

### Reference

Clayton DB, Brock 3rd JW. Lower urinary tract obstruction in the fetus and neonate. *Clin Perinatol*. 2014;41:643-659.

### Cross-reference

Walters MM, Robertson RL. *Pediatric Radiology: The Requisites*. 4th ed. Philadelphia: Elsevier; 2017:155-156.

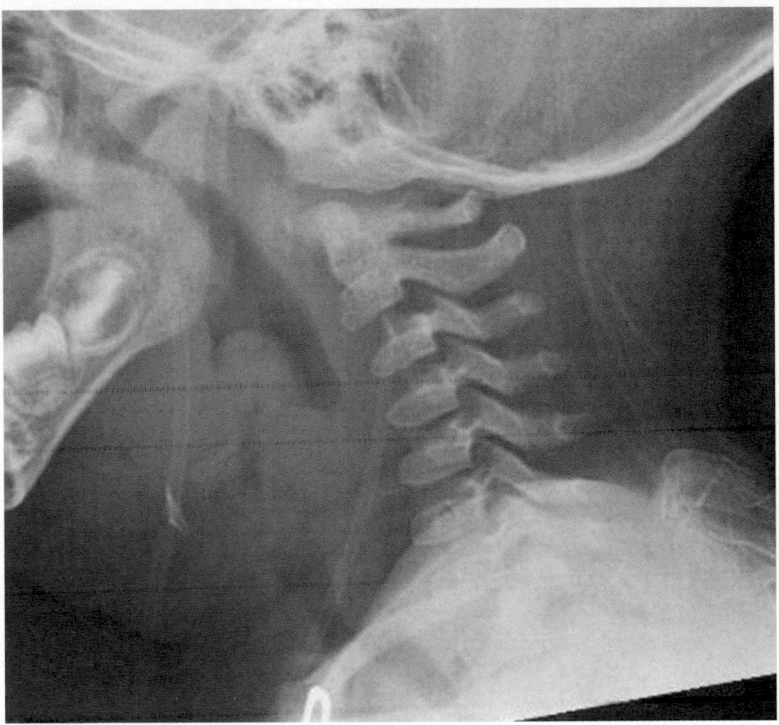

Fig. 20.1

**HISTORY:** 8-year-old girl presents with throat pain, difficulty breathing, and drooling.

1. Based on the image, what is the best diagnosis?
   A. Tonsillitis
   B. Epiglottitis
   C. Exudative tracheitis
   D. Swallowed foreign body

2. Since the introduction of vaccines, what is the mean age at which patients develop epiglottitis?
   A. 3.5 years
   B. >12 years
   C. 5.6 years
   D. 7.4 years

3. In a patient with suspected epiglottitis with drooling, but with the ability to maintain an airway, what is the best way to obtain confirmatory imaging?
   A. Computed tomography (CT) with contrast to rule out abscess
   B. Plain radiograph, lateral projection, in the upright position
   C. Plain radiograph, lateral projection, in the supine position
   D. Magnetic resonance imaging (MRI) of the neck to reduce radiation exposure

4. Which of the following is the most common organism associated with epiglottis?
   A. *Haemophilus influenzae* type B
   B. Group A beta-hemolytic *Streptococcus pneumoniae*
   C. *Klebsiella pneumoniae*
   D. *Moraxella catarrhalis*

## CASE 20

### Epiglottitis

1. B

2. B

3. B

4. A

### Comment

Epiglottitis is most commonly caused by *Haemophilus influenzae* type B (HIB). Now that immunization against HIB has become routine, the incidence of epiglottitis has dramatically decreased. Classically, the peak incidence was said to occur at 3.5 years, but since the introduction of the HIB vaccine, the average age has increased significantly, and epiglottitis is now more common in older children and adults. If the patient is stable and imaging is needed, lateral and anteroposterior (optional, especially if epiglottitis is strongly suspected) views of the neck are obtained with the patient in a comfortable upright position. The epiglottis appears markedly swollen and thickened ("thumb sign"). Computed tomography (CT) does not play a role in the diagnosis of epiglottitis. Exudative (or bacterial) tracheitis is also rare and a potentially life-threatening disease, but, unlike epiglottitis, occurs in the subglottic airway. It is typically seen in children who are older than those with croup, and on imaging, one can see intraluminal filling defects, plaque-like irregularity of the tracheal wall, and asymmetric subglottic narrowing.

### Reference

Darras KE, Roston AT, Yewchuk LK. Imaging acute airway obstruction in infants and children. *Radiographics*. 2015;35(7):2064–2079.

### Cross-reference

Walters MM, Robertson RL. *Pediatric Radiology: The Requisites*. 4th ed. Philadelphia: Elsevier; 2017:15–16.

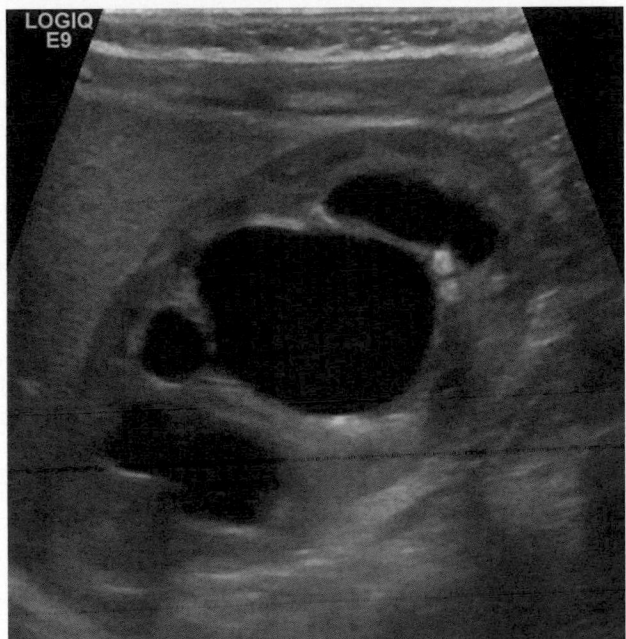

Fig. 21.1

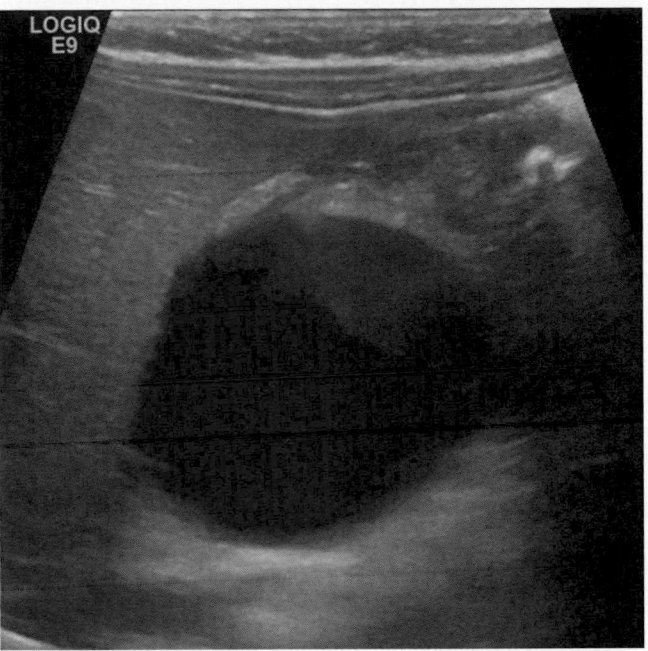

Fig. 21.2

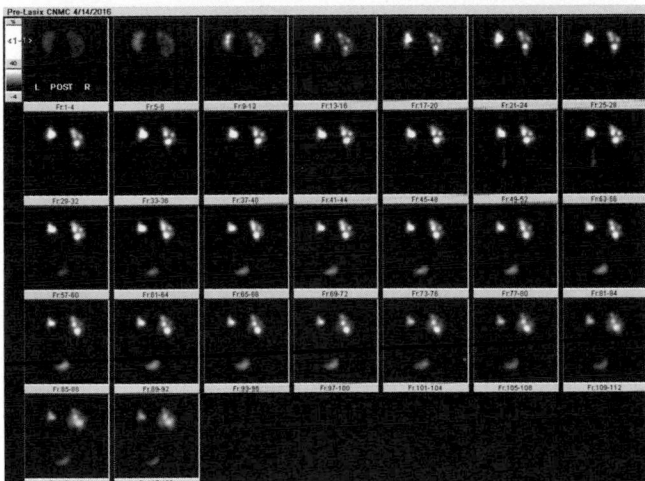

Fig. 21.3

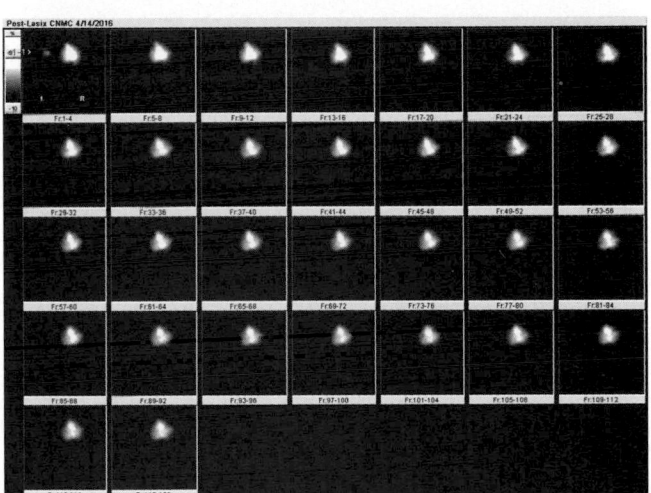

Fig. 21.4

**HISTORY:** Newborn girl with known prenatal diagnosis, withheld

1. What is the best diagnosis?
   A. Multicystic dysplastic kidney
   B. Hydronephrosis
   C. Megaureter
   D. Ureteropelvic junction (UPJ) obstruction

2. What is the most common imaging strategy for UPJ obstruction?
   A. Perform magnetic resonance imaging (MRI) immediately after birth, then follow up with semiannual ultrasounds.
   B. Perform ultrasound first, then do a nuclear renal scan to grade the degree of obstruction and determine when/if surgical intervention is necessary.
   C. Perform a voiding cystourethrogram (VCUG) first, then do an ultrasound if the VCUG is positive for reflux.
   D. Perform a retrograde urethrogram.

3. Which option describes the classic imaging finding of UPJ obstruction?
   A. Moderate to marked hydronephrosis, calyceal dilation that is disproportionate to pelviectasis, and abrupt tapering of the pelvis without hydroureter.
   B. Pelvicaliectasis may persist for years following successful surgery.
   C. Delayed contrast excretion can be seen in a contrast-enhanced computed tomography (CT) scan or MRI.
   D. All of the above

4. True or false?
   A. In patients with UPJ obstruction, nuclear renal scans are typically performed with a diuretic challenge and show hydronephrosis with poor drainage despite hydration and diuretic washout.
   B. In patients with UPJ obstruction, nerve fibers are depleted in the muscular layers in the ureteric wall.

## CASE 21

### Ureteropelvic Junction Obstruction

1. D

2. B

3. D

4. A) True, B) False

### *Comment*

Ureteropelvic junction (UPJ) obstruction is the most common cause of abdominal mass in a newborn. It occurs in about 1 in 1000 live births, more often in boys, and on the left side.

Most cases are diagnosed prenatally. Similar to their adult counterparts, older children presenting with UPJ obstruction are likely to have extrinsic compression from crossing vessels.

Ultrasound demonstrates a very large renal pelvis, with dilation that is disproportionately large compared to the calyces. Pre- and post-Lasix mercaptoacetyltriglycine (MAG3) nuclear medicine studies are helpful in determining the level of obstruction and differential function. Magnetic resonance urography is an emerging modality for evaluation of UPJ obstruction; however, its use is not as common compared to the modalities described earlier. The surgical approach to this entity has evolved over time, and recent data indicate that correction may not be necessary in all children.

### References

González R, Schimke CM. Ureteropelvic junction obstruction in infants and children. *Pediatr Clin North Am.* 2001;48(6):1505–1518.

Houben CH, Wischermann A, Börner G, Slany E. Outcome analysis of pyeloplasty in infants. *Pediatr Surg Int.* 2000;16(3):189–193.

### Cross-reference

Walters MM, Robertson RL. *Pediatric Radiology: The Requisites.* 4th ed. Philadelphia: Elsevier; 2017:149–152.

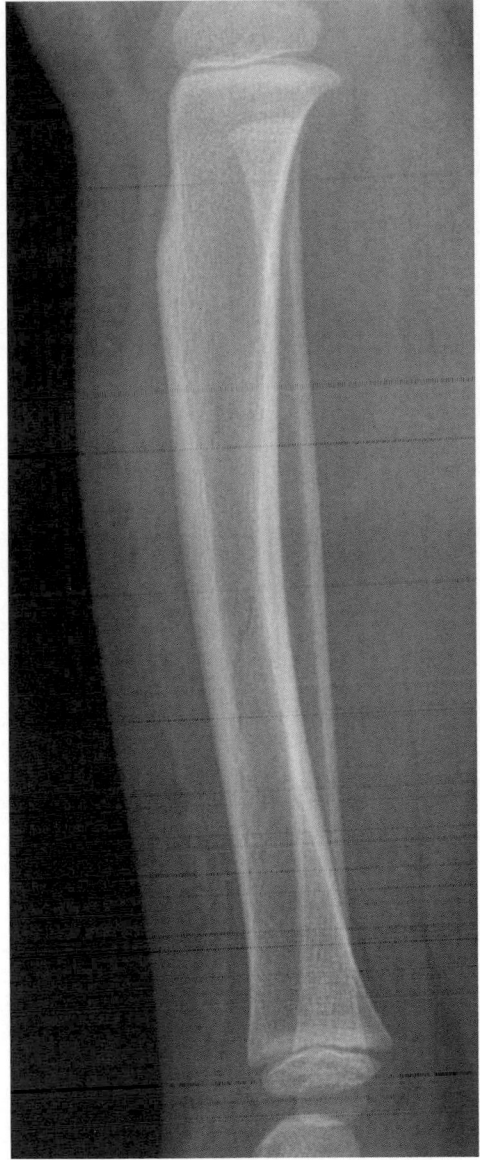

Fig. 22.1

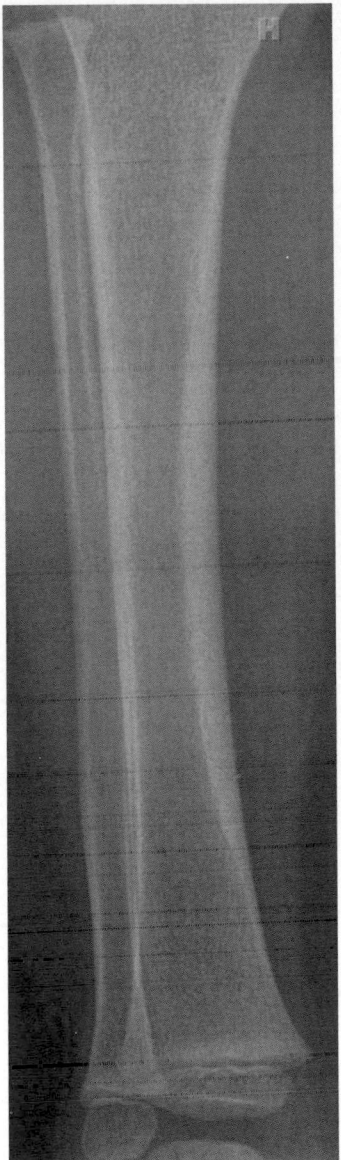

Fig. 22.2

**HISTORY:** Refusal of weight bearing in the lower extremity of a toddler.

1. What is your diagnosis?
   A. Toddler's fracture
   B. Child abuse
   C. Neuroblastoma metastasis
   D. Osteomyelitis

2. What is the most common location for toddler's fractures?
   A. Tibial midshaft
   B. Proximal femoral epiphysis
   C. Distal femoral diaphysis
   D. Metatarsal, especially the fifth ray

3. Which of the following describes the typical clinical presentation of a toddler's fracture?
   A. 2-year-old normally ambulating child suddenly refuses to bear weight or limps
   B. 4-year-old child presenting with fever and refusal to bear weight

   C. 10-year-old presents with lower limb pain after jumping on a trampoline
   D. 2-month-old infant brought to emergency department with bruising over the lower extremities

4. Which option describes the classic imaging finding of toddler's fracture?
   A. Spiral nondisplaced lucent fracture line in the distal tibia
   B. Sclerotic fracture line parallel to the calcaneal apophysis
   C. Buckle or bowing deformity of the distal shaft of the fibula
   D. All of the above

## CASE 22

### Toddler's Fracture

1. A

2. A

3. A

4. D

### Comment

Toddler's fracture is a stress fracture of the lower extremity in a newly ambulating child usually after minor trauma. The most common clinical presentation is the child's refusal to walk or bear weight in the affected lower extremity. Physical exam reveals pain to direct palpation. The peak age of presentation is 1 to 3 years of age. The diagnosis can be difficult at the initial evaluation because of negative radiography findings. In cases with strong clinical suspicion, conservative treatment with casting is recommended with a follow-up radiography performed in 10 days. The femur, tibia, fibula, talus, calcaneus, cuboid, and metatarsals can be affected. These are typically nondisplaced hairline fractures and can sometimes present with buckling, especially in the tibia and fibula. In the hindfoot, cuboid fractures can present with a sclerotic band. These fractures heal without deformity.

### Reference

Sapru K, Cooper JG. Management of the toddler's fracture with and without initial radiographic evidence. *Eur J Emerg Med*. 2012;21(6):451–454.

### Cross-reference

Walters MM, Robertson RL. *Pediatric Radiology: The Requisites*. 4th ed. Philadelphia: Elsevier; 2017:255.

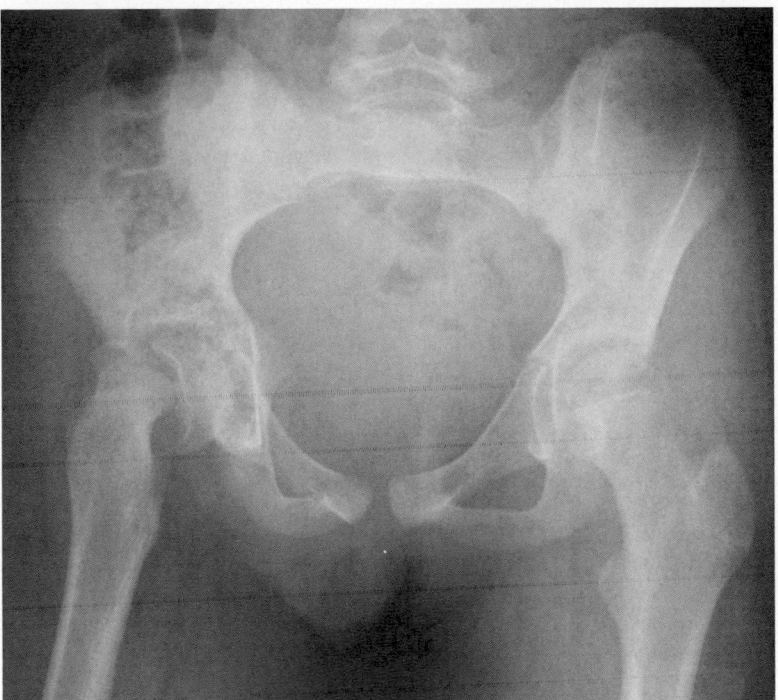

Fig. 23.1

**HISTORY:** 11-year-old obese male presenting with hip pain

1. Based on the imaging findings, what is the best diagnosis? (Choose all that apply.)
   A. Legg-Calve-Perthes disease
   B. Septic hip
   C. Transient synovitis of the hip
   D. Slipped capital femoral epiphysis (SCFE)

2. How often is SCFE bilateral at initial presentation?
   A. 20% to 30%
   B. 40% to 50%
   C. 60% to 70%
   D. >80%

3. What type of a Salter-Harris fracture does this represent?
   A. Type I
   B. Type II
   C. Type III
   D. Type IV

4. Which option is *not* a risk factor for SCFE?
   A. Hypothyroidism
   B. Excessive growth hormone production
   C. Renal osteodystrophy
   D. Rickets

## CASE 23

### Slipped Capital Femoral Epiphysis

1. D

2. A

3. A

4. B

## Comment

Slipped capital femoral epiphysis (SCFE) is an idiopathic Salter-Harris type I fracture. At initial presentation, it is bilateral in up to 20% to 30% of cases. Conditions that weaken the physis and/or predispose to Salter-Harris type I fractures also increase the risk for SCFE, including thyroid or growth hormone deficiency (both are necessary for growth and maturation of the physeal cartilage, with subsequent calcification and replacement by mineralized osteoid), renal osteodystrophy, rickets, poor nutrition, and rapid growth spurts. Peak incidence occurs between 10 and 16 years (these years coincide with growth spurts). Boys are affected more commonly than girls. Also more commonly affected are African Americans and overweight patients. Treatment is with pinning of the epiphysis with minimal or no reduction. Long-term complications include femoroacetabular impingement (FAI), osteoarthrosis, and avascular necrosis. Diagnosis is best made on a frog-leg lateral radiograph or via magnetic resonance imaging (MRI). On the radiograph, a line drawn through the lateral aspect of the femoral neck should normally bisect the lateral aspect of the epiphysis. On MRI, widening of the physis with or without normal anatomical alignment is diagnostic. Bone marrow edema is often seen in the adjacent metaphysis. A normal radiograph does not exclude SCFE.

### Reference

Jarrett DY, Matheney T, Kleinman PK. Imaging SCFE: diagnosis, treatment and complications. *Pediatr Radiol*. 2013;43(suppl 1):S71–S82.

### Cross-reference

Walters MM, Robertson RL. *Pediatric Radiology: The Requisites*. 4th ed. Philadelphia: Elsevier; 2017:220.

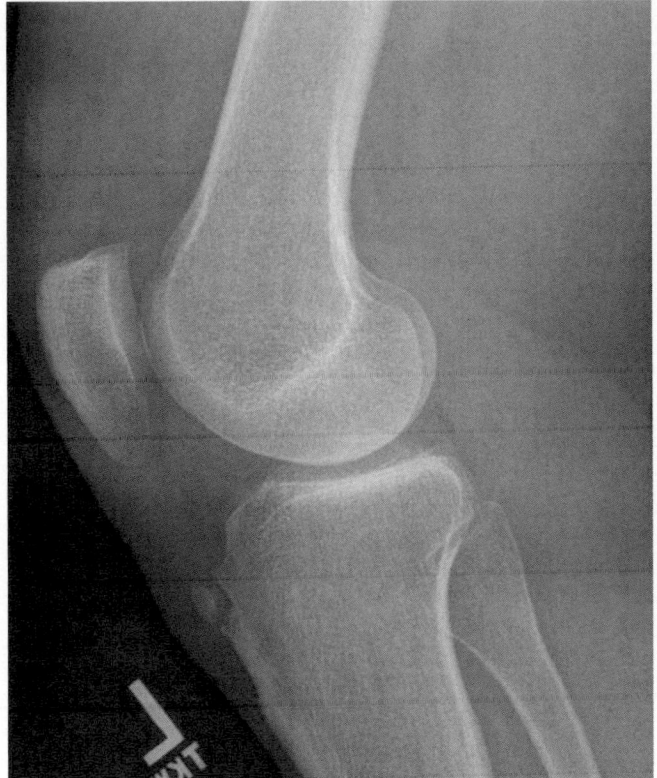

**Fig. 24.1**

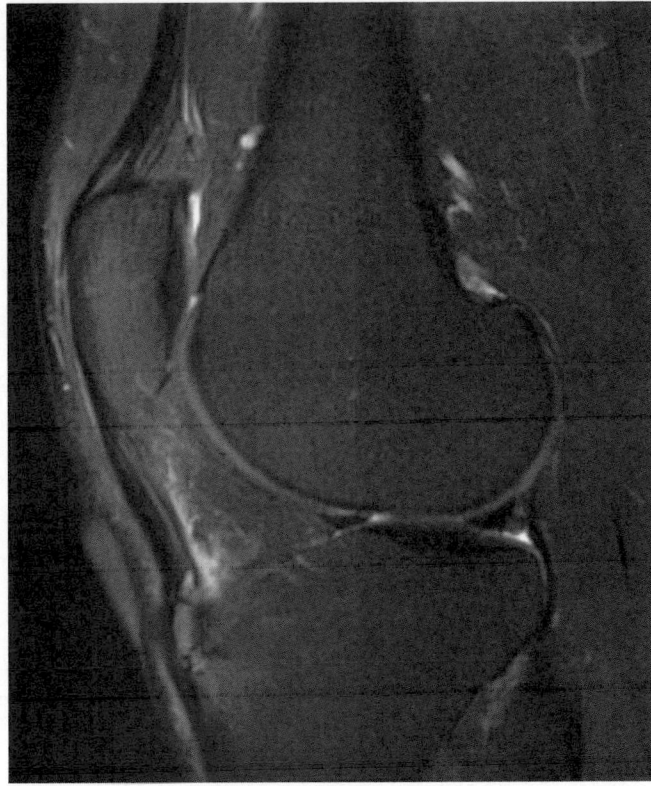

**Fig. 24.2**

**HISTORY:** 17-year-old male presenting with tenderness and pain in his knee

1. Given the imaging findings, which of the following would you include in your differential diagnosis? (Choose all that apply.)
   A. Normal variant irregular ossification center of the tibial tuberosity
   B. Sinding-Larsen-Johansson disease
   C. Osgood Schlatter disease
   D. Patellar tendonitis

2. In what percentage of patients is Osgood Schlatter disease found bilaterally?
   A. <15%
   B. 15% to 25%
   C. 25% to 50%
   D. >50%

3. Which of the following statements about Osgood Schlatter disease is *incorrect*?
   A. It is usually self-limited.
   B. It affects girls more than boys.
   C. It is due to repetitive microtrauma during the phase of skeletal maturation of the tibial tubercle.
   D. Irregular fragmented ossification of the tibial tubercle often remains following resolution of clinical symptoms, but the soft tissue swelling resolves.

4. True or false?
   A. Osgood Schlatter disease is primarily a clinical diagnosis.

## CASE 24

### Osgood Schlatter Disease

1. C

2. B

3. B

4. True

### Comment

Osgood Schlatter disease, also known as tibial osteochondrosis, represents a traction apophysitis of the patellar tendon insertion on the tibial tubercle. It is bilateral in about 25% to 50% of patients and affects boys more often than girls. It is caused by repetitive microtrauma during the phase of skeletal maturation of the tibial tubercle, typically between 10 and 15 years of age in males, and between 8 and 13 years of age in girls. Patients classically present with a painful and visible area of swelling anterior to the proximal tibial metaphysis, and diagnosis is made based on clinical findings and the patient's history. Imaging is performed to confirm the diagnosis and to rule out other causes of knee pain. Plain radiographs reveal characteristic soft tissue swelling adjacent to the patellar tendon insertion on the tibial tubercle, with ossification and thickening of the patellar tendon insertion site. The tibial tubercle itself is typically irregular and fragmented, and fragmentation commonly remains after resolution of clinical symptoms, but soft tissue swelling should resolve. On magnetic resonance imaging (MRI), a T2-hyperintense edema pattern is typically seen within bone fragments and in the adjacent tibial tubercle. The distal patellar tendon shows thickening and T2 hyperintensity along with soft tissue edema pattern in the adjacent soft tissues. The clinical course is usually self-limited, and treatment is conservative with rest and nonsteroidal antiinflammatory medications. Distinguishing this entity from a normal variant irregular ossification center of the tibial tubercle are the clinical presentation with pain and the associated soft tissue swelling. Sinding-Larsen-Johansson disease has a similar etiology but affects the proximal patellar tendon origin at the inferior pole of the patella. Patellar tendonitis typically affects the proximal patellar tendon rather than the distal insertion.

### Reference

Dupuis CS, Westra SJ, Makris J, Wallace EC. Injuries and conditions of the extensor mechanism of the pediatric knee. *Radiographics*. 2009;29(3):877–886.

### Cross-reference

Walters MM, Robertson RL. *Pediatric Radiology: The Requisites*. 4th ed. Philadelphia: Elsevier; 2017:252.

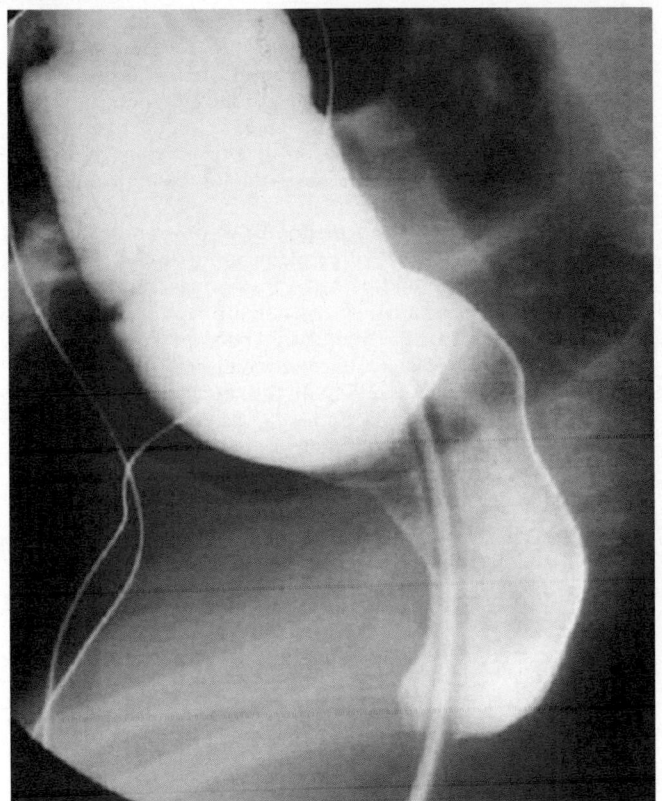

Fig. 25.1

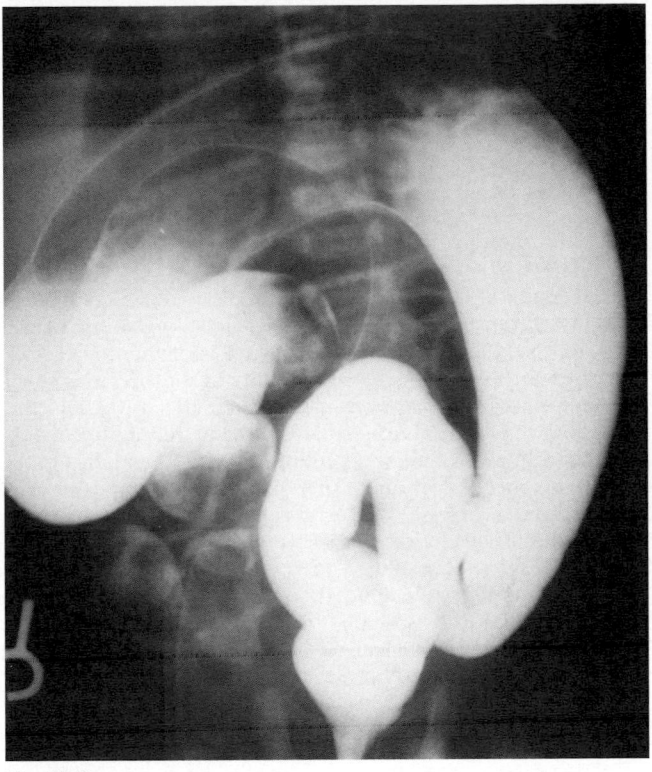

Fig. 25.2

**HISTORY:** Newborn female infant presents at the radiology suite with failure to pass meconium in the first 48 hours of life.

1. What is the most likely diagnosis?
   A. Meconium plug syndrome
   B. Meconium ileus
   C. Anal atresia
   D. Hirschsprung disease (HD)

2. What is the classic imaging finding on enema in this entity?
   A. Rectosigmoid ratio (RSR) >1
   B. RSR <1
   C. Narrowing of the unaffected bowel
   D. Short colon

3. Which option describes the affected bowel segment in this entity?
   A. Overpopulation of Meissner plexus
   B. Lacking of Meissner and Auerbach plexuses
   C. Overpopulation of Auerbach plexus
   D. Normal Meissner and Auerbach plexuses

4. Which of the following is true regarding imaging of Hirschsprung disease (HD)?
   A. Magnetic resonance imaging (MRI) is increasingly used to image the bowel wall.
   B. Ultrasonography is superior to MRI and computed tomography (CT) for initial diagnosis.
   C. Despite concerns for radiation, CT is the gold standard for diagnosis.
   D. Plain radiograph followed with enema is the imaging algorithm for HD.

## Hirschsprung Disease

1. D
2. B
3. B
4. D

### Comment

The diagnosis of Hirschsprung disease (HD) relies on identification of the absence of ganglion cells at the myenteric (Auerbach) and submucosal (Meissner) plexuses of the bowel wall. The disease results in decreased motility in the affected bowel segment, lack of propagation of the peristaltic waves into the aganglionic colon, and abnormal or absent relaxation of this segment. Failure to pass meconium and abdominal distention in the newborn, or chronic constipation in older infants and children are the classic clinic presentation. Dr. Hirschsprung initially described the disease in 1886 when, at the time, the dilated colon was considered to be the abnormality, thus the term *congenital megacolon*. HD is 4 times more common in males. HD is usually sporadic, although familial occurrence is reported in 5% to 20% of patients. There is strong association with Down syndrome; 5% to 15% of HD patients have Down syndrome. Other associations include Waardenburg syndrome, congenital deafness, malrotation, gastric diverticulum, and intestinal atresias. Approximately 75% of cases are classic short-segment HD, in which the aganglionic segment does not extend beyond the upper sigmoid. Long-segment involvement can be seen in up to 20% of cases. Total colonic aganglionosis is possible, but is luckily quite rare and affects approximately 5% of patients.

An enema is usually performed with water-soluble contrast and is the study of choice after plain radiography. The rectosigmoid ratio (RSR) should be 1; the transverse diameter of the rectum should be equal to or larger than the sigmoid. An RSR of <1 is concerning for HD and should prompt a rectal suction biopsy for definitive diagnosis. Identification of the transition zone, RSR <1, irregular contour of the affected segment, and delayed evacuation of the barium are the imaging findings, and when two or more of these findings are present, diagnosis of HD becomes a stronger suspicion. Complications include toxic megacolon, chronic constipation, and anemia. There is no known increased risk for malignancy in the colon.

### Reference

Tam PK. Hirschsprung's disease: a bridge for science and surgery. *J Pediatr Surg*. 2016;51(1):18–22.

### Cross-reference

Walters MM, Robertson RL. *Pediatric Radiology: The Requisites*. 4th ed. Philadelphia: Elsevier; 2017:96–97.

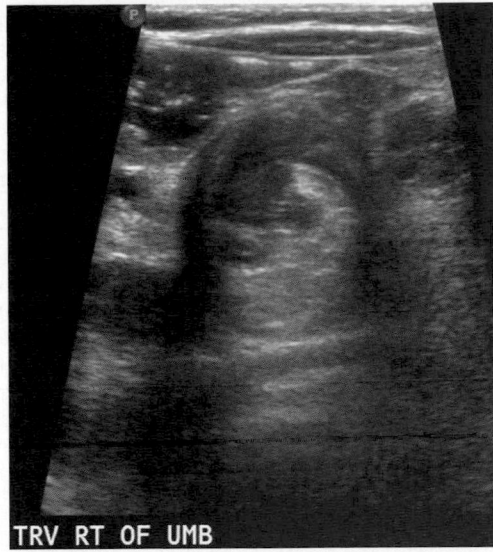

TRV RT OF UMB

Fig. 26.1

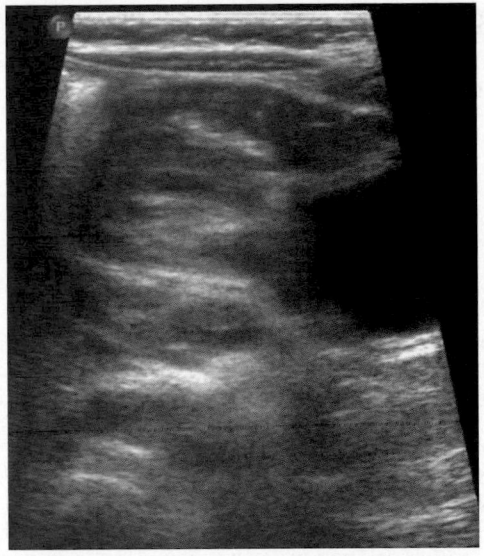

Fig. 26.2

See Supplemental Figures section for additional figures for this case.

**HISTORY:** 4-year-old presenting with abdominal pain

1. Based on the imaging findings, what is the best diagnosis?
   A. Intussusception secondary to a Meckel diverticulum or duplication cyst
   B. Idiopathic intussusception
   C. Hypertrophic pyloric stenosis
   D. Burkitt lymphoma

2. What is the most common location of idiopathic intussusception?
   A. Ileocolic
   B. Colocolic
   C. Jejunoileal
   D. Duodenojejunal

3. Which of the following is a contraindication to image-guided pressure reduction?
   A. Pneumoperitoneum
   B. Prolonged history of symptoms
   C. Decreased vascularity of the intussusceptum on ultrasound (US)
   D. Documented cystic mass such as a Meckel diverticulum or duplication cyst within the intussusceptum

4. Which of the following statements about idiopathic intussusception is correct?
   A. Alternating lethargy and irritability is a common presenting sign.
   B. Boys are 7 times more commonly affected than girls.
   C. Currant jelly stools are the most sensitive and specific presenting sign.
   D. Treatment of choice for idiopathic intussusception is surgery.

## Intussusception

1. A

2. A

3. A

4. A

## *Comment*

Idiopathic intussusception occurs in children between the ages of about 4 months and 4 years, most commonly 4 to 12 months, with males and females affected similarly. Outside of that age range, a lead point causing the intussusception is more likely, and treatment is then surgical. Causes of lead points include a Meckel diverticulum (as shown in this case), duplication cyst, polyp, lipoma, hematoma, and lymphoma (e.g., Burkitt lymphoma). Ultrasound is the modality of choice to diagnose intussusception and typically shows a target sign (transverse image) or a pseudokidney sign (longitudinal image), with alternating layers of hyper- and hypoechogenicity in the right lower quadrant. Occasionally the intussusception may progress more proximally, in which case, all four quadrants need to be surveyed. Typically, the transverse diameter of the intussusception measures 2.5 to 5 cm. Alternating lethargy and irritability, colic/crampy abdominal pain, and palpable right-sided abdominal mass are common presenting symptoms. Bloody diarrhea, "red currant jelly" stools, and vomiting can also be seen.

For idiopathic intussusception, image-guided pressure reduction, with air insufflation or liquid contrast, is the treatment of choice. The likelihood of successful reduction of the intussusception decreases with prolonged history of symptoms (>24 to 72 hours) as well as decreased vascularity and interloop fluid in the intussusceptum. Contraindications to image-guided pressure reduction include pneumoperitoneum and peritonitis. Small bowel intussusception is less common than ileocolic intussusception in the pediatric age group and typically measures less than 2 cm in transverse diameter. Most of these are transient and resolve on their own. When persistent or recurrent, however, a lead point may be present, for example, polyps in Peutz-Jeghers syndrome, intramural hematoma in Henoch-Schoenlein purpura, or a nodal mass in lymphoma, and the treatment is then surgical.

### Reference

Di Giacomo V, Trinci M, van der Byl G, Catania VD, Calisti A, Miele V. Ultrasound in newborns and children suffering from non-traumatic acute abdominal pain: imaging with clinical and surgical correlation. *J Ultrasound*. 2014;18(4):385–393.

### Cross-reference

Walters MM, Robertson RL. *Pediatric Radiology: The Requisites*. 4th ed. Philadelphia: Elsevier; 2017:108–112.

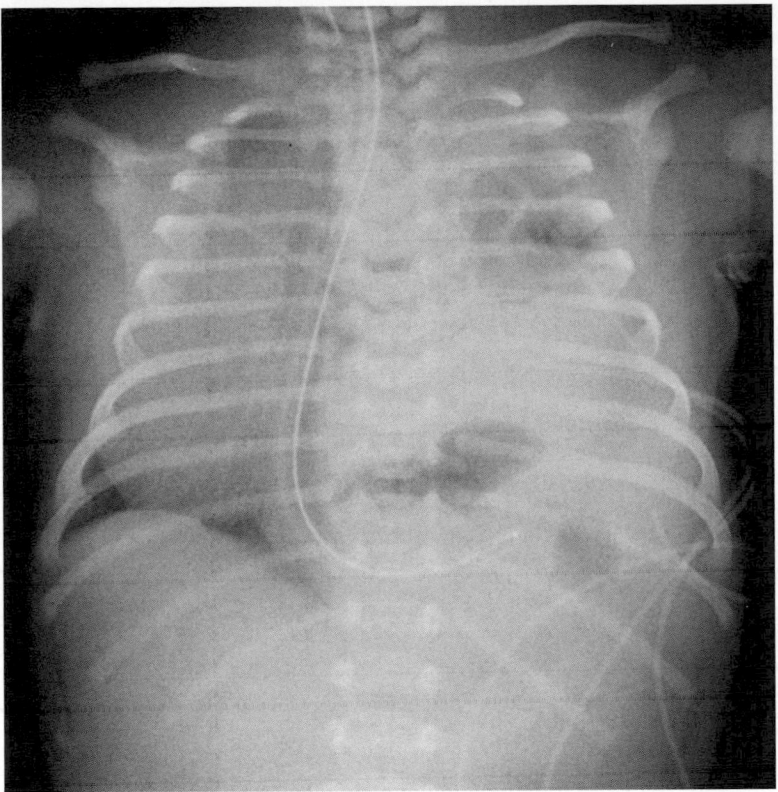

Fig. 27.1

**HISTORY:** Neonatal infant presents with respiratory distress.

1. What is the most common location of a congenital diaphragmatic hernia?
   A. Anterior on the right
   B. Posterior on the right
   C. Anterior on the left
   D. Posterior on the left

2. What is the most important predictor of morbidity and mortality?
   A. Presence of liver herniation
   B. Degree of pulmonary hypoplasia
   C. Presence of colonic herniation
   D. Presence of stomach herniation

3. Which of the following has been found to be most influential in reducing mortality rates?
   A. Delivery and postnatal care in a high-volume extracorporeal membrane oxygenation (ECMO) center
   B. Definitive surgical correction in the first few days of life
   C. Absence of stomach herniation

4. Which option describes the best diagnostic clue to suggest this diagnosis over its mimickers?
   A. Solid mass near diaphragm
   B. Hyperlucent lung near the diaphragm
   C. Bubbly lesion with multiple air-fluid levels
   D. Abnormal position of support devices

## CASE 27

### Congenital Diaphragmatic Hernia

1. D
2. B
3. A
4. D

### Comment

Congenital diaphragmatic hernia (CDH) occurs in 1 of every 2000 to 3000 live births and accounts for 8% of all major congenital anomalies. The most common location is posteriorly (Bochdalek) on the left. It is usually diagnosed prenatally with ultrasound. Initial postnatal radiograph may not show the herniated bowel loops due to lack of air in the bowel early on. Mediastinal shift with displacement of the heart to the opposite side of the hernia is typical. Abnormal position of support devices, if present, can help point to CDH as the correct diagnosis.

The hernia may contain stomach, small bowel, colon, or liver. Herniation of the liver into the right chest is associated with a worse prognosis, but the most important prognostic factor is the degree of pulmonary hypoplasia. The mortality rate associated with CDH ranges from approximately 10% to 50%, with the lowest rates observed in high-volume centers with extracorporeal membrane oxygenation (ECMO) capabilities. Treatment is surgical and can be performed during pregnancy (ex utero intrapartum treatment [EXIT] procedure) or after birth once the infant is stable. Many infants born with CDH have major associated abnormalities, including congenital heart disease and malrotation. Lesions that can have a similar appearance on imaging include congenital pulmonary airway malformation, congenital lobar hyperinflation, and pulmonary sequestration, which can resemble CDH prior to aeration of the bowel.

### References

Alamo L, Gudinchet F, Meuli R. Imaging findings in fetal diaphragmatic abnormalities. *Pediatr Radiol*. 2015;45(13):1887–1900.

McHoney M. Congenital diaphragmatic hernia, management in the newborn. *Pediatr Surg Int*. 2015;31(11):1105–1113.

### Cross-reference

Walters MM, Robertson RL. *Pediatric Radiology: The Requisites*. 4th ed. Philadelphia: Elsevier; 2017:14–15.

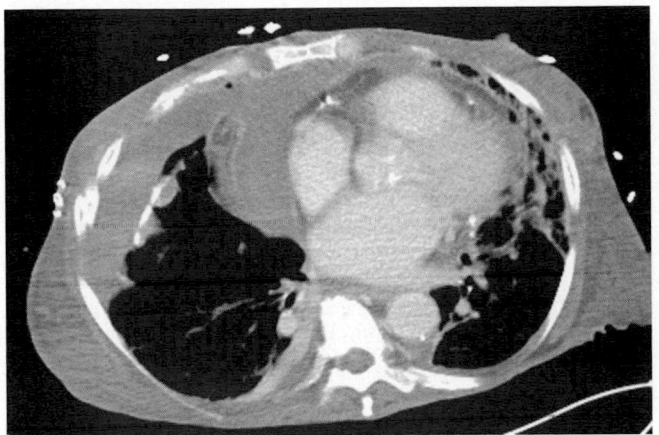

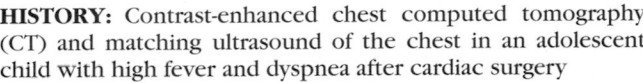

**Fig. 28.1**

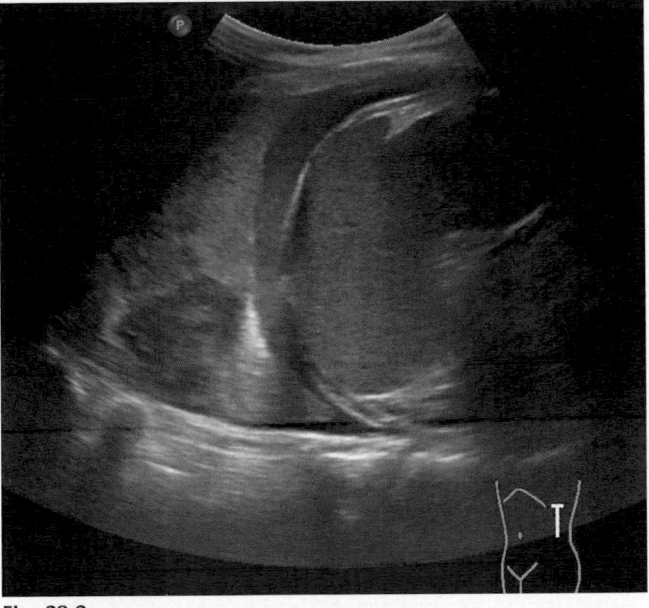

**Fig. 28.2**

**HISTORY:** Contrast-enhanced chest computed tomography (CT) and matching ultrasound of the chest in an adolescent child with high fever and dyspnea after cardiac surgery

1. Which signature pathological imaging finding do you see on the chest CT?
   A. Pleural effusion with atelectasis
   B. Pleural free air with atelectasis
   C. Pleural hemorrhage with atelectasis
   D. Chylothorax with atelectasis

2. Which option describes additional findings in the chest ultrasound study that allow you to narrow your differential diagnosis?
   A. Hypodense pleural fluid, adjacent atelectasis, and intrapulmonary infiltrate/abscess
   B. Hypodense pleural fluid, adjacent atelectasis, and pneumatocele
   C. Hyperdense pleural fluid, adjacent atelectasis, and intrapulmonary infiltrate/abscess
   D. None of the above.

3. What is the most likely final diagnosis?
   A. Infected intrapulmonary hematoma
   B. Fluid-filled intrapulmonary pneumatocele with pleural effusion
   C. Pneumonia with abscess formation and parapneumonic pleural empyema
   D. Pneumonia with intrapulmonary necrosis and clear pleural effusion

4. Which statement is correct?
   A. Pleural effusions/transudates are typically nonsterile.
   B. Pleural empyemas are frequently related to congestive heart failure.
   C. Chylothorax often results from an injury to the thoracic duct.
   D. Blood in the pleural space usually results from necrotizing pneumonia.

## CASE 28

### Empyema in Pneumonia

1. A
2. C
3. C
4. D

## Comment

Parapneumonic pleural empyema refers to the accumulation of purulent exudate or pus in the pleural space secondary to pneumonia. Pleural empyemas may also be seen secondary to pleuritis, secondary to sepsis, or after a penetrating chest wall injury. Pleural empyemas should be differentiated from reactive sterile pleural effusions/transudates because of significant differences in clinical management. Pleural empyemas require a more aggressive antibiotic treatment, and in rare cases a surgical evacuation may become necessary. Parapneumonic transudates typically resolve spontaneously when the pneumonia is treated. Transudates may also be seen in a variety of other disease processes including congestive heart disease, nephrotic syndromes, autoimmune conditions, or liver disease. Excessive amounts of ascites may also leak into the pleural space. Differential diagnosis includes a chylothorax secondary to an injury to the thoracic duct, a hematothorax after trauma, or a malignant pleural effusion in a metastasizing malignant process.

Finally, excessive pleural fluid may result from a ventriculo-pleural shunt.

In most instances, pleural empyemas are first suspected on chest radiography as a nonspecific pleural fluid collection adjacent to a pneumonic infiltrate. Differentiation from a pleural transudate on chest radiography is limited. Pleural empyemas are typically more contained/loculated, limiting the redistribution of the fluid in various patient positions.

Pleural ultrasound is usually diagnostic. In contrast to sterile pleural transudate, pleural empyemas usually show multiple septations/strands, internal debris, and an increased echogenicity of the fluid. Occasionally a thickening and hyperemia of the pleural leaves are seen. Pleural calcifications may be noted in chronic cases.

Computed tomography (CT) can easily identify the amount of pleural fluid, however the internal septations/strands may remain undetected. Contrast-enhanced CT can easily show the complexity of the pneumonia, allows detection of intrapulmonary abscesses, and can show the pleural thickening and possible calcifications.

### References

McCauley L, Dean N. Pneumonia and empyema: causal, casual or unknown. *J Thorac Dis*. 2015;7:992–998.

Newman B. Ultrasound body applications in children. *Pediatr Radiol*. 2011;41(suppl 2):555–561.

### Cross-reference

Walters MM, Robertson RL. *Pediatric Radiology: The Requisites*. 4th ed. Philadelphia: Elsevier; 2017:36–37.

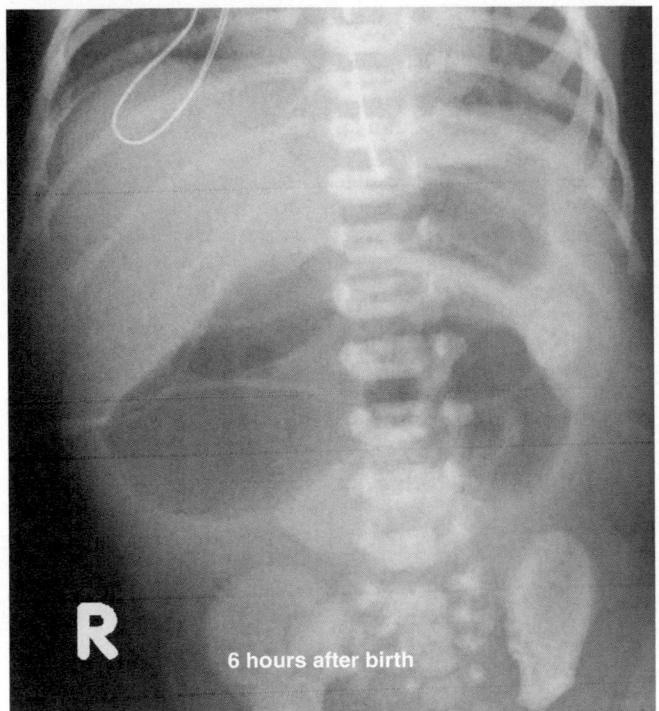

6 hours after birth

Fig. 29.1

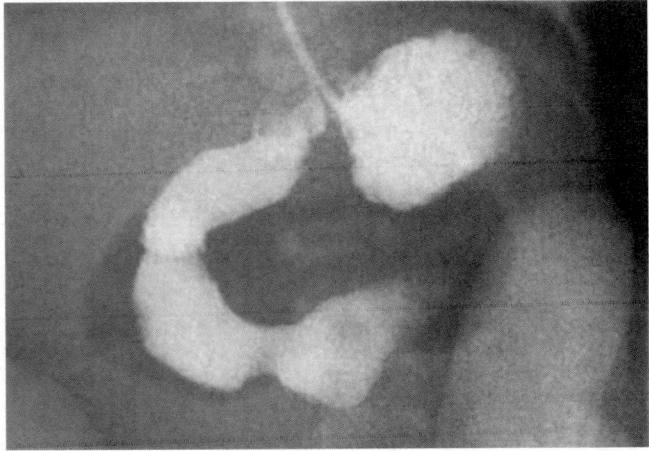

Fig. 29.2

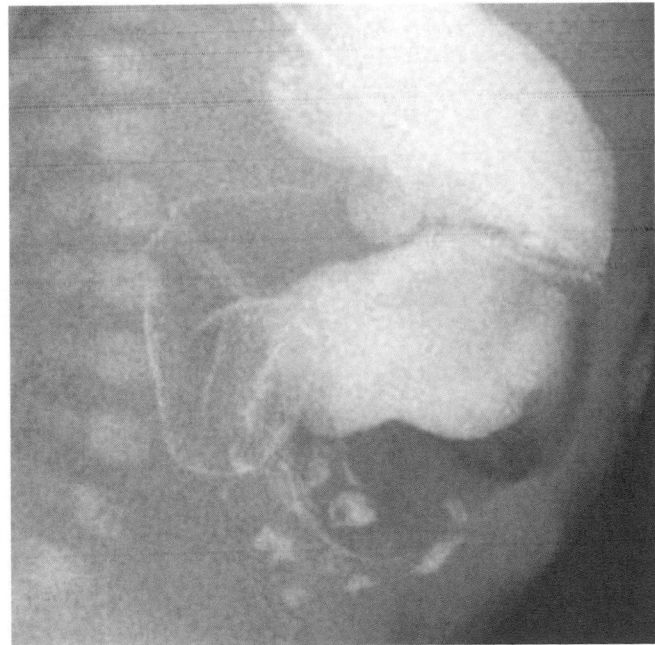

Fig. 29.3

**HISTORY:** Newborn with a suspected gastrointestinal (GI) abnormality prenatally. Details of prenatal imaging withheld.

1. What is the most likely presenting symptom in this infant?
   A. Bilious emesis
   B. Failure to pass meconium
   C. Respiratory distress
   D. Large for gestational age

2. Based on the plain radiograph, which of the following should be suspected?
   A. Upper GI obstruction
   B. Lower GI obstruction
   C. Hirschsprung disease
   D. Meconium plug syndrome

3. What is the most likely diagnosis based on the upper GI exam?
   A. Proximal jejunal atresia
   B. Distal jejunal atresia
   C. Ileal atresia
   D. Anal atresia

4. What is the most common cause of this entity?
   A. Intrauterine vascular obstruction involving the mesenteric vessels
   B. Chromosome 6 deletion
   C. Trauma
   D. Congenital infection

## CASE 29

### Jejunal Atresia

1. A

2. A

3. A

4. A

## Comment

Intestinal atresias are believed to result from in utero vascular accident due to compression, twisting, or embolic occlusion. The mortality rate is low, especially in isolated cases, however patients are still affected by comorbidities such as sepsis, short bowel syndrome, need for prolonged total parenteral nutrition, and hospital stay. Jejunoileal atresia is the most common type of intestinal atresia, and jejunal atresia is more common than ileal atresia. One-third of these children are born prematurely, and <1% have associated chromosomal abnormalities. Associations have been reported with gastroschisis: 10% of patients with gastroschisis have jejunoileal atresia and 10% of patients with jejunoileal atresia will have cystic fibrosis. Jejunal atresias can be multiple, and concurrent duodenal or colonic atresias may occur in 6% of patients. Approximately 20% have malrotation. A combination of dilated bowel loops (diameter >7 mm) and polyhydramnios can be suggestive of atresia in prenatal evaluations. The presenting symptom depends on how proximal the atresia is. If the atresia is proximal, then bilious emesis is present; if the atresia is distal, then delayed passage of meconium occurs. These conditions can have variable degrees of abdominal distention. Patients with delayed partial or incomplete jejunal atresia can present with a failure to thrive. Plain abdominal radiography alone can be diagnostic because swallowed air acts as a negative contrast. In proximal atresia, a small number of distended bowel loops are seen with absence of distally aerated bowel loops, as shown in this case. Distal ileal obstruction generally manifests with multiple, diffuse, similarly dilated loops of bowel proximal to the level of obstruction. The presence of a soft tissue mass or curvilinear calcification suggests a complicated obstruction such as perforation with meconium peritonitis, pseudocyst formation, and segmental volvulus.

In the presented case, an upper gastrointestinal (GI) study was performed to confirm a suspected diagnosis of proximal small bowel atresia and rule out malrotation. The atresias that allow passage of contrast material are incomplete as shown here. Water-soluble enema studies are performed when distal bowel obstruction is suspected to confirm diagnosis and rule out meconium ileus, Hirschsprung disease, or small left colon syndrome. The size of the colon is helpful in determining a differential diagnosis. Microcolon can be seen in distal obstructions such as ileal atresia, meconium ileus, or total colonic Hirschsprung disease. A normal- or near-normal–sized colon can be seen in jejunal or proximal ileal atresias or ileal duplications. The earlier the timing of the insult, the smaller the caliber of the colon. Prognosis depends on the amount of residual functional small bowel.

### References

Adams SD, Stanton MP. Malrotation and intestinal atresias. *Early Hum Dev.* 2014;990(12):921–925.

Berrocal T, Torres I, Gutiérrez J, Prieto C, del Hoyo ML, Lamas M. Congenital anomalies of the upper gastrointestinal tract. *Radiographics.* 1999;19(4):855–872.

### Cross-reference

Walters MM, Robertson RL. *Pediatric Radiology: The Requisites.* 4th ed. Philadelphia: Elsevier. 2017:101–103.

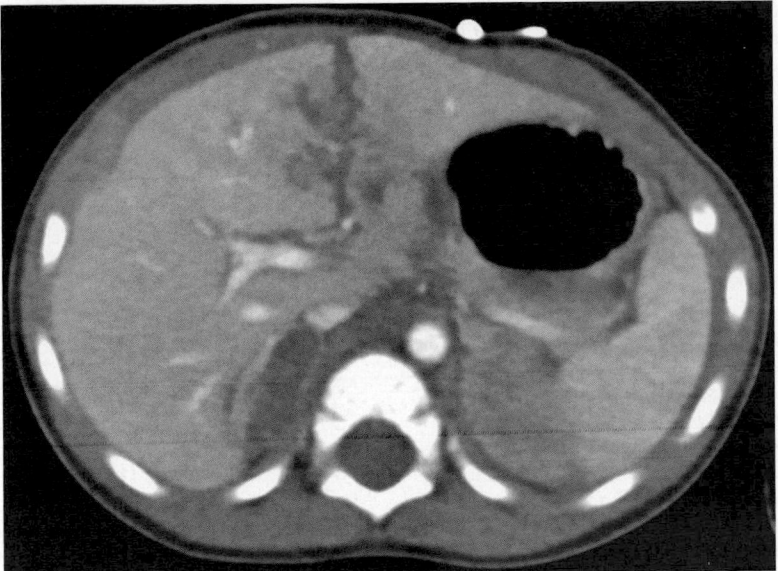

**Fig. 30.1**

**HISTORY:** 4-year-old presenting with right upper quadrant pain after sustaining blunt trauma

1. What is the second most frequently injured solid organ in children after blunt trauma?
   A. Spleen
   B. Kidney
   C. Liver
   D. Pancreas

2. What is the best management strategy in this hemodynamically stable patient?
   A. Surgery due to clear imaging evidence of liver laceration, subcapsular hematoma, retroperitoneal hematoma.
   B. Clinical follow-up as an inpatient and repeat imaging if necessary.
   C. Discharge to home now and have imaging follow-up in three weeks.
   D. Call interventional radiology for consult and plan a portal vein embolization.

3. What is the most common cause of death in the pediatric age group taken as a whole?
   A. Cancer
   B. Congenital anomalies
   C. Trauma
   D. Influenza and pneumonia

4. True or false?
   The grade of injury as determined by the American Association for the Surgery of Trauma (AAST) grading system determines the management of the patient.

## CASE 30

### Liver Trauma

1. C
2. B
3. C
4. False

### Comment

Trauma is the leading cause of death in the pediatric population by a wide margin. The liver is the second most commonly injured solid organ after spleen in the pediatric age group following blunt abdominal trauma. Mortality related to liver trauma is about 25%. Some of the most common accompanying findings, in decreasing order of frequency, are hemoperitoneum, splenic injury, rib fractures, duodenal injury, and pancreatic injury. Types of injury to the liver include parenchymal lacerations, subcapsular and parenchymal hematomas, and vascular avulsions. The most popular liver trauma grading system is the American Association of Surgery of Trauma (AAST) grading system, which ranges from grade I, small subcapsular hematoma or small capsular tear/laceration, to grade VI, hepatic vascular avulsion. However, management is guided primarily by the patient's hemodynamic status and whether or not active extravasation is seen on imaging rather than the grade of the injury. More than 90% of initially hemodynamically stable patients can be successfully treated conservatively. Complications to be on the lookout for after liver trauma include biloma, delayed hemorrhage, hemobilia, hepatic infarcts, and pseudoaneurysms.

### Reference

Kokabi N, Shuaib W, Xing M. Intra-abdominal solid organ injuries: an enhanced management algorithm. *Can Assoc Radiol J.* 2014;65(4):301–309.

### Cross-reference

Walters MM, Robertson RL. *Pediatric Radiology: The Requisites.* 4th ed. Philadelphia: Elsevier; 2017:137–138.

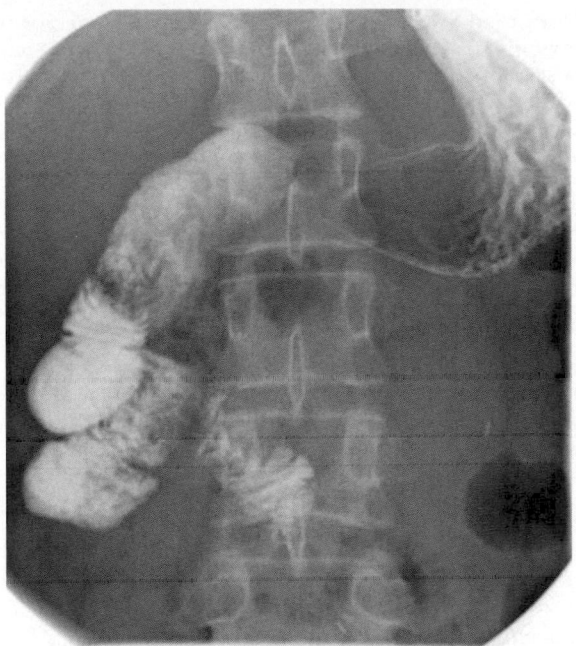

**Fig. 31.1**

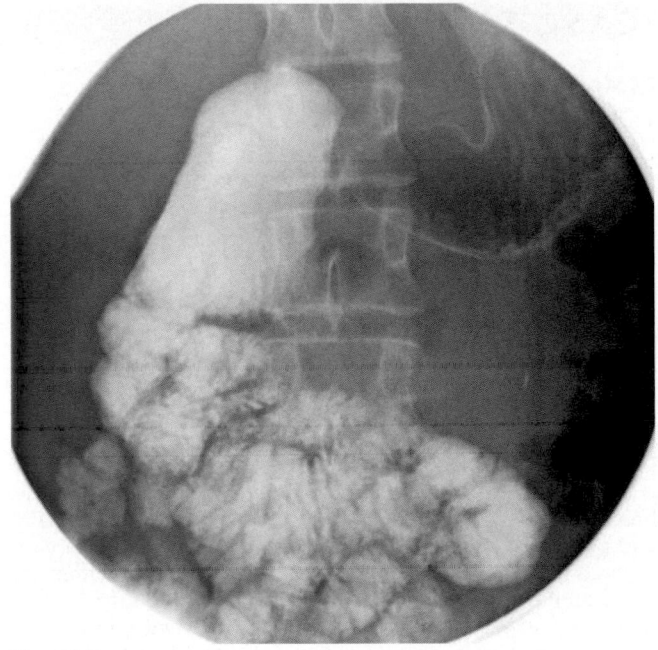

**Fig. 31.2**

**HISTORY:** 6-year-old boy with history of intermittent episodes of vomiting, abdominal pain, and weight loss. An upper gastrointestinal (GI) study was performed to rule out reflux or a gastric outlet obstruction.

1. Which signature pathological imaging finding do you see on the upper GI study?
   A. Gastric outlet obstruction
   B. Duodenal obstruction
   C. Malposition of the stomach and duodenal loop
   D. Malposition of the duodenal loop and small bowel

2. What is your most likely diagnosis based upon the upper GI study?
   A. Duodenal web
   B. Duodenal obstruction due to Ladd's bands
   C. Intestinal malrotation
   D. Heterotaxia

3. During fetal life, the bowel rotates how many degrees around the omphalomesenteric axis?
   A. Clockwise 180 degrees
   B. Counterclockwise 180 degrees
   C. Clockwise 270 degrees
   D. Counterclockwise 270 degrees

4. Which statement is correct?
   A. Children with an omphalocele have a higher incidence of intestinal malrotation.
   B. Malrotation typically presents with nonbilious vomiting.
   C. Hypertrophic pyloric stenosis increases the risk of malrotation.
   D. The cecum is malpositioned in 100% of children with intestinal malrotation.

## Malrotation

1. D
2. C
3. D
4. A

## *Comment*

Intestinal malrotation is characterized by a congenital anomalous position of the small and possibly the large bowel within the abdomen. Malrotation results from an absent or incomplete rotation of the bowel during intrauterine life. The progressive growth and lengthening of the bowel during intrauterine life requires a complex 270-degree rotation and migration of the bowel within the abdominal cavity. The cecum will eventually end in the right lower abdomen, and the small bowel is well secured due to a long mesenteric attachment. This anatomical setup minimizes the risk of acute rotations around the mesenteric vascular pedicle. Consequently, children with a congenital malpositioned small and large bowel are at higher risk for an acute volvulus.

Next to the potentially life-threatening midgut volvulus, malrotation may become apparent in the neonatal period because of bilious vomiting associated with duodenal obstruction. The risk for malrotation is increased if there is a history of an omphalocele, gastroschisis, or congenital diaphragmatic hernia. Furthermore, malrotation may be seen together with duodenal and jejunal atresia, annular pancreas, Hirschsprung disease, and heterotaxy syndrome.

The primary imaging modality of choice is an upper gastrointestinal (GI) series. The normal position of the duodenojejunal junction (DDJ) should be at or to the left of the left-sided vertebral pedicle and at the level of the duodenal bulb on frontal views, and posterior to the stomach on lateral views. Variations of the normal DDJ position may mimic malrotation. If the position of the DDJ is undetermined on the upper GI series, a small-bowel follow-through examination should be considered to localize the exact position of the small bowel and ileocecal junction. The cecum is abnormally positioned in 80% of patients with malrotation.

### Reference

Applegate KE, Anderson JM, Klatte EC. Intestinal malrotation in children: a problem-solving approach to the upper gastrointestinal series. *Radiographics*. 2006;26(5):1485–1500.

### Cross-reference

Walters MM, Robertson RL. *Pediatric Radiology: The Requisites*. 4th ed. Philadelphia: Elsevier; 2017:100–101.

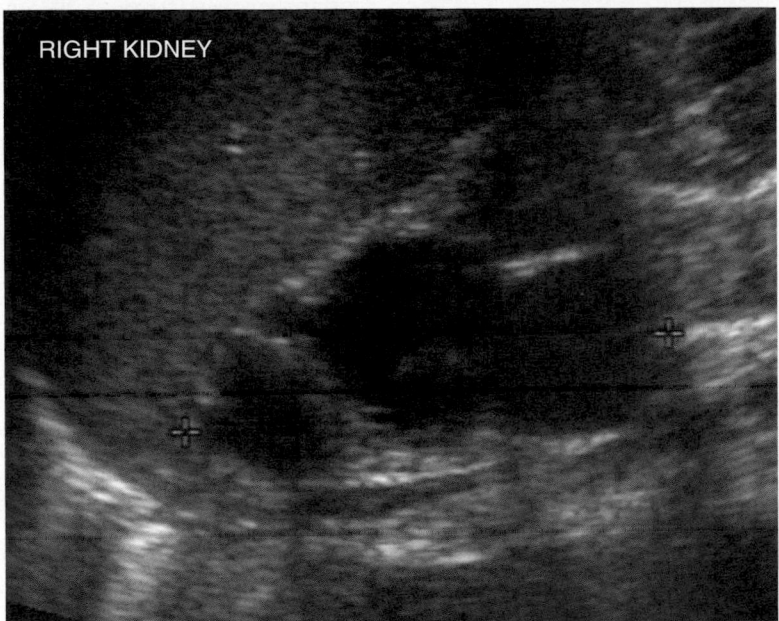

**Fig. 32.1**

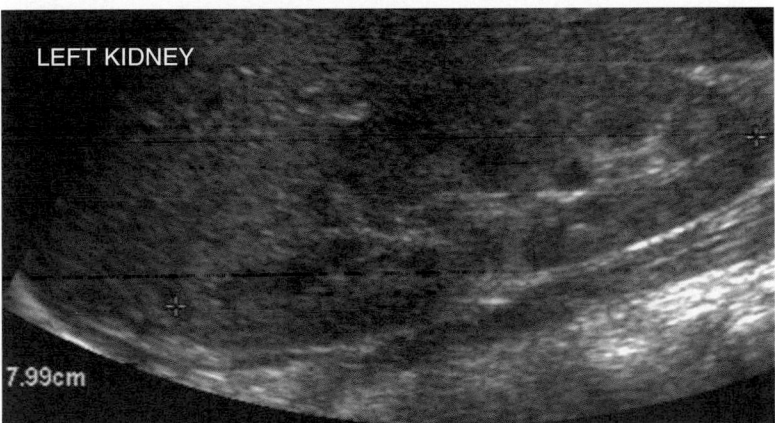

7.99cm

**Fig. 32.2**

**HISTORY:** Kidney abnormality detected during 20 gestational week ultrasound in an otherwise healthy infant.

1. Which of the following is true for the entity shown on the images?
   A. Autosomal recessive penetrance
   B. Probably due to atresia of the ureter or ureteropelvic junction during the metanephric stage of intrauterine development
   C. The most common abdominal mass in a newborn
   D. 80% of cases have anomalies in the contralateral kidney

2. Which syndrome can be associated with multicystic dysplastic kidney (MCDK)?
   A. Turner syndrome
   B. Trisomy 21
   C. Chromosome 22 deletions
   D. All of the above

3. Typical imaging features of MCDK include all of the following except:
   A. Cysts of varying size that do not interconnect
   B. Segmentation in duplicated kidneys
   C. MAG3 scintigraphy demonstrates perfusion of the MCDK on initial images; however, sequential images document lack of any excretory function.
   D. Approximately 50% of cases develop Wilms tumor.

4. True or false?
   A. Annual follow-up ultrasounds are helpful to monitor involution of MCDK.
   B. Typically, MCDK does not have a reniform shape and the intervening parenchyma between the cysts is echogenic and fibrous tissue.

## Multicystic Dysplastic Kidney

1. B
2. D
3. D
4. (A) True, (B) True

## Comment

Multicystic dysplastic kidney (MCDK) probably results from atresia of the ureter or ureteropelvic junction during the metanephric stage of intrauterine development. It is the second most common abdominal mass in a neonate and the most common cause of cystic disease in children. MCDK is characterized by multiple noncommunicating cysts of various sizes with no identifiable functioning kidney parenchyma. Ultrasound reveals cysts of varying sizes that do not interconnect (unlike massive hydronephrosis). The outer contour of the kidney is often lobulated, with outer cyst walls forming margins of the mass. The intervening parenchyma tends to be echogenic, representing fibrous tissue, without a recognizable corticomedullary tissue. MCDK most commonly affects the left side. Associated genitourinary abnormalities are seen in 25% to 40% of cases: approximately 40% of patients have contralateral abnormality such as ureteropelvic junction obstruction (UPJO) and vesicoureteral reflux. Among the nonurologic abnormalities, the heart and musculoskeletal system are most commonly affected. Associated syndromes are Turner syndrome, trisomy 21, chromosome 22 deletion, and Waardenburg syndrome. MCDK is unilateral because bilateral involvement is not compatible with life. Approximately 50% of cases involute by 10 years of age. The smaller the size of MCDK (<5 to 6 cm), the more likely it is to involute. Although slight increased risk of Wilms tumor was a concern, recent studies suggest no increased risk of Wilms tumor in these patients. Technetium sestamibi mercaptoacetyltriglycine (Tc-99m MAG3) or dimercaptosuccinic acid (DMSA) scan can be done to confirm nonfunctioning renal tissue to conform diagnosis, however ultrasound (US) has been shown to have 100% sensitivity in all cases.

## Reference
Cardona-Grau D, Kogan BA. Update on multicystic dysplastic kidney. *Curr Urol Rep*. 2015;16(10):67.

## Cross-reference
Walters MM, Robertson RL. *Pediatric Radiology: The Requisites*. 4th ed. Philadelphia: Elsevier; 2017:149.

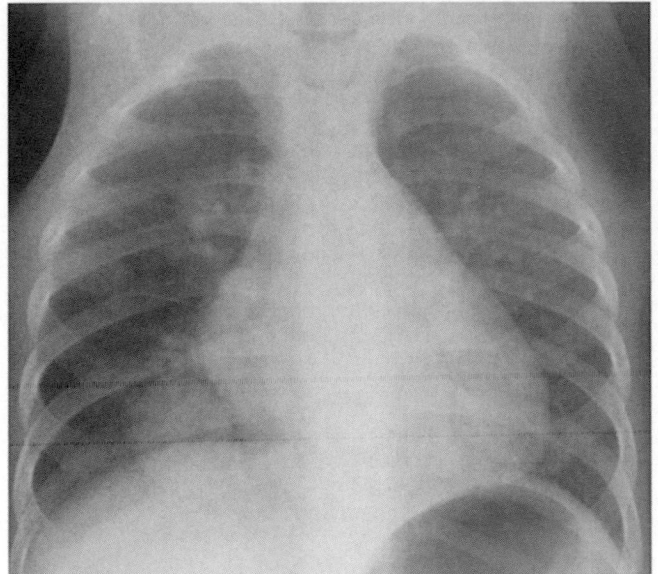

Fig. 33.1

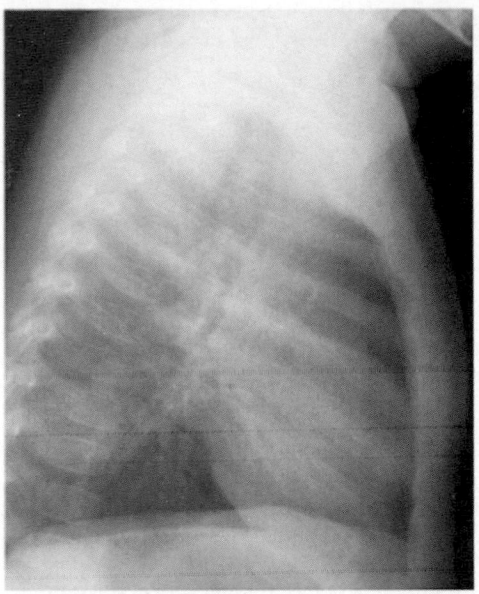

Fig. 33.2

**HISTORY:** Anteroposterior (AP) and lateral chest film of a 6-year-old child with an unremarkable previous history who now presents with high fever and cough

1. Which signature pathological imaging finding do you see?
   A. Focal lesion in the right lower lobe
   B. Focal lesion in the right pleural space
   C. Focal lesion in the right paravertebral space
   D. Focal lesion in the right chest wall

2. What is your most likely diagnosis for this 6-year-old?
   A. Congenital pulmonary airway malformation
   B. Pulmonary sequestration
   C. Tuberculoma
   D. Round pneumonia

3. What is the most frequent causative agent in round pneumonia?
   A. *Streptococcus influenzae* or *Haemophilus pneumoniae*
   B. *Streptococcus pneumoniae* or *Haemophilus influenzae*
   C. *Staphylococcus influenzae* or *Mycobacterium avium*
   D. *Staphylococcus avium* or *Mycobacterium influenzae*

4. Which statement is correct?
   A. Computed tomography (CT) imaging may be considered to exclude an underlying pathology.
   B. Round pneumonia typically occurs in the second decade of life.
   C. Round pneumonia is usually multifocal.
   D. CT imaging may be considered to evaluate the pores of Kohn and canals of Lambert.

## CASE 33

### Round Pneumonia

1. A
2. D
3. B
4. A

### Comment

Nomen est omen, or "the name is a sign"; round pneumonia is defined as a bacterial pneumonia that appears like a round or oval, frequently well-defined opacity on a chest radiograph mimicking a focal mass lesion. Round pneumonias are typically seen in young children within the first 8 years of life. Children present with nonspecific signs of infection including fever, cough, shortness of breath, and malaise. The etiologic agent is typically *Streptococcus pneumoniae* or *Haemophilus influenzae*. Round pneumonias are most often seen in the lower lobes in a posterior location and occur as a solitary focal pneumonia.

There are various explanations for this child-specific presentation of round pneumonia. It is currently believed that the immature interalveolar communications (pores of Kohn) and lack of collateral airways (canals of Lambert) contain the infection, respectively preventing rapid spread of infection between the lung subsegments throughout a lobe.

Chest radiography is usually diagnostic. If the lesion does not resolve under adequate antibiotic treatment, then cross-sectional imaging should be considered to rule out a bronchogenic cyst, congenital pulmonary airway malformation (CPAM), pulmonary sequestration, hydatid disease, or neuroblastoma. Pulmonary blastoma is an exquisitely rare differential diagnosis. Metastatic lesions may look like a round pneumonia; however, the multifocality of metastatic lesions suggests the correct diagnosis.

### Reference

Liu YL, Wu PS, Tsai LP, Tsai WH. Pediatric round pneumonia. *Pediatr Neonatol*. 2014;55:491–494.

### Cross-reference

Walters MM, Robertson RL. *Pediatric Radiology: The Requisites*. 4th ed. Philadelphia: Elsevier; 2017:35–36.

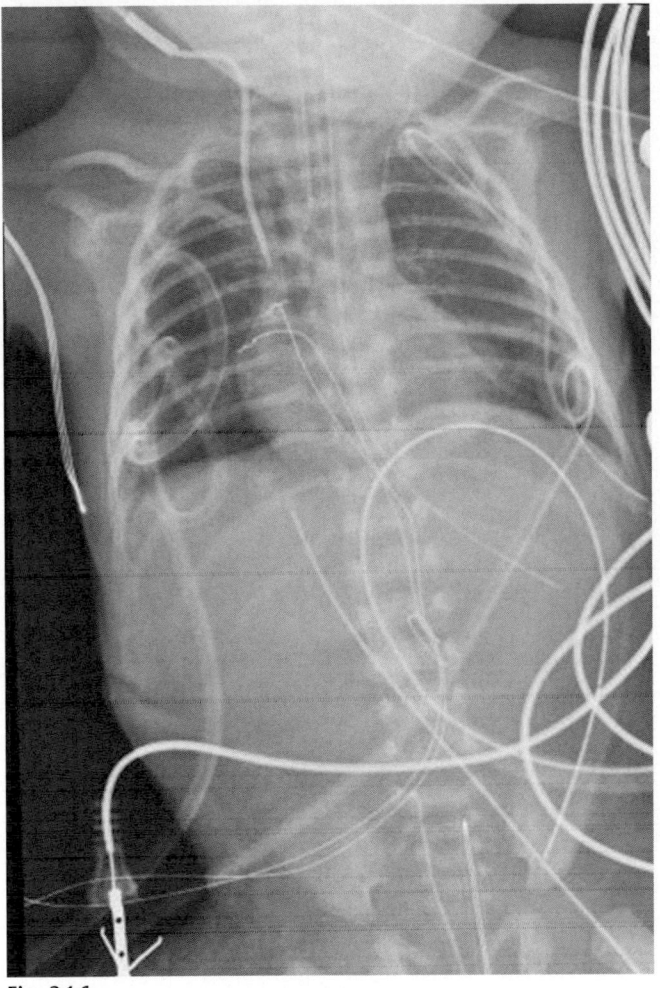

Fig. 34.1

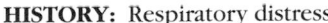

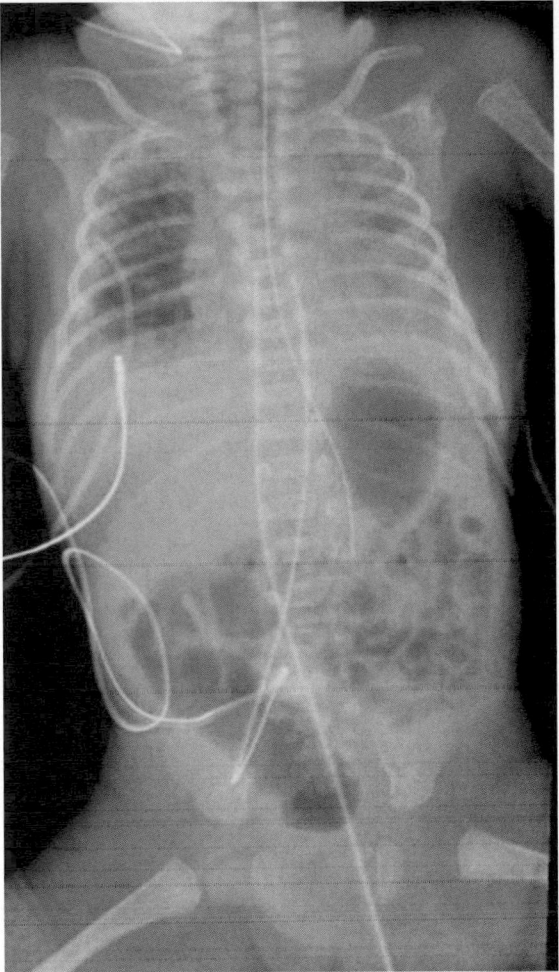

Fig. 34.2

**HISTORY:** Respiratory distress

1. Which levels are acceptable for positioning of an umbilical arterial catheter? (Choose all that apply.)
   A. T7
   B. T11
   C. L2
   D. L4

2. Which statement correctly describes the movement of the tip of the endotracheal tube in relation to the movement of the neck?
   A. Neck extension moves the tip caudally
   B. Neck rotation moves the tip cranially
   C. Neck flexion has no impact on the tip location
   D. Neck flexion moves the tip caudally

3. Which option correctly describes proper tip positioning of a peripherally inserted central catheter (PICC)?
   A. Right atrium
   B. Superior vena cava or inferior vena cava close to the right atrium
   C. Brachiocephalic vein
   D. Superior vena cava or right atrium

4. Which option is *not* a correct statement about the use of extracorporeal membrane oxygenation (ECMO) catheters?
   A. The venous cannula should be positioned with the tip in the right atrium, at about the eighth or ninth rib level posteriorly.
   B. An arterial cannula placed via the right common carotid artery should be positioned with the tip in the innominate artery at the origin of the common carotid artery.
   C. Generalized opacification ("whiteout") of the lungs after commencement of ECMO indicates malfunction of the catheters.
   D. Widening of interhemispheric fissure and extraaxial cerebrospinal fluid (CSF) spaces on head ultrasound is a common finding that typically reverses after discontinuation of ECMO.

## CASE 34

### Support Devices in the Neonate

1. A, D
2. D
3. B
4. C

### *Comment*

The umbilical arterial catheter (UAC) is introduced from the umbilical stump and then follows the umbilical artery, the common iliac artery, and the aorta. The initial downward looping near the umbilicus is characteristic and helps differentiate it from the umbilical venous catheter (UVC). For high approach UAC line placement, the distal tip should be between T6 and T10 to avoid major aortic branches. For low UAC placement, the distal tip should be below the L3 level. Due to its aortic placement, the UAC typically superimposes the left pedicle of the vertebral bodies. The distal tip of the UVC should be at or just above the diaphragm, at the inferior cavoatrial junction. High positioning of the UVC in the right atrium can cause fibrillations and endocardial injury/tamponade because the tips of these catheters are sharp. An oblique view allows better viewing of the superficial course of the UVC.

Endotracheal tubes (ETs) should have their tip between the thoracic inlet and the carina, which is typically located at about T4/T5 in a neonate. Neck flexion moves the ET tube caudally, and extension moves the ET tube cranially. Remember that the tip of the ET tube goes with the chin, that is, if the chin moves down, the ET tube moves down.

PICC lines should have their tip in the superior vena cava (SVC) or inferior vena cava (IVC) near the junction to the right atrium, not within the right atrium itself. Because of their small caliber, these tips can cause laceration of the atrial wall, leading to cardiac tamponade.

It is important to see the entry site of the catheters to enable differentiation between the UVC and lower extremity PICC lines.

### References

Barnacle AM, Smith LC, Hiorns MP. The role of imaging during extracorporeal membrane oxygenation in pediatric respiratory failure. *AJR Am J Roentgenol.* 2006;186(1):58–66.

Lobo L. The neonatal chest. *Eur J Radiol.* 2006;60(2):152–158.

### Cross-reference

Walters MM, Robertson RL. *Pediatric Radiology: The Requisites.* 4th ed. Philadelphia: Elsevier; 2017:12–14.

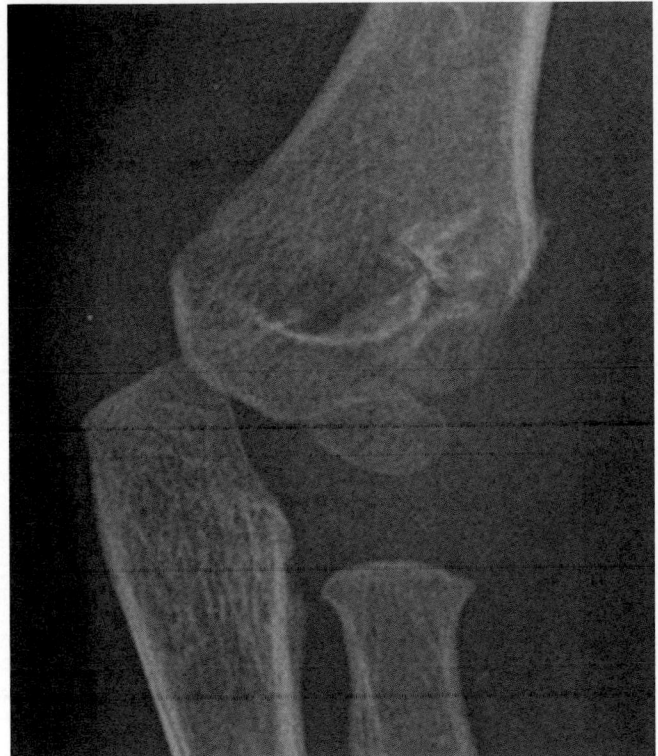

Fig. 35.1

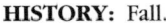

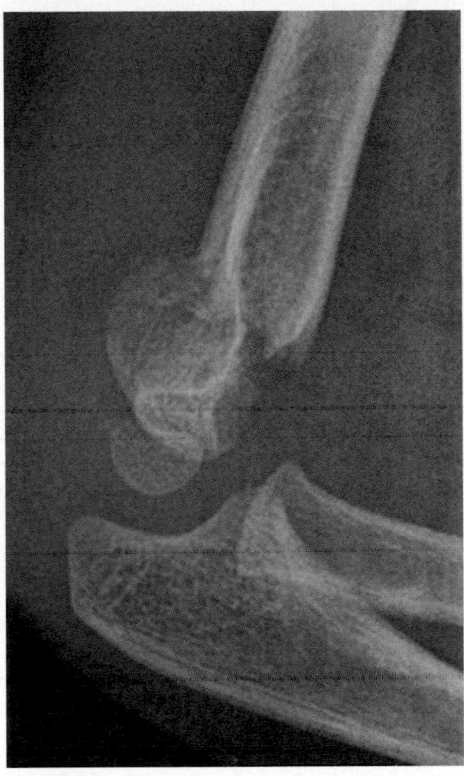

Fig. 35.2

**HISTORY:** Fall.

1. What kind of fracture do you see?
   A. Supracondylar elbow fracture
   B. Galeazzi fracture
   C. Colles fracture
   D. Barton fracture

2. Which of the following is not an expected complication of this type of fracture?
   A. Cubitus varus
   B. Cubitus valgus
   C. Nerve injury
   D. Limb-length discrepancy

3. Which option illustrates the continuum from the most common to the least common elbow fractures in children?
   A. Supracondylar humerus>medial epicondyle>lateral epicondyle>radius>ulna

   B. Supracondylar humerus>lateral epicondyle>medial epicondyle>radius>ulna
   C. Medial epicondyle>lateral epicondyle>supracondylar humerus>ulna>radius
   D. Lateral epicondyle>medial epicondyle>supracondylar humerus>ulna>radius

4. True or false?
   A. Flexion injuries are the most common cause of supracondylar elbow fractures in children
   B. CRITOE is the mnemonic for ossification centers in the elbow: Capitellum (1), radial head (3), internal (medial) epicondyle (5), trochlea (7), olecranon (9), external (lateral) epicondyle (11) (numbers in parenthesis refer to the age of ossification)

## CASE 35

### Supracondylar Elbow Fracture

1. A
2. D
3. B
4. (A) False, (B) False

## Comment

Approximately 70% of traumatic fractures involve the upper extremity and 8% to 10% involve the distal humerus, proximal radius, or ulna. Supracondylar elbow fractures are the most common pediatric elbow fracture. Extension-type injuries resulting from a fall onto an outstretched hand (FOOSH) account for 97% of supracondylar fractures. Flexion injuries are rare and often result from a direct blow to the posterior elbow, which usually requires stabilization and open reduction. Supracondylar fractures are typically seen in skeletally immature patients in the first decade of life with high incidence of complications such as nerve injury or malunion leading to cubitus varus or valgus.

Elbow radiographs are performed in two standard planes: the anteroposterior view, with the elbow fully extended and the forearm in supination, and the lateral view, with the elbow in 90-degree flexion and the forearm in neutral position. Many radiologic landmarks and lines are defined to help describe and diagnose elbow fractures. The anterior humeral line is defined in the lateral view as a longitudinal line drawn along the anterior cortex of the humerus and should traverse the middle third of the capitulum. The radiocapitellar line is defined in the lateral view as a line along the center of the radius and should intersect the capitulum. The articular surfaces of the elbow are contained within the joint capsule. Three fat pads lie over the capsule: the anterior over the coronoid fossa, the posterior over the olecranon fossa, and the third over the supinator as it wraps around the radius. Fracture, hematoma, and effusion into an intact capsule can cause capsular distention, improving the visibility of the fat pads and identifying the occult fractures. In the setting of acute trauma, a visible posterior fat pad should be regarded as abnormal, particularly posterior to the radial head or to a nondisplaced supracondylar fracture. The anterior fat pad can be seen in normal conditions; if the pad is displaced anteriorly, then it is regarded as abnormal.

### References

Little KJ. Elbow fractures and dislocations. *Orthop Clin N Am.* 2014;45(3):327–340.

Omid R, Choi PD, Skaggs DL. Supracondylar humeral fractures in children. *J Bone Joint Surg Am.* 2008;90(5):1121–1132.

### Cross-reference

Walters MM, Robertson RL. *Pediatric Radiology: The Requisites.* 4th ed. Philadelphia: Elsevier; 2017:245–247.

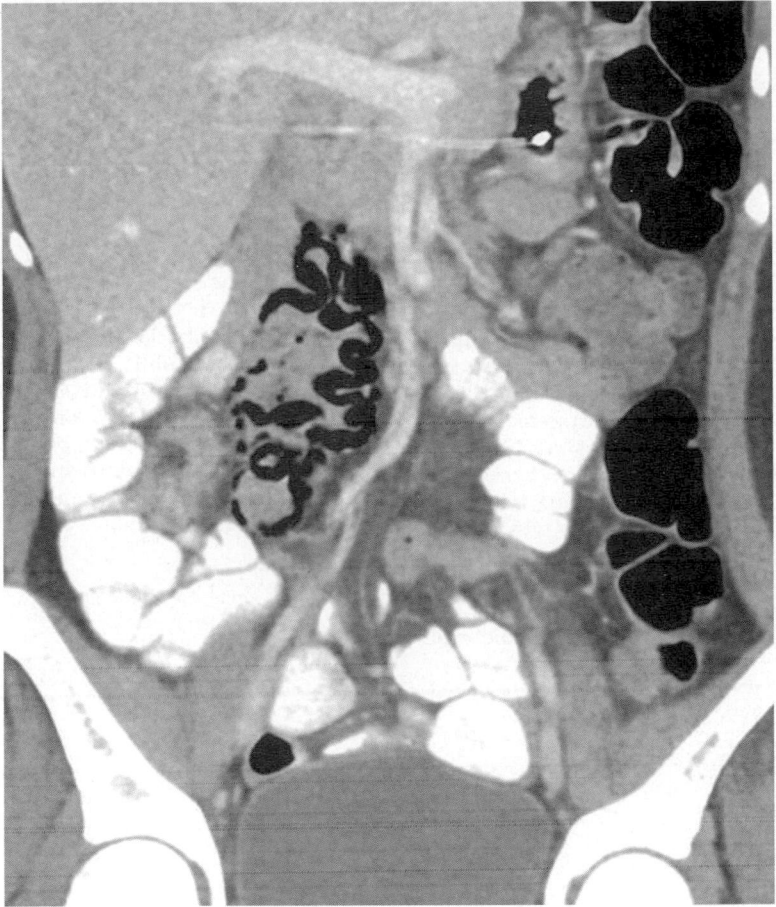

**Fig. 36.1**

**HISTORY:** 16-year-old patient presenting with neutropenia.

1. What is your diagnosis?
   A. Crohn disease
   B. Ischemic colitis
   C. Typhlitis
   D. Graft-versus-host disease

2. What is the classic imaging finding of neutropenic colitis?
   A. Massive mural thickening of the cecum and ascending colon wall
   B. Marked colonic submucosal edema causing wall thickening and nodularity over a long colonic segment
   C. Diffuse bowel abnormality from duodenum to rectum with mucosal enhancement
   D. None of the above

3. Which imaging study is the best for diagnosis?
   A. Fluoroscopy
   B. Positron emission tomography-computed tomography (PET-CT)
   C. Contrast-enhanced magnetic resonance imaging (MRI)
   D. Contrast-enhanced CT

4. Which of the following is the synonym of typhlitis?
   A. Ileocecal syndrome
   B. Cecitis
   C. Necrotizing enteropathy
   D. All of the above

## CASE 36

### Typhlitis (Neutropenic Enterocolitis)

1. C
2. A
3. D
4. D

## Comment

Typhlitis, also known as neutropenic enterocolitis, is an inflammatory/necrotizing process typically affecting the cecum and ascending colon, and sometimes involving the terminal ileum as well. It is typically seen in the setting of neutropenia, initially described in children with acute myelogenous leukemia (AML) and acute lymphocytic leukemia (ALL); however, other entities like aplastic anemia, immunosuppression due to transplant, high-dose chemotherapy treatment, myelodysplastic syndrome, or infectious processes like acquired immune deficiency syndrome (AIDS), cytomegalovirus (CMV), *Pseudomonas*, *Clostridium*, *Escherichia coli*, *Enterobacter*, or *Candidiasis* can be predisposing factors. Patients present with fever and right lower quadrant pain. Plain radiographs demonstrate dilated cecum and ascending colon with air-fluid levels, and thumb-printing of the cecum/ascending colon due to edema. Most cases are diagnosed with contrast-enhanced computed tomography (CT) exam of the abdomen (recommended oral contrast is water), which demonstrates mural wall thickening in the cecum and ascending colon, with heterogeneous bowel wall enhancement. Pneumatosis intestinalis can be seen as shown in this case. The surrounding fat is usually inflamed with stranding and mild contrast enhancement and fluid in the paracolic gutter can also be seen. Dilated small bowel loops are usually due to paralytic ileus. Clinical history and the region of involvement in the bowel help differentiate typhlitis from pseudomembranous colitis (pancolitis due to *Clostridium difficile* infection), Crohn disease (primary involvement in the terminal ileum and skip lesions in the colon), or other infectious causes. Complications are sepsis, abscess, perforation, or death. Prognosis is related to degree of neutropenia. Late stage at the time of diagnosis, wall thickness >10 mm, and use of cytarabine is associated with higher mortality.

### Reference

Baker ME. Acute infectious and inflammatory enterocolitides. *Radiol Clin N Am.* 2015;53(6):1255–1271.

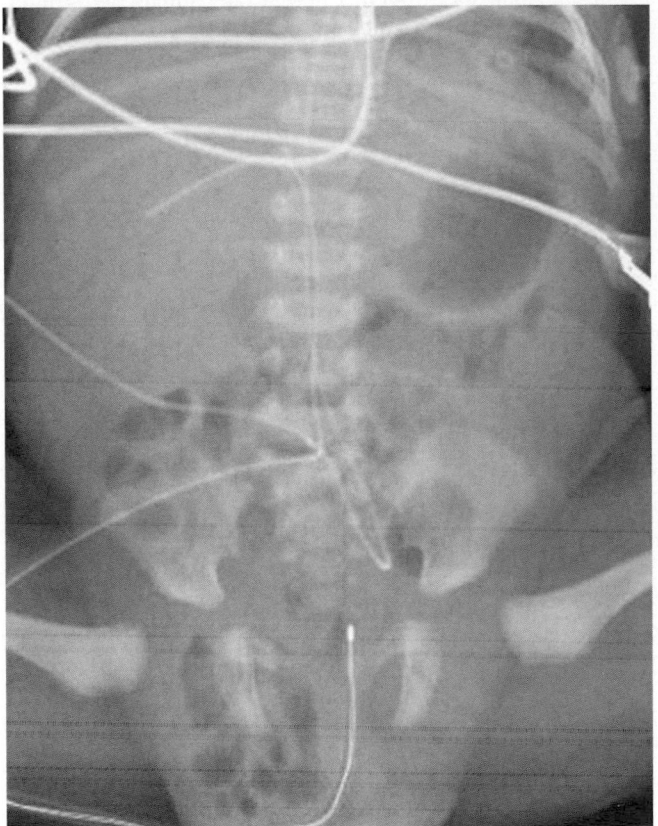

Fig. 37.1

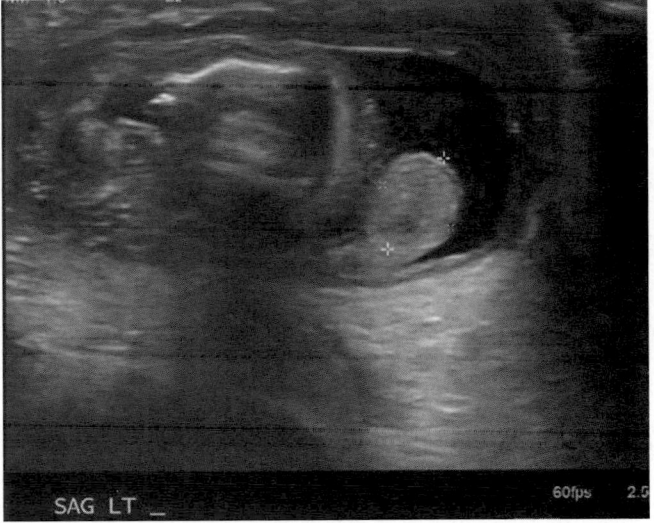

Fig. 37.2

**HISTORY:** Preterm male infant, babygram ordered to evaluate line placement

1. What is the incidental finding?
   A. Noncentral placement of umbilical arterial catheter terminating in the left portal vein
   B. Noncentral placement of umbilical venous catheter terminating in the right portal vein
   C. Bilateral inguinal hernia
   D. Right inguinal hernia

2. True or false?
   A. Girls are more commonly affected than boys.
   B. Bilateral hernias are more common in females.

3. Which statement is accurate?
   A. Congenital inguinal hernias are indirect hernias.
   B. Congenital inguinal hernias are direct hernias.
   C. Infants have a lower incidence of incarceration compared to older children.
   D. Although incarcerated, congenital hernias do not present a surgical emergency.

4. True or false?
   A. Congenital inguinal hernias have a high incidence of solid organ herniation.
   B. In male infants, processus testicularis fails to obliterate, leading to inferior herniation of bowel loops in congenital inguinal hernias.

## CASE 37

### Congenital Inguinal Hernia

1. A

2. D

3. A

4. A) False, B) False

## Comment

The incidence of pediatric inguinal hernia is approximately 4%. Most pediatric inguinal hernias are indirect hernias. Overall, inguinal defects are 10-fold more common in males than in females. Prematurity is associated with increased incidence. Most inguinal hernias (60% to 75%) are on the right side and are most likely secondary to later descent of the right testicle. Female gender, prematurity, and presence of a left-sided inguinal hernia are risk factors for bilateral involvement.

Congenital inguinal hernia occurs when processus vaginalis fails (female equivalent is canal of Nuck) to obliterate, resulting in inferior herniation of a variable combination of fat/omentum, bowel, or, rarely, other abdominal organs.

Most infants with inguinal hernias are initially asymptomatic, and radiography demonstrates the hernia as an incidental finding, as shown in this case. The rate of incarceration is higher in neonates compared to other age groups, reaching 30% in preterm infants. The most common clinical presentation is intermittent bulging in the groin, scrotum, or labia, exacerbated by increased intraabdominal pressure when the infant cries and strains during bowel movement.

The diagnosis can be established based on the presenting symptoms and physical exam alone in most cases. Anteroposterior radiographs can demonstrate aerated bowel loops in the groin and/or scrotum (or labia in females). Ultrasonography is the preferred imaging modality for evaluation of herniated contents. Differential diagnoses include undescended testicle and hydrocele.

Some advocate repair of inguinal hernias in infants prior to their discharge from the intensive care unit given the higher risk of incarceration. Term and older children are usually treated electively.

### Reference

Kelly B, Ponsky TA. Pediatric abdominal wall defects. *Surg Clin North Am.* 2013;93(5):1255–1267.

### Cross-reference

Walters MM, Robertson RL. *Pediatric Radiology: The Requisites.* 4th ed. Philadelphia: Elsevier; 2017:179.

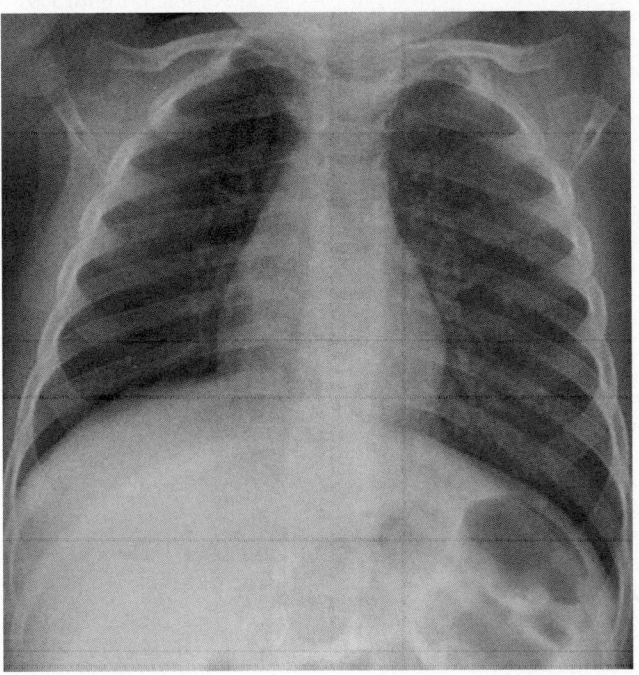

Fig. 38.1

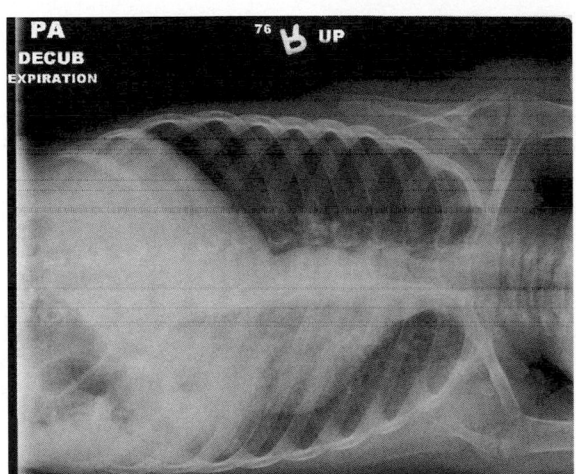

Fig. 38.2

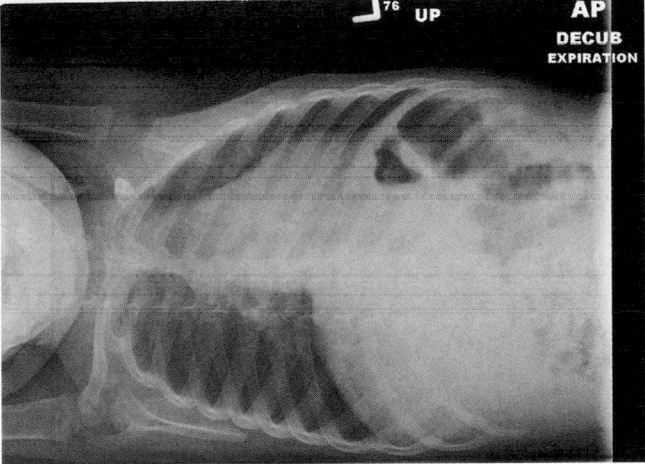

Fig. 38.3

**HISTORY:** 23-month-old male presenting with wheezing

1. Given the imaging findings, which of the following is the best diagnosis?
   A. Swyer-James
   B. Extrinsic compression of the airway
   C. Intrinsic obstruction of the airway by a foreign body
   D. Pulmonary sling

2. After foreign body aspiration to the right main bronchus with air trapping, which of the following imaging findings would you expect to see when compared to the anteroposterior (AP) supine view? (Choose all that apply.)
   A. Decrease in lung volume on the right with right-sided decubitus view
   B. Unchanged lung volume on the left with left-sided decubitus view
   C. Unchanged lung volume on the right with right-sided decubitus view
   D. Decreased lung volume on the left with left-sided decubitus view

3. Which of the following is the most common location for an aspirated foreign body to lodge?
   A. Trachea
   B. Larynx
   C. Left main bronchus
   D. Right main bronchus

4. Which statement about aspirated foreign bodies is *not* correct?
   A. Most aspirated foreign bodies are not radiopaque.
   B. The volume of affected lung segments may be normal, increased, or decreased.
   C. There is typically oligemia in the affected lung segments.
   D. Most cases are seen in infants younger than 1 year.

## CASE 38

### Foreign Body Aspiration

1. C

2. C, D

3. D

4. D

### Comment

Aspirated foreign bodies most commonly lodge in the right main bronchus due to its more direct continuation of (decreased angulation with respect to) the trachea and its larger size compared to the left main bronchus. Most aspirated foreign bodies are not radiopaque. Although extrinsic compression may cause similar lung findings, the symptoms are usually more gradual in onset, and imaging shows a soft tissue mass in the mediastinum or hilum. Patients with pulmonary sling typically present with respiratory distress at birth. Patients with Swyer-James typically have a hyperlucent area of lung that is hypoplastic and is believed to result from postinfectious bronchiolitis obliterans. Patients may develop a chronic cough, wheezing, and recurrent pneumonia.

If the patient can follow commands, inspiratory and expiratory views can be obtained to look for an asymmetric static lung volume on both views, indicating air trapping due to foreign body aspiration in the right clinical context. Because most cases of foreign body aspiration occur in toddlers and young children between the ages of 1 and 3, patients will not be able to consistently follow commands. In those cases, anteroposterior (AP) and bilateral decubitus views are obtained to look for a lack of "compression" of the dependent lung related to air trapping. Thus, in the setting of a foreign body lodged in the right main bronchus, AP and right lateral decubitus views will show no change in volume of the obstructed right lung despite its dependent position. The left lateral decubitus view will show decreased volume of the normal left lung in the dependent position. Although we typically look for air trapping and hyperexpansion in the affected lung, it should be remembered that the affected lung may show normal volume, increased volume, or decreased volume, and that the salient finding is lack of change between inspiration and expiration or between AP and decubitus views. Reactive oligemia can be observed on the affected side.

### Reference

Pugmire BS, Lim R, Avery LL. Review of ingested and aspirated foreign bodies in children and their clinical significance for radiologists. *Radiographics*. 2015;35(5):1528–1538.

### Cross-reference

Walters MM, Robertson RL. *Pediatric Radiology: The Requisites*. 4th ed. Philadelphia: Elsevier; 2017:18–19.

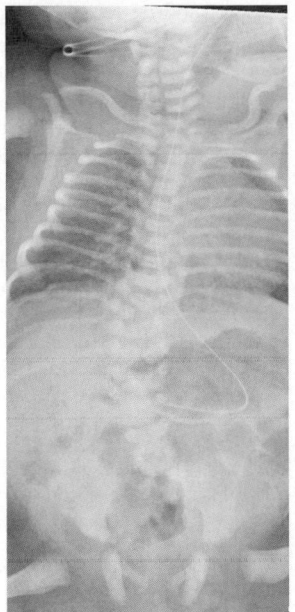

Fig. 39.1          Fig. 39.2

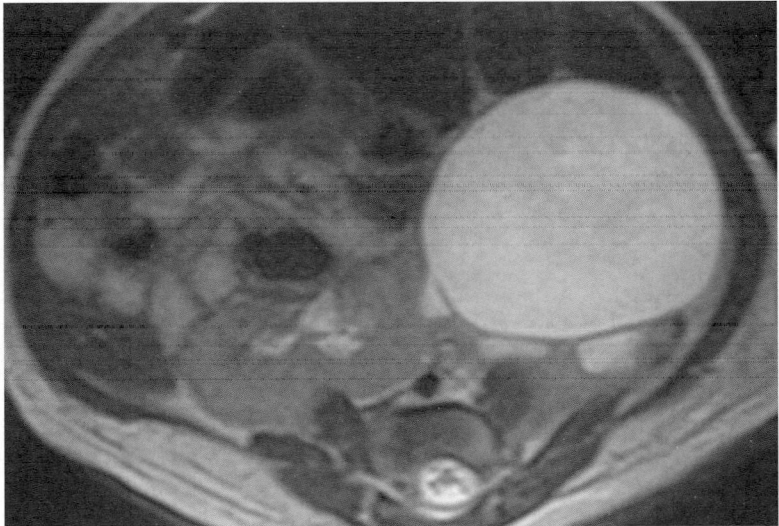

Fig. 39.3

**HISTORY**: Prenatal echocardiogram demonstrated ventricular septal defect (VSD) and left renal agenesis

1. What is the most likely diagnosis in this newborn?
   A. Vertebral defects, anal atresia, cardiac defects, tracheo-esophageal fistula, renal anomalies, and limb abnormalities (VACTERL) association
   B. Trisomy 21
   C. Holt-Oram syndrome
   D. Congenital scoliosis

2. Which of the following best describes the renal anomaly?
   A. Crossed fused ectopic kidney
   B. Horseshoe kidney
   C. Malrotated left kidney with possible ureteropelvic junction (UPJ) obstruction
   D. Left multicystic dysplastic kidney

3. Which option represents the correct order of frequency of anomalies in this association?
   A. Cardiac>renal>anal>tracheoesophageal>vertebral
   B. Cardiac>tracheoesophageal>renal>anal>vertebral
   C. Vertebral>cardiac>tracheoesophageal>renal>anal
   D. Vertebral>tracheoesophageal>cardiac>renal>anal

4. Which malformation is *not* seen in VACTERL?
   A. Brain malformation
   B. Lung agenesis
   C. Renal agenesis
   D. Duodenal atresia

## CASE 39

### VACTERL Association

1. A

2. B

3. A

4. A

### Comment

VACTERL is a nonrandom association of anomalies involving multiple organ systems (except brain): vertebral defects, anal atresia, cardiac defects, tracheoesophageal fistula, renal anomalies, and limb abnormalities. When three or more of these anomalies are present, the diagnosis is established. This is an association rather than a syndrome because no specific genetic or chromosomal defect has been identified. The best diagnostic clue is vertebral anomalies in the presence of other malformations. Vertebral anomalies can be related to abnormal formation (such as hemi- or butterfly vertebrae) or segmentation defects. Absence of the sacrum (as seen in this case) and caudal regression syndrome can be seen. There can be tethered cord (as seen in this case, terminating in an intradural lipoma).

The frequency of anomalies in VACTERL association is as follows: cardiac (77%), renal (72%), anal (63%), radial ray (58%), tracheoesophageal fistula (40%), and vertebral (37%). Concurrence of three or more anomalies is 95% more likely to be VACTERL association than by chance. In addition to the previously mentioned anomalies, patients with VACTERL association may have lung agenesis, kidney agenesis, horseshoe lungs, horseshoe kidneys (as shown in this case), microgastria, duodenal atresia, and malrotation.

The management of patients with VACTERL/VATER association typically centers on surgical correction of the specific congenital anomalies (typically anal atresia, certain types of cardiac malformations, and/or tracheoesophageal fistula) in the immediate postnatal period, followed by long-term medical management of sequelae of the congenital malformations.

### Reference

Solomon BD. VACTERL/VATER association. *Orphanet J Rare Dis*. 2011;6:56–67.

### Cross-reference

Walters MM, Robertson RL. *Pediatric Radiology: The Requisites*. 4th ed. Philadelphia: Elsevier; 2017:208, 334.

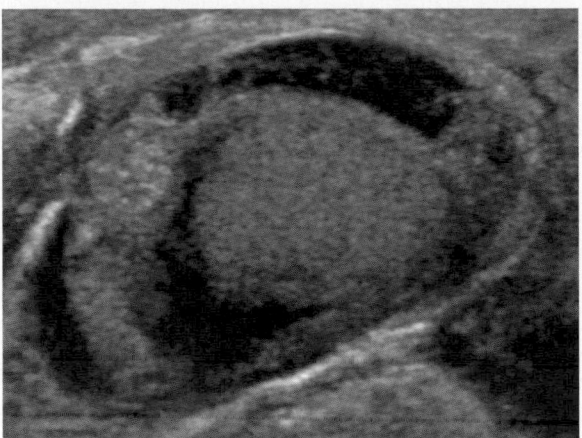

Fig. 40.1

See Supplemental Figures section for additional figures for this case.

**HISTORY:** 10-year-old boy presenting with acute scrotal pain and swelling.

1. What is your diagnosis?
   A. Epididymoorchitis
   B. Scrotal cellulitis
   C. Testicular torsion
   D. Torsion of the testicular appendage

2. Choose the correct statement regarding the entity shown.
   A. Testicular torsion is far more common than torsion of the testicular appendage.
   B. Torsion of the testicular appendage is commonly seen in toddlers.
   C. Hydrocele is uncommon.
   D. None of the above.

3. Which statement is accurate regarding testicular appendage(s)?
   A. The only remnant is the paramesonephric duct of the testis located between the superior pole of the testis and the epididymis.
   B. There are multiple remnants, all originating from the Müllerian duct.
   C. The epididymal remnant originates from the Wolffian duct.
   D. None of the above.

4. Which statement is correct regarding diagnosis and management of torsion of testicular remnants?
   A. Surgery is mandatory within the first 6 hours after diagnosis.
   B. It is a self-limiting disease that can be supported with analgesics and antiinflammatory agents for symptomatic relief.
   C. It is a self-limiting disease that can be supported with antibiotics.
   D. None of the above.

## CASE 40

### Torsion of the Testicular Appendage

1. D
2. D
3. C
4. B

## Comment

Torsion of the intrascrotal appendages is the most common cause of an acute scrotum in children and represents 40% to 60% of the underlying causes of this entity. The incidence is far more common than epididymoorchitis and testicular torsion. The most common appendage to twist is a testicular remnant of the paramesonephric (Müllerian) duct located between the superior pole of the testis and the epididymis. Appendix epididymis is a remnant of the mesonephric (Wolffian) duct, most often seen projecting from the head of epididymis. The cause of testicular appendage torsion is unknown but may be related to anatomy, trauma, and/or prepubertal enlargement.

The most common clinical presentation is acute scrotal pain and swelling, a tender and palpable nodule at the superior testicular pole, and rarely a "blue-dot" sign corresponding to the necrotic appendage, in the presence of a preserved cremasteric reflex. The best imaging tool is ultrasound (US) with Doppler, which reveals an enlarged appendage (spherical as opposed to normal vermiform shape and >6 mm diameter), heterogeneous echogenicity with internal microcystic changes, an avascular appendage with increased peripheral vascularity, and normal vascular flow to the testis. Edema, vascular congestion, and lymphatic dilation and necrosis may be contributing to microcystic changes. Hydrocele is common. Analgesic and antiinflammatory medications are used for relief of symptoms. The pain usually resolves within a week. The prognosis is excellent, because this is a self-limiting disease.

### Reference

Lev M, Ramon J, Mor Y, Jacobson JM, Soudack M. Sonographic appearances of torsion of the appendix testis and appendix epididymis in children. *J Clin Ultrasound*. 2015;43(8):485–489.

### Cross-reference

Walters MM, Robertson RL. *Pediatric Radiology: The Requisites*. 4th ed. Philadelphia: Elsevier; 2017:177–178.

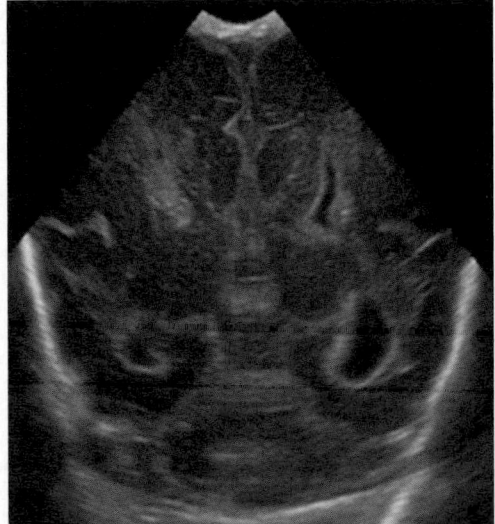

Fig. 41.1

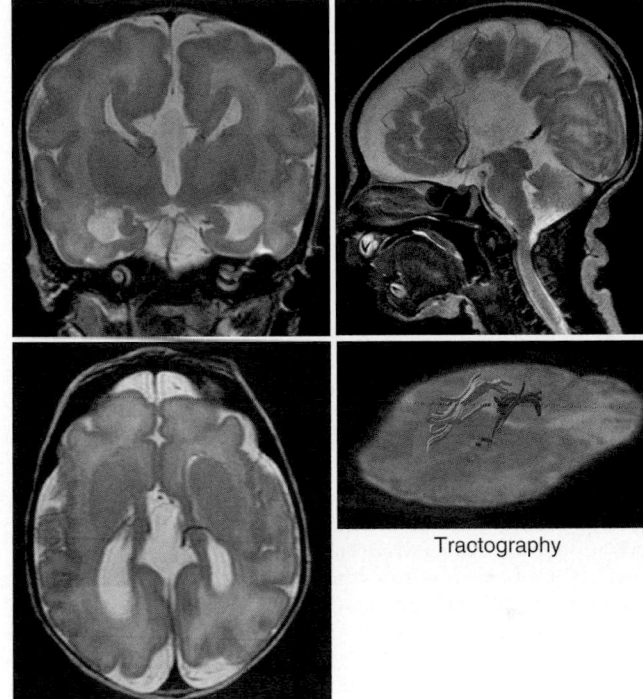

Tractography

Fig. 41.2

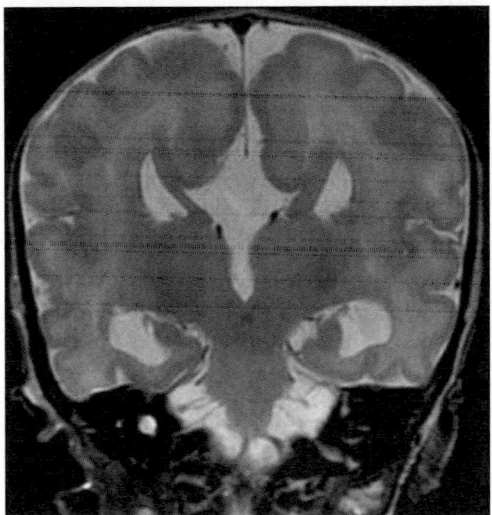

Fig. 41.3

**HISTORY:** Newborn child with a suspected brain malformation on a prenatal ultrasound

1. Which signature pathological imaging finding do you see on the cranial ultrasound study?
   A. Widely separated lateral ventricles
   B. Parallel course of the lateral ventricles
   C. Texas longhorn configuration of the lateral ventricles
   D. All of the above

2. Which key finding is present in the multiplanar magnetic resonance imaging (MRI)?
   A. Complete agenesis of the corpus callosum
   B. Fused thalami
   C. Cortical polymicrogyria
   D. Duplicated anterior commissure

3. What are the T2-hypointense white matter tracts along the medial contour of the lateral ventricles called?
   A. Bourneville bundles
   B. Joubert bundles
   C. Probst bundles
   D. Alexander bundles

4. Which syndrome is characterized by corpus callosum agenesis?
   A. Sturge-Weber-Dimitri syndrome
   B. Aicardi Goutieres syndrome
   C. Aicardi syndrome
   D. Prader-Willi syndrome

## Corpus Callosum Agenesis

1. D
2. A
3. C
4. C

## Comment

The corpus callosum may be completely absent (agenesis) or partially formed (hypogenesis). Anomalies of the corpus callosum are often associated with additional cerebral or cerebellar abnormalities such as interhemispheric cysts, malformations of the cortical development, cerebellar dysgenesis, cephaloceles, or hypothalamic anomalies. Callosal anomalies may be isolated or part of complex syndromes such as Aicardi syndrome, fetal alcohol syndrome, Chiari II malformation, or Dandy Walker malformation. Although asymptomatic isolated corpus callosum agenesis has been reported, the vast majority of affected children present with seizures, macrocephaly, developmental delay, cognitive impairment, or hypothalamic dysfunction.

Corpus callosum anomaly is the most common commissural malformation. Corpus callosum anomalies are typically suspected on prenatal imaging (ultrasound or fetal magnetic resonance imaging [MRI]). Most frequently the posterior part and inferior genu and rostrum are absent; however, many degrees and variations of hypogenesis/agenesis may occur. In addition to the missing corpus callosum, an absent or incomplete inversion of the cingulate gyrus is noted with the mesial sulci extending in a radiating pattern toward the third ventricle on midline sagittal images (as shown in this case). The third ventricle may extend between cerebral hemispheres (high-riding ventricle) along the cerebral falx. Additional interhemispheric cysts (the most common associated finding) or lipomas (rare) can be seen. On axial and coronal imaging, the interhemispheric fissure is widened, and the lateral ventricles are displaced laterally and course in a typical parallel fashion. The posterior/occipital horns of the lateral ventricles are usually wide (colpocephaly). The T2 hypointense aberrant white matter tracts (Probst bundle) run along the medial contour of the ventricles and induce the characteristic Texas longhorn configuration of the lateral ventricles on coronal imaging. Finally, additional commissural anomalies may include hypoplasia of the anterior and hippocampal commissures with malrotation of the hippocampi and absence of the inferior cingulum.

### Reference

Poretti A, Meoded A, Rossi A, Raybaud C, Huisman TA. Diffusion tensor imaging and fiber tractography in brain malformations. *Pediatr Radiol*. 2013;43(1):28–54.

### Cross-reference

Walters MM, Robertson RL. *Pediatric Radiology: The Requisites*. 4th ed. Philadelphia: Elsevier; 2017:267–268.

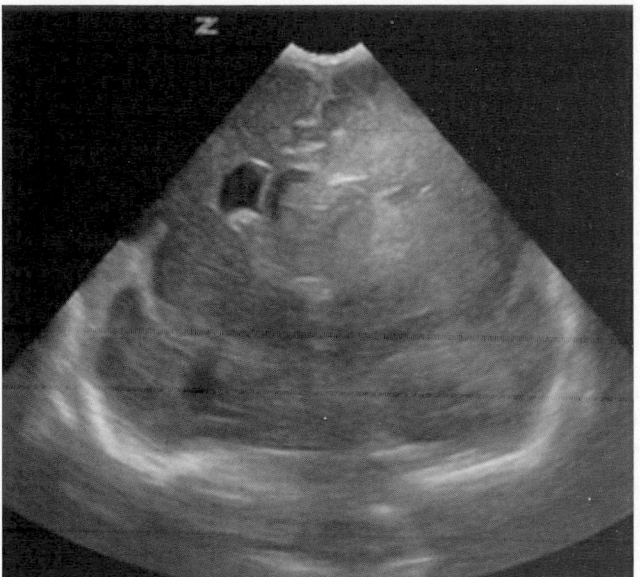

Fig. 42.1

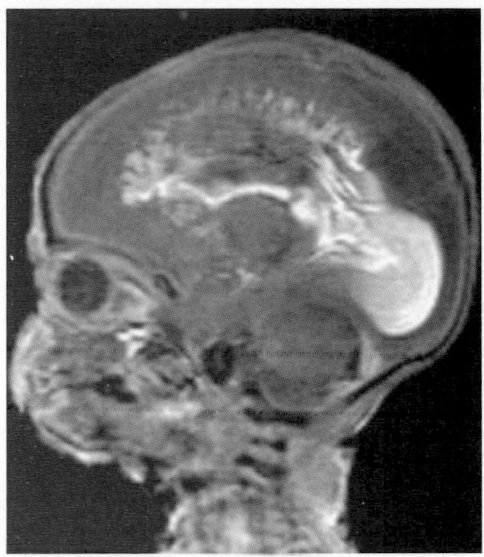

Fig. 42.2

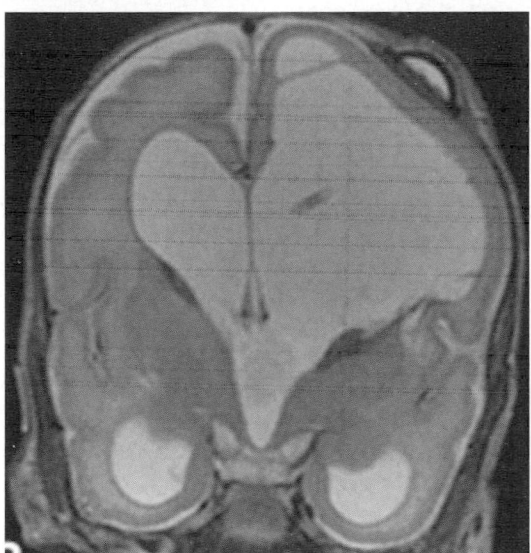

Fig. 43.3

**HISTORY:** Biplanar ultrasound (US) and matching sagittal T1- and follow-up axial T2-weighted magnetic resonance (MR) images of a preterm neonate with acute drop in hematocrit

1. What is the best description of the findings on coronal ultrasound (US)?
   A. Intraventricular hemorrhage without hydrocephalus
   B. Intraventricular hemorrhage with adjacent arterial infarct
   C. Intraventricular hemorrhage with adjacent venous infarct
   D. Intraventricular hemorrhage with hydrocephalus

2. Which option best describes the diagnosis in this case?
   A. Periventricular venous infarction
   B. Periventricular hemorrhagic venous infarction
   C. Grade 3 germinal matrix hemorrhage
   D. Grade 4 germinal matrix hemorrhage

3. Which statement is correct?
   A. Grade 1 germinal matrix hemorrhage is frequently complicated by a secondary obstructive hydrocephalus.
   B. Grade 2 germinal matrix hemorrhage is characterized by intraventricular blood products combined with ventriculomegaly.
   C. Grade 3 germinal matrix hemorrhage is characterized by intraventricular blood products combined with ventriculomegaly.
   D. Grade 4 germinal matrix hemorrhage is characterized by cerebellar hemorrhage.

4. Which option describes the follow-up imaging after periventricular hemorrhagic venous infarction (PVHI)?
   A. The periventricular white matter is preserved.
   B. Porencephalic cyst develops in the area of PVHI.
   C. The ipsilateral ventricle is typically compressed.
   D. The basal ganglia and thalami are typically infarcted.

## Germinal Matrix Hemorrhage

1. C
2. B
3. C
4. B

## Comment

Germinal matrix hemorrhage (GMH) refers to focal bleedings within the germinal matrix (GM), which is considered to be the birthplace of the cortical neurons before they migrate toward the cortical ribbon. The GM is a highly vascular gelatinous structure with little architectural support for its immature capillary bed extending along the entire ventricle early in embryonic life. The GM progressively involutes with advancing gestational age (GA), and final remnants of the GM can still be found after 32 weeks GA in the region of the caudothalamic groove.

GMH occurs primarily, but not exclusively, in preterm neonates with very low birth weight. The incidence of GMH is nearly 45% in these infants. Anticoagulation and thrombocytopenia during extracorporeal membrane oxygenation (ECMO) and prenatal exposure to cocaine, which alters the blood pressure, increase the risk of GMH even in full-term infants.

GMHs are clearly seen on head ultrasound (US) studies as hyperechoic focal lesions and are graded according to the Papile classification. GMH grade 1 involves hemorrhage confined to the GM. Grade 2 GMHs are complicated by extension of the hemorrhage into a normal-sized ventricular system, whereas GMHs with a concomitant ventricular dilation are classified as GMH grade 3. If the focal GMH obstructs the normal deep venous drainage, resultant periventricular venous stasis can be complicated by a periventricular venous infarction with or without hemorrhagic conversion (periventricular hemorrhagic infarction [PVHI]). Grade 4 is not preferred terminology because it implies opening of the intraventricular hemorrhage to the parenchyma, which is not the case. On follow-up, a porencephalic cyst may develop that communicates with the ventricular system (as shown on the T2-weighted image). Grade 1 GMHs usually resolve without long-lasting complications. Grade 2 and 3 GMHs may be complicated by obstructive hydrocephalus, partially due to adhesions at the level of the Sylvian aqueduct.

Magnetic resonance imaging, and in particular susceptibility-weighted imaging, easily shows the blood products within the GM and ventricles. Diffusion-weighted imaging is helpful to identify the ischemic brain tissue.

### Reference

Orman G, Benson JE, Kweldam CF, et al. Neonatal head ultrasonography today: a powerful imaging tool! *J Neuroimaging.* 2015;25(1):31-55.

### Cross-reference

Walters MM, Robertson RL. *Pediatric Radiology: The Requisites.* 4th ed. Philadelphia: Elsevier; 2017:308-309.

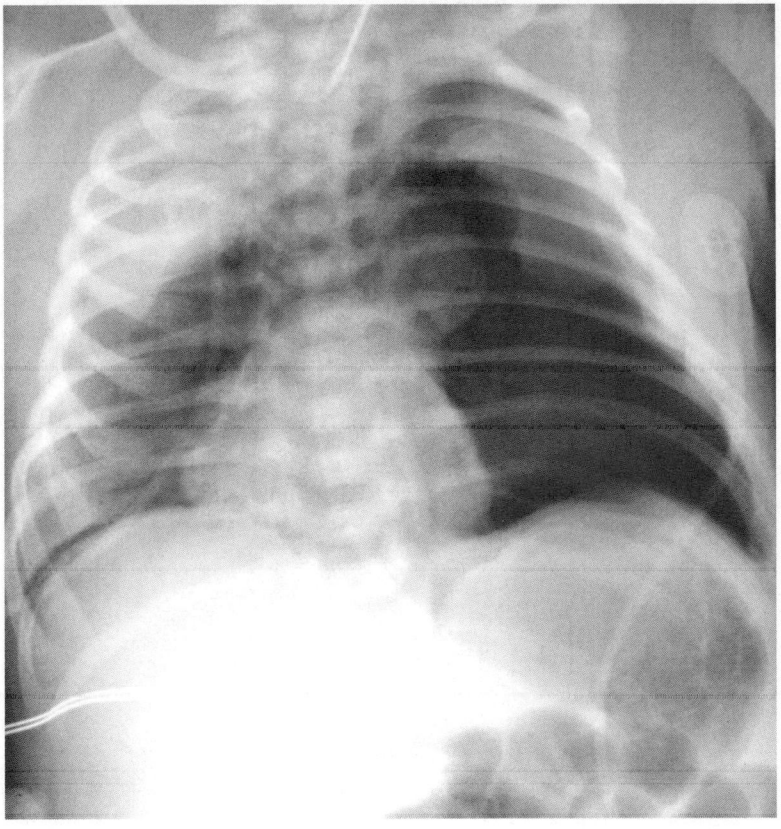

**Fig. 43.1**

**HISTORY:** Intubated neonate presenting with respiratory distress

1. Based on the imaging findings, what is the best diagnosis? (Choose all that apply.)
   A. Pneumothorax
   B. Pneumomediastinum
   C. Pneumopericardium
   D. Subcutaneous emphysema

2. Which of the following accounts for the appearance of the Spinnaker sail/angel wings sign?
   A. Mediastinal air dissecting into the pleural space
   B. Mediastinal air dissecting along pulmonary arteries
   C. Mediastinal air dissecting along the anterior junction line between the lungs
   D. Mediastinal air dissecting underneath the thymus

3. Which option should *not* be considered as a common cause of pneumomediastinum?
   A. Surfactant deficiency disease/interstitial emphysema
   B. Asthma
   C. Foreign body
   D. Rupture of a bronchial duplication cyst

4. True or false?
   A. Pneumomediastinum is an emergency that requires surgical intervention in most cases.

## CASE 43

### Pneumomediastinum

1. A and B

2. D

3. D

4. False

### *Comment*

Pneumomediastinum can be seen in the setting of birth-related trauma, or when interstitial emphysema develops in newborn infants with surfactant deficiency disease or meconium aspiration who are on positive pressure ventilation. In these patients, high-pressure ventilation with oxygen-rich air injures the fragile alveolar walls and allows air to leak into the interstitial spaces and lymphatics, from which it can dissect centrally to the mediastinum. In newborns and infants, the Spinnaker sail sign (or angel wings sign) can be encountered, which is due to mediastinal air lifting up the thymus. In older children, asthma is a common cause of pneumomediastinum, and in toddlers, one should keep in mind foreign body aspiration as a common cause. Especially in older children with pneumomediastinum, air is commonly seen to track into the neck as subcutaneous emphysema. Trauma and iatrogenic causes should also be considered in the evaluation. Pneumomediastinum can be asymptomatic or may be associated with tachypnea. Pneumomediastinum is typically self-limiting and resolves spontaneously over the course of a few days to a few weeks.

### Cross-reference

Walters MM, Robertson RL. *Pediatric Radiology: The Requisites.* 4th ed. Philadelphia: Elsevier; 2017:54–55.

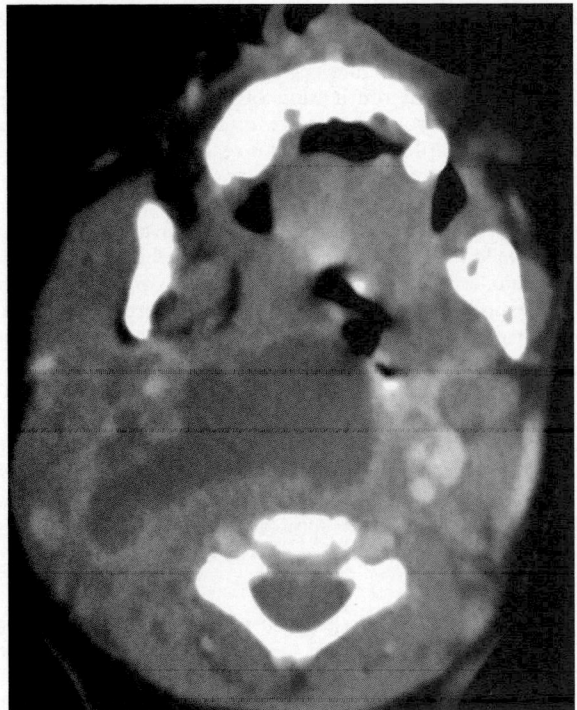

Fig. 44.1

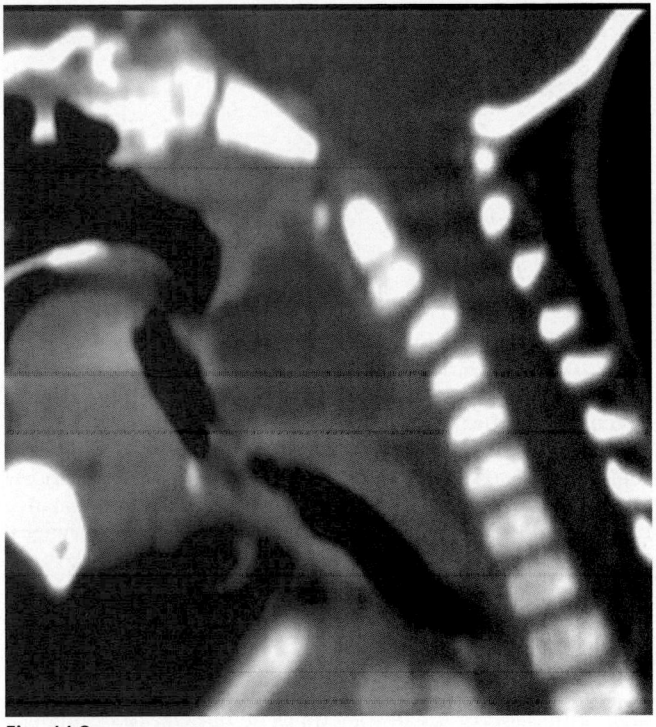

Fig. 44.2

**HISTORY:** 9-month-old presenting with increased fussiness and low oral intake

1. What space is involved in the abnormality depicted on these images (initial image on the left and short-term follow-up image on the right)?
   A. Prevertebral space
   B. Retropharyngeal space
   C. Parapharyngeal space
   D. Cannot tell

2. What is the best diagnosis for the findings shown on the follow-up image?
   A. Retropharyngeal edema
   B. Retropharyngeal abscess
   C. Suppurative adenitis
   D. Retropharyngeal phlegmon

3. The danger space is part of which space and how far does it extend caudally?
   A. Prevertebral space; extends inferiorly to the diaphragm
   B. Retropharyngeal space; extends inferiorly to the diaphragm
   C. Prevertebral space; extends inferiorly to T1–T6
   D. Retropharyngeal space; extends inferiorly to the diaphragm

4. Which statement about the retropharyngeal space and retropharyngeal space collections is false?
   A. Collections associated with suppurative adenitis typically do not cross the midline.
   B. The alar fascia, which is visible on magnetic resonance imaging (MRI), separates the true retropharyngeal space anteriorly from the danger space more posteriorly.
   C. Common causes of reactive retropharyngeal edema include radiation therapy, pharyngitis, internal jugular vein thrombosis, and longus coli tendonitis.
   D. The true retropharyngeal space extends from the skull base to about T1–T6.

## CASE 44

### Retropharyngeal Abscess

1. B
2. B
3. D
4. B

### Comment

The retropharyngeal space is bounded by the prevertebral fascia (anterior to the longus coli and longus capitis muscles) posteriorly, the visceral fascia anteriorly, and the carotid space laterally on either side. It extends from the skull base to the mediastinum and is separated by the alar fascia into the true retropharyngeal space anteriorly, and the danger space posteriorly. These spaces are not distinguishable by magnetic resonance imaging (MRI) in a healthy patient. The true retropharyngeal space extends from the skull base variably to T1–T6, where the alar fascia fuses with the visceral fascia to obliterate the true retropharyngeal space. Dorsally, the danger space continues down further into the posterior mediastinum to the level of the diaphragm.

Nodes in the retropharyngeal space are often large in children until puberty. It can sometimes be difficult to distinguish reactive edema or phlegmon from an abscess and suppurative adenitis, but the following guidelines may help. Reactive edema uniformly fills the retropharyngeal space, has smooth margins, and is tapered along its superior and inferior margins on the sagittal view. It has no mass effect and no wall enhancement and may be seen in the setting of radiation treatment, internal jugular vein thrombosis, calcific tendinitis, and pharyngitis. Retropharyngeal phlegmon, unlike reactive edema, may show mass effect on prevertebral muscles or the posterior pharyngeal wall. Suppurative adenitis occurs in reactive lymph nodes that have undergone liquefactive necrosis contained by the nodal capsule. Retropharyngeal nodes do not cross the midline, so the fluid is located laterally in the retropharyngeal space and is rounded or oval in configuration. There may be a thin hyperdense or enhancing rim, and associated reactive retropharyngeal edema is commonly seen. Treatment is typically with antibiotics. Retropharyngeal abscess is frequently caused by rupture of a suppurative node into the retropharyngeal space with moderate mass effect, resulting in flattening of the prevertebral muscles and anterior displacement of the pharynx. There is commonly an enhancing wall. A trial of antibiotics may initially be attempted, but surgical drainage may be required, especially if there is associated airway compromise.

### Reference

Hoang J, Branstetter 4th BF, Eastwood J, Glastonbury CM. Multiplanar CT and MRI of collections in the retropharyngeal space: is it an abscess? *AJR Am J Roentgenol.* 2011;196(4):W426–W432.

### Cross-reference

Walters MM, Robertson RL. *Pediatric Radiology: The Requisites.* 4th ed. Philadelphia: Elsevier; 2017:387–388.

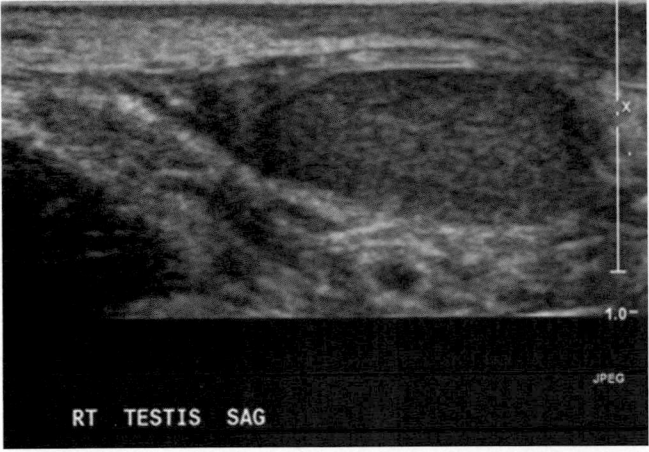

Fig. 45.1

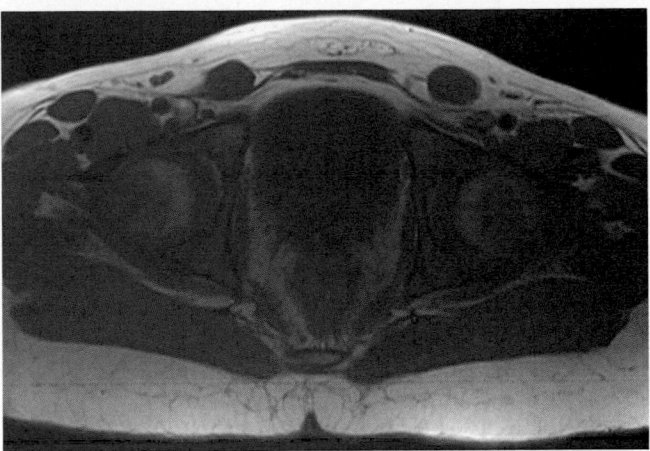

Fig. 45.2

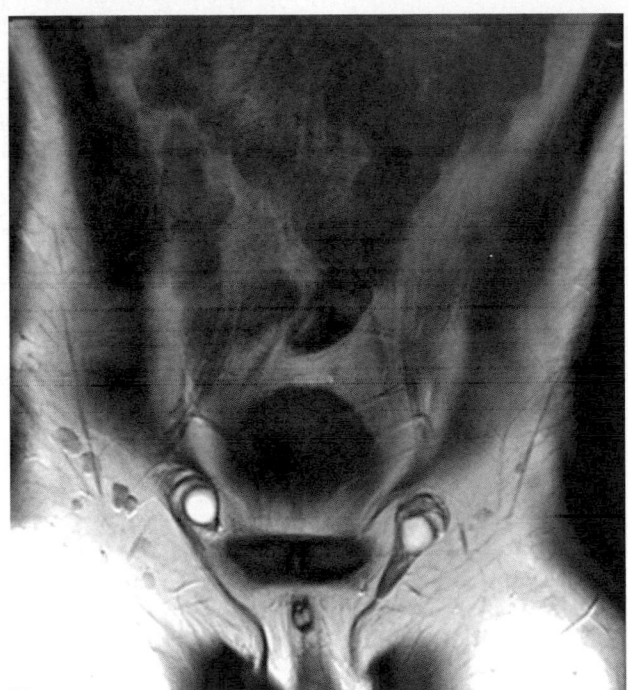

Fig. 45.3

**HISTORY:** Ultrasound and T1/T2-weighted magnetic resonance imaging (MRI) scans of a boy with nonpalpable testicles

1. Where are the testicles?
   A. Peritoneal cavity
   B. Inner opening of the inguinal canal
   C. Outside of the inguinal canal in the prepubic region
   D. High in the scrotal sac

2. What are the imaging characteristics of the testicles?
   A. T1 hypointense, T2 hypointense
   B. T1 hypointense, T2 hyperintense
   C. T1 hyperintense, T2 hypointense
   D. T1 hyperintense, T2 hyperintense

3. What is the official term for undescended testicles?
   A. Cryptorchidism
   B. Monorchism
   C. Anorchism
   D. Cryptodism

4. Which options are causes and risk factors for undescended testicles?
   A. Severe prematurity
   B. Congenital malformation syndromes (Down, Prader-Willi)
   C. Diabetes and obesity of the mother
   D. All of the above

## CASE 45

### Undescended Testicles

1. C
2. B
3. A
4. D

### Comment

Cryptorchidism or undescended testicle(s) refers to uni- or bilateral failed or incomplete descent of the testicle(s) from the peritoneal cavity through the inguinal canal into the scrotum. Cryptorchidism is clinically asymptomatic and is typically diagnosed on routine pediatric screening examination because of an "empty scrotum" on palpation. Cryptorchidism is more common among premature infants than term babies. Spontaneous descent into the scrotum may be delayed and can be seen to occur well into the first year of life.

In true cryptorchidism the testicles can be seen in various locations along the natural path of descent. In the most incomplete descent, the testicle(s) remain inside the abdominal cavity below the kidneys, usually in close proximity to the inner opening of the inguinal canal. Alternatively, they are located within the inguinal canal or just outside the inguinal canal in the prescrotal or prepubic region. In rare instances the testicles can be found in a true ectopic location subcutaneously along the thigh, or in the perineal region. Undescended testicles are often smaller or hypoplastic and are at higher risk for testicular torsion. Many publications have suggested that undescended testicles are at higher risk for testicular germ cell tumors; however, this has not yet been proven. Cryptorchidism may be seen in a variety of syndromes including Down syndrome, Noonan syndrome, or Prader-Willi syndrome as well as in multiple endocrine abnormalities.

Ultrasound is the first-line imaging modality to localize the undescended testicles. Ultrasound is, however, limited for the evaluation of intraabdominal testicles and in those cases where the testicles are hypoplastic. Alternatively, the high soft tissue resolution of magnetic resonance imaging (MRI) may allow localization of the T2-hyperintense testicles with higher sensitivity.

### Reference

Tasian GE, Copp HL, Baskin LS. Diagnostic imaging in cryptorchidism: utility, indications, and effectiveness. *J Pediatr Surg*. 2011;46: 2406-2413.

### Cross-reference

Walters MM, Robertson RL. *Pediatric Radiology: The Requisites*. 4th ed. Philadelphia: Elsevier; 2017:175-176.

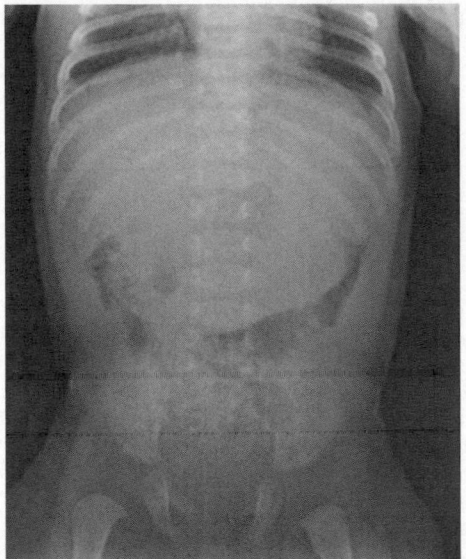

Fig. 46.1

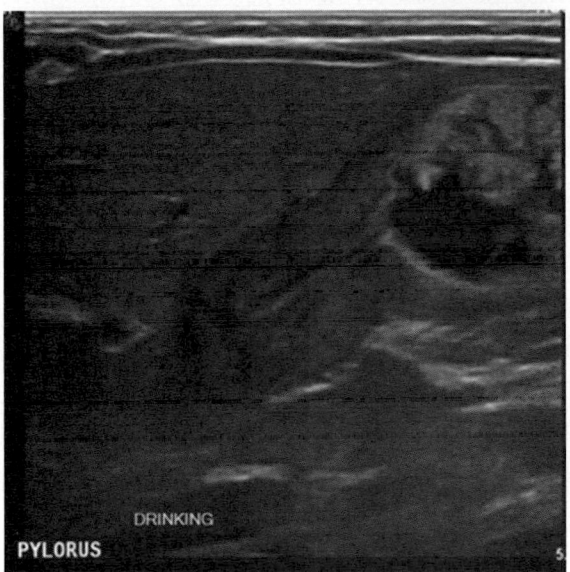

Fig. 46.2

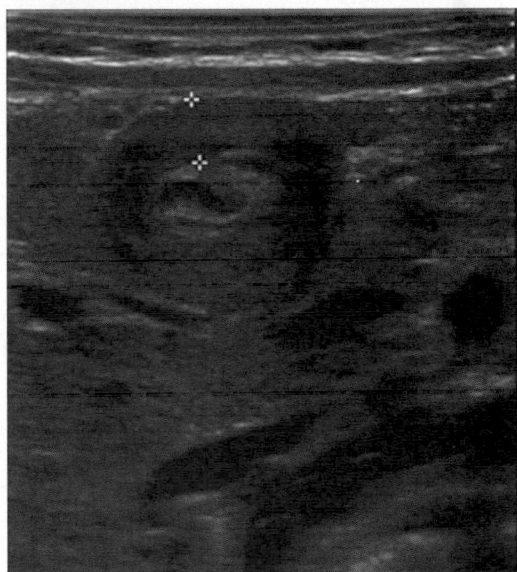

Fig. 46.3

**HISTORY:** 8-week-old male infant with failure to thrive and projectile vomiting

1. Which signature pathological imaging finding do you see on the abdominal radiography?
   A. Significantly enlarged spleen
   B. Significantly enlarged/fluid-filled stomach
   C. Large renal mass lesion
   D. Calcified retroperitoneal mass lesion

2. What does the ultrasonography study show?
   A. Normal-sized pyloric channel
   B. Thickened and elongated pyloric muscle
   C. Fluid within/passing the pyloric channel
   D. Intussusception of the stomach into the duodenum

3. What is the most likely diagnosis?
   A. Hypertrophic pyloric stenosis
   B. Hypotrophic pyloric stenosis
   C. Duodenal atresia
   D. Duodenal web

4. Which statement is correct?
   A. Hypertrophic pyloric stenosis is more common in males than females.
   B. Hypertrophic pyloric stenosis is more common in females than males.
   C. Hypertrophic pyloric stenosis is typically seen between 0 and 4 weeks of age.
   D. Hypertrophic pyloric stenosis is typically seen between 4 and 6 months of age.

## Hypertrophic Pyloric Stenosis

1. B
2. B
3. A
4. A

### Comment

Hypertrophic pyloric stenosis refers to an idiopathic hypertrophy/hyperplasia of the pyloric muscle typically seen in neonates 4 to 12 weeks of age. The hypertrophic muscle obstructs the gastric outlet with resultant projectile, nonbilious vomiting after feeding. Failure to pass or very limited passage of fluid/milk across the pyloric channel results in progressive dehydration, often initially detected by less wet diapers followed by weight loss and lethargy. Electrolyte derangement with low serum chloride and potassium and elevated bicarbonate (hypochloremic alkalosis) may be seen. On physical examination, the hypertrophic pylorus may be palpated and is typically described as an epigastric "olive."

Abdominal radiography can show a gas-distended stomach while the remainder of the abdomen appears gas-free. Diagnosis relies on epigastric high-resolution linear ultrasound examination, which allows direct visualization and measurement of the pyloric muscle. The pyloric channel is typically elongated beyond 15 mm, the thickness of the pyloric muscle exceeds 3 mm, the overall transverse diameter of the pylorus is more than 13 mm, and the pyloric muscle appears hypoechoic. For functional evaluation, a small amount of water may be given at the end of the study. Subsequent dynamic ultrasound may show a trickle of water pass the pyloric channel or no passage at all. In addition, gastric hyperperistalsis is often noted. Occasionally, on initial ultrasound study, the measurements do not fulfill the criteria for diagnosis. Follow-up studies may be necessary because the pyloric muscle hypertrophy may mature over time. Fluoroscopic studies and computed tomography are currently considered unnecessary.

Differential diagnosis includes severe gastroesophageal reflux, malrotation with or without midgut volvulus, duodenal web or stenosis, annular pancreas, or extrinsic masses compressing the pyloric channel.

### Reference

Ranells JD, Carver JD, Kirby RS. Infantile hypertrophic pyloric stenosis: epidemiology, genetics, and clinical update. *Adv Pediatr.* 2011;58:195–206.

### Cross-reference

Walters MM, Robertson RL. *Pediatric Radiology: The Requisites.* 4th ed. Philadelphia: Elsevier; 2017:107–108.

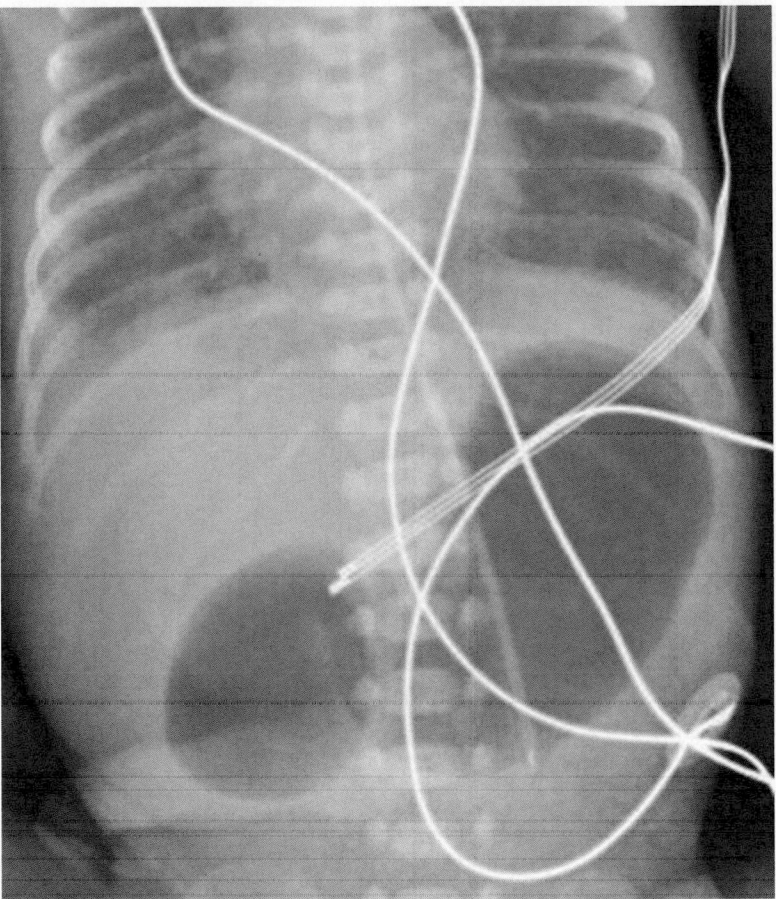

**Fig. 47.1**

**HISTORY:** newborn with history of Down Syndrome, presenting with bilious emesis.

1. What is your diagnosis in this newborn infant?
   A. Hypertrophic pyloric stenosis
   B. Malrotation
   C. Gastrointestinal (GI) duplication cyst
   D. Duodenal atresia

2. Which statement is most accurate concerning duodenal atresia?
   A. It is the most common upper GI obstruction in neonates.
   B. Approximately 50% of cases have additional anomalies.
   C. The survival rate is quite high with surgical treatment.
   D. All of the above.

3. Which statement is most accurate regarding the imaging findings of duodenal atresia?
   A. A double bubble sign with no distal gas on radiography is classic.
   B. Vomiting and/or a nasogastric tube may hide the double bubble sign on the initial radiographs.
   C. A "corkscrew" configuration of narrowed bowel beyond the obstruction is classic.
   D. A and B.

4. Which statement regarding the imaging workup of suspected duodenal atresia is correct?
   A. All patients with the double bubble sign should have an upper GI examination with barium.
   B. An upper GI exam is necessary only if gas is present distal to the bubble.
   C. Computed tomography (CT) is best for the initial imaging diagnosis.
   D. None of the above.

## Duodenal Atresia

1. D
2. D
3. D
4. B

## *Comment*

Duodenal atresia (DA) occurs in 1 in 10,000 live births and represents 60% of intestinal atresias. The etiology of DA was believed to be different than other intestinal atresia, which is based on vascular compromise theory, rather than failure of the duodenal lumen recanalization during the second gestational month. Most DAs present in the second portion of the duodenum. Up to 45% have Down syndrome. Additional gastrointestinal (GI) anomalies can be seen: malrotation and annular pancreas in up to 30% of cases; second duodenal web in 1% to 3% of cases; choledochal cyst, preduodenal portal vein, esophageal atresia, and tracheoesophageal fistula in up to 18% of cases; and imperforate anus. Diagnosis is usually established during prenatal ultrasound (US). Postnatally bilious emesis, dehydration, and weight loss can be presenting symptoms. The classic imaging finding is the double bubble sign. Distal gas can be present if obstruction is incomplete, such as in patients with duodenal stenosis or annular pancreas. Alternatively, acute midgut volvulus or collateral pathway by variant biliary/pancreatic duct may present with distal gas and double bubble. In patients with DA, the duodenal bubble is usually markedly dilated indicating chronic in utero obstruction. True double bubble with no distal bowel gas is essentially diagnostic for DA. An upper GI exam is necessary only if distal gas is present. The windsock anomaly can be seen in patients with duodenal webs, where the obstructing membrane distends distally and results in dilation beyond the level of actual obstruction. The survival rate of patients with DA is 90% with surgical treatment.

### Reference

Adams SD, Stanton MP. Malrotation and intestinal atresia. *Early Hum Dev.* 2014;90(12):921–925.

### Cross-reference

Walters MM, Robertson RL. *Pediatric Radiology: The Requisites.* 4th ed. Philadelphia: Elsevier; 2017:99–100.

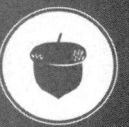

# Fair Game

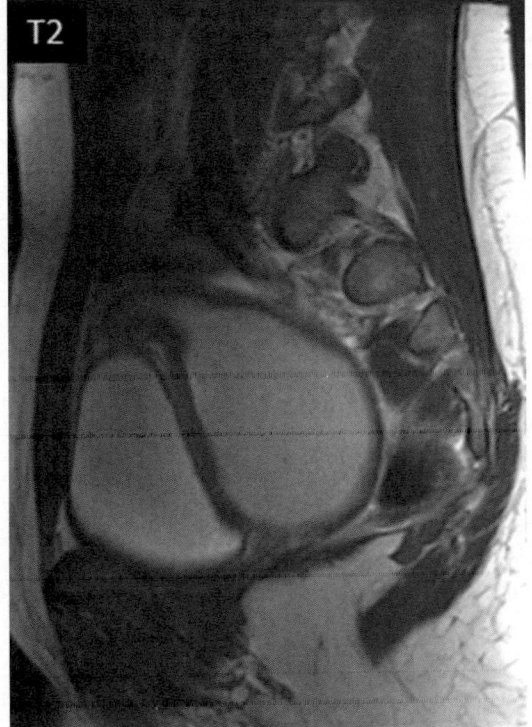

Fig. 48.1

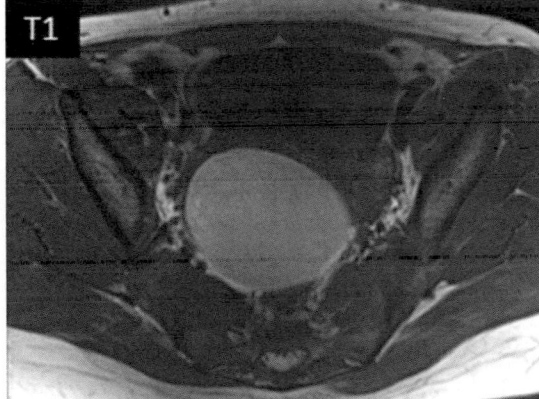

Fig. 48.2

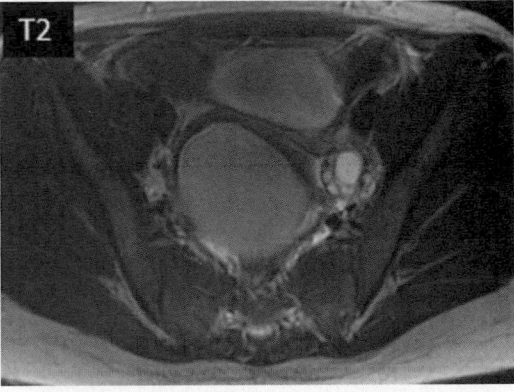

Fig. 48.3

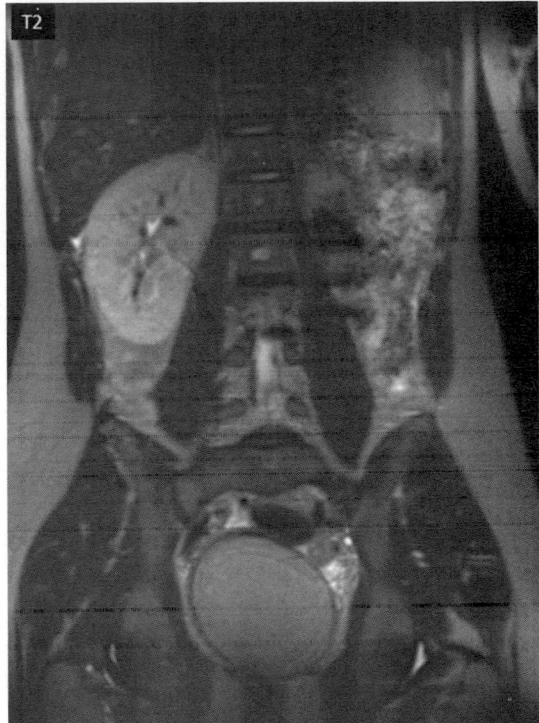

Fig. 48.4

**HISTORY:** 12-year-old girl presented with first episode of urinary tract infection and abdominal pain. She had not yet started menstruation.

1. Which finding is seen on magnetic resonance imaging (MRI)?
   A. Blood in the uterus/vagina
   B. Clear fluid in the uterus/vagina
   C. Blood in the rectum
   D. Blood in the urinary bladder

2. What is the most likely diagnosis?
   A. Cloacal malformation
   B. Hydrometrocolpos
   C. Ovarian teratoma
   D. Pelvic abscess

3. What is the most likely cause of the hydrometrocolpos?
   A. Distal vaginal atresia
   B. Imperforate hymen
   C. Transverse vaginal septum
   D. Vaginal duplication

4. Which additional anatomical structures are missing?
   A. Left kidney and left ovary
   B. Right kidney and right ovary
   C. Left kidney and right ovary
   D. Right kidney and left ovary

## CASE 48

### Hydrometrocolpos

1. A

2. B

3. A

4. C

### Comment

Hydrometrocolpos is characterized by a fluid- or fluid/blood-filled cystic dilation of the vagina or vagina and uterus. The dilation can be secondary to distal vaginal stenosis, vaginal atresia, transverse vaginal septum, or an imperforate hymen. Vaginal septums are most commonly located between the middle and upper third of the vagina. Children may present with a focal pelvic mass lesion displacing or compressing adjacent structures. Obstruction of the distal ureter, ureterovesical junction, or urethra increases the risk of recurrent urinary tract infections. Furthermore, absent or delayed menarche, cyclic pelvic pain, or a prolapsing interlabial mass lesion can be seen.

On imaging, a well-circumscribed dilation of the superior vagina and uterus is seen. The vagina is usually more dilated than the muscular uterus. The fluid within the vagina/uterus is typically heterogeneous on ultrasound with layering debris. On magnetic resonance imaging (MRI), the blood products typically appear T1 hyperintense. The urinary bladder and rectum may be compressed.

Renal, uterine, ovarian, or intestinal anomalies may coexist. Identification of the uterus is essential to exclude Mayer-Rokitansky-Küster-Hauser (MRKH) syndrome, which is characterized by failure of the uterus and the vagina to develop properly in women who have normal ovarian function and normal external genitalia. Occasionally, hydrometrocolpos may be diagnosed on prenatal imaging.

### References

Ameh EA, Mshelbwala PM, Ameh N. Congenital vaginal obstruction in neonates and infants: recognition and management. *J Pediatr Adolesc Gynecol*. 2011;24:74–78.

Mazir Z, Rizvi RM, Qureshi RN, Khan ZS, Khan Z. Congenital vaginal obstructions: varied presentation and outcome. *Pediatr Surg Int*. 2006;22:749–753.

### Cross-reference

Walters MM, Robertson RL. *Pediatric Radiology: The Requisites*. 4th ed. Philadelphia; Elsevier: 2017:183–185.

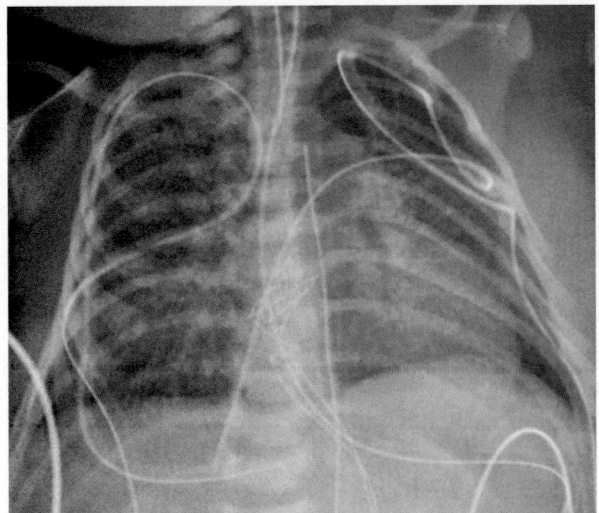

Fig. 49.1

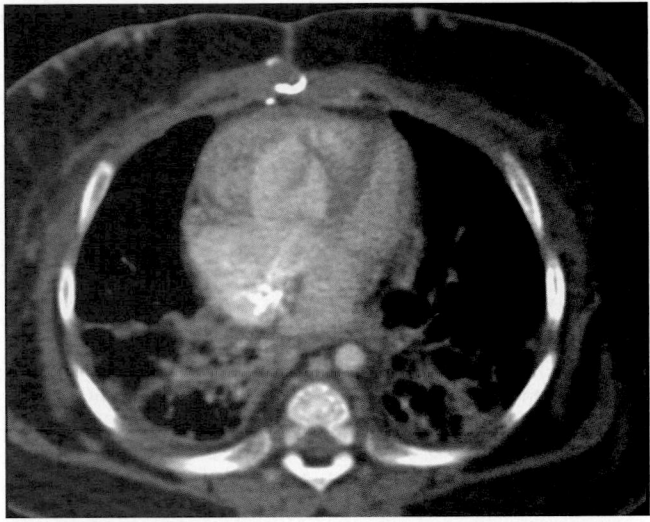

Fig. 49.2

**HISTORY:** Newborn presenting with cardiogenic shock

1. Based on the imaging findings, which of the following would you include in your differential diagnosis? (Choose all that apply.)
   A. Rhabdomyoma
   B. Aortic stenosis
   C. Hypoplastic left heart
   D. Cor triatriatum

2. Which statement about hypoplastic left heart syndrome is false?
   A. It is entirely compatible with fetal life.
   B. Prostaglandins are contraindicated in the neonatal period to allow the ductus arteriosus to close naturally.
   C. Balloon septostomy is performed if the atrial septum is inadequately allowing blood to pass from the left to the right atrium.
   D. It is uniformly fatal within days to weeks without treatment.

3. What is the most commonly performed surgical procedure used to treat patients with hypoplastic left heart syndrome?
   A. Waterston-Cooley
   B. Mustard/Senning
   C. Glenn
   D. Norwood

4. Which of the following is the first step of the Norwood procedure?
   A. Superior vena cava to pulmonary artery anastomosis
   B. Inferior vena cava to right pulmonary artery anastomosis
   C. Atrial septectomy and creation of a neoaorta from the pulmonary artery
   D. Switch of aorta and pulmonary artery with coronary artery reanastomosis

## CASE 49

### Hypoplastic Left Heart Syndrome

1. C

2. B

3. D

4. C

### *Comment*

In hypoplastic left heart syndrome, patients develop a combination of hypoplasia or atresia of the ascending aorta, aortic valve, left ventricle, and mitral valve. It is entirely compatible with fetal life because the inadequate systemic cardiac chambers and outflow tract are bypassed in the setting of high fetal pulmonary vascular resistance, a patent foramen ovale, and wide open ductus arteriosus. The first steps in treatment are to ensure continued patency of the ductus arteriosus with prostaglandins and to ensure that the atrial septum is patent to allow admixture of the systemic and pulmonary circulation in the right atrium. Balloon septostomy or interatrial stent placement (as seen on the plain radiograph in this case) is performed if necessary. Without treatment, this condition is uniformly fatal within days to weeks after birth. On imaging, shunt vascularity, an enlarged heart (from right ventricle enlargement), an enlarged right atrium, and an enlarged main pulmonary artery are typically seen. The first stage of the Norwood procedure is performed as soon as the patient is stable and consists of an atrial septectomy and creation of a neoaorta from the pulmonary artery, which is anastomosed to the thoracic aorta. Pulmonary circulation is maintained via a Blalock-Taussig shunt from the subclavian artery to the right pulmonary artery. The second stage, which is typically performed between 4 and 6 months of age, consists of replacing the Blalock-Taussig shunt with a bidirectional Glenn (superior vena cava to right pulmonary artery anastomosis), and then later adding a Fontan shunt (inferior vena cava to right pulmonary artery anastomosis).

### Reference

Fonseca BM. Perioperative imaging in hypoplastic left heart syndrome. *Semin Cardiothorac Vasc Anesth*. 2013;17(2):117–127.

### Cross-reference

Walters MM, Robertson RL. *Pediatric Radiology: The Requisites*. 4th ed. Philadelphia: Elsevier; 2017:84–86.

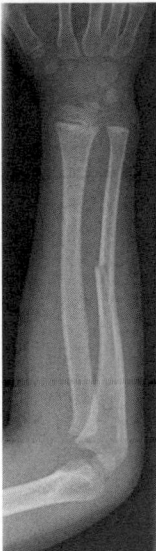

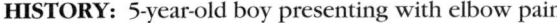

**Fig. 50.1**

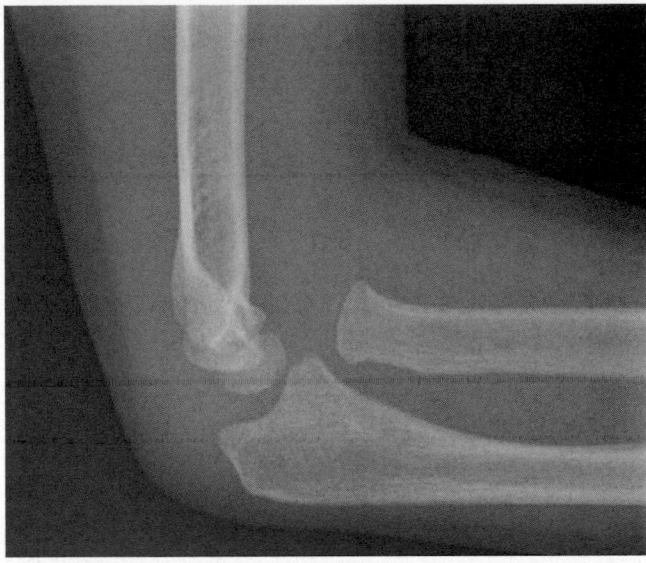

**Fig. 50.2**

**HISTORY:** 5-year-old boy presenting with elbow pain

1. Based on the images provided, what is the best diagnosis?
   A. Galeazzi fracture
   B. Monteggia fracture
   C. Isolated ulnar shaft fracture
   D. Isolated radiocapitellar joint dislocation

2. Which statement about Monteggia fractures is false?
   A. They involve a fracture of the ulnar shaft.
   B. They involve dislocation of the radiocapitellar joint.
   C. They are 3 times more common than Galeazzi fractures.
   D. They occur more commonly in adults than in children.

3. What is the most common type of radiocapitellar joint dislocation in Monteggia fractures?
   A. Posterior
   B. Lateral
   C. Anterior
   D. Medial

4. Which statement about Galeazzi fractures is false?
   A. They involve a fracture of the radial shaft.
   B. They involve proximal ulna dislocation at the elbow.
   C. They involve disruption of the distal radioulnar joint.
   D. The most common mechanism is a fall on an outstretched hand (FOOSH).

## CASE 50

### Monteggia Fracture

1. B
2. B
3. C
4. B

### *Comment*

Similar to the pelvis or mandible, the forearm can be thought of as a ring, with fracture and displacement of one component requiring dislocation or fracture and displacement of an additional component of the ring. In a Monteggia fracture, there is a displaced fracture of the ulnar shaft, which is accompanied by a dislocation of the radiocapitellar joint. In the Galeazzi fracture, which is more common than the Monteggia fracture, a radial shaft fracture is accompanied by a dislocation of the distal radioulnar joint. In Monteggia fractures, anterior dislocation of the radiocapitellar joint is most common. Associated radial head fractures can rarely occur. Because forearm fracture is the more obvious injury, the dislocation of the radiocapitellar joint can be missed, which can lead to limited mobility.

### Reference

Eathiraju S, Mudgal CS, Jupiter JB. Monteggia fracture-dislocations. *Hand Clin*. 2007;23(2):154–177.

### Cross-reference

Walters MM, Robertson RL. *Pediatric Radiology: The Requisites*. 4th ed. Philadelphia: Elsevier; 2017:249.

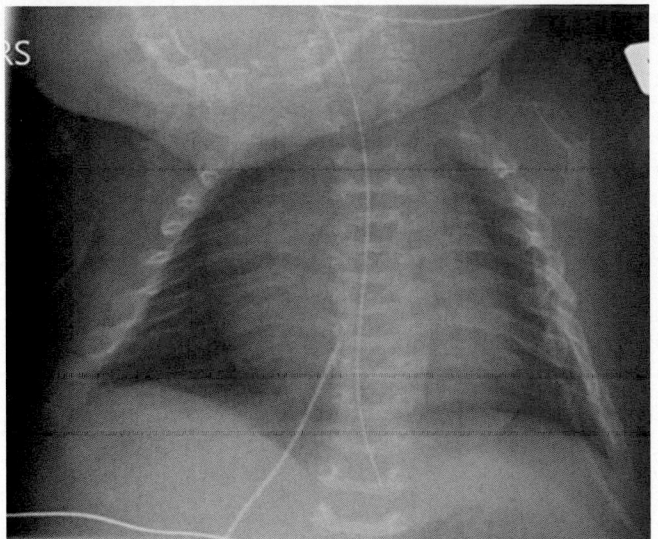

Fig. 51.1

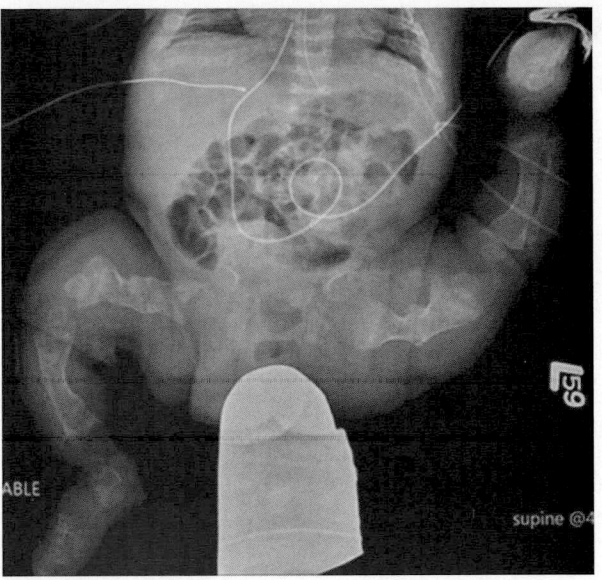

Fig. 51.2

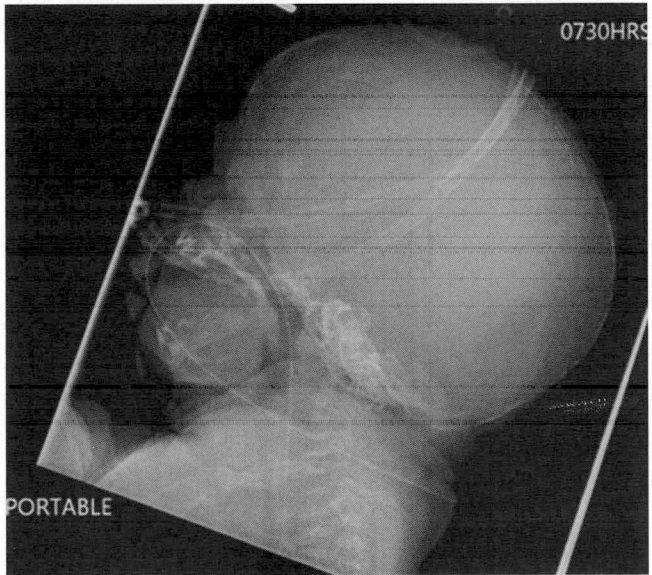

Fig. 51.3

**HISTORY:** Full-term male delivered by C-section. Prenatal ultrasound revealed severe shortening of long bones and multiple fractures. After an initial cry at delivery, cessation of breathing was noted and intubation was performed

1. Which findings are seen on the radiographs?
   A. Multiple rib and long bone fractures
   B. Thin calvarium and basilar impression
   C. Platyspondyly
   D. All of the above

2. What is the most likely diagnosis?
   A. Neurofibromatosis type 1
   B. Rickets
   C. Osteogenesis imperfecta
   D. Nonaccidental injury

3. Which statement is incorrect?
   A. Platyspondyly is associated with Chiari II malformation.
   B. Platybasia and basilar invagination may result in brain stem compression, ventriculomegaly, and syringohydromyelia.
   C. Rib fractures and a small chest cavity may result in respiratory distress.
   D. Wormian bones are typically seen in osteogenesis imperfecta.

4. Which subtype of osteogenesis imperfecta is typically lethal in the perinatal period?
   A. Type I
   B. Type II
   C. Type III
   D. Type IV

## CASE 51

### Osteogenesis Imperfecta

1. D
2. C
3. A
4. B

## Comment

Osteogenesis imperfecta (OI), or brittle bone disease, is a genetic disorder impacting normal bone development. OI is characterized by increased bone fragility, which may be associated with additional connective tissue abnormalities. OI results from a reduction of the normal type 1 collagen production or from abnormal collagen synthesis. Currently up to 11 different, partially overlapping subtypes have been defined. Prognosis varies widely based upon the subtype. OI affects 6 to 7 of 100,000 people at birth. The characteristic clinical features allow diagnosis in most cases. Biochemical (collagen) or molecular (DNA) tests may help to confirm diagnosis. Most patients with OI (about 90%) follow an autosomal dominant pattern of inheritance.

Type I is the most frequent form. Clinical symptoms are usually mild; the incidence of fractures varies from none to numerous. Type II is the most severe form. The vast majority of children die intrauterine; some survive into the immediate postnatal time period. On prenatal imaging, multiple fractures are noted, which may affect almost every bone. The chest cavity is typically small secondary to multiple rib fractures with associated pulmonary hypoplasia. Intracranial hemorrhages are often seen. Type I and II patients usually have blue sclera.

Next to the obvious fractures in various stages of healing, skeletal manifestations may include diffuse osteopenia, markedly thinned calvarium, delayed closure of fontanelles/sutures, excessive Wormian bone formation, flattened vertebral bodies, shortened and deformed extremities, short stature, and progressive skeletal deformities (scoliosis, kyphosis). In addition, platybasia with secondary basilar invagination may result in brain stem compression, ventriculomegaly, and syringohydromyelia. Osseous changes may be identified by prenatal ultrasound. A reduced acoustic shadowing of the long bones is observed as well as an increased nuchal translucency.

### References

Cheung MS, Glorieux FH. Osteogenesis imperfecta: update on presentation and management. *Endocr Metab Disord*. 2008;9(2):153–160.

Barnes AM, Chang W, Morello R, et al. Deficiency of cartilage-associated protein in recessive lethal osteogenesis imperfecta. *N Engl J Med*. 2006;355(26):2757–2764.

### Cross-reference

Walters MM, Robertson RL. *Pediatric Radiology: The Requisites*. 4th ed. Philadelphia: Elsevier; 2017:206–207.

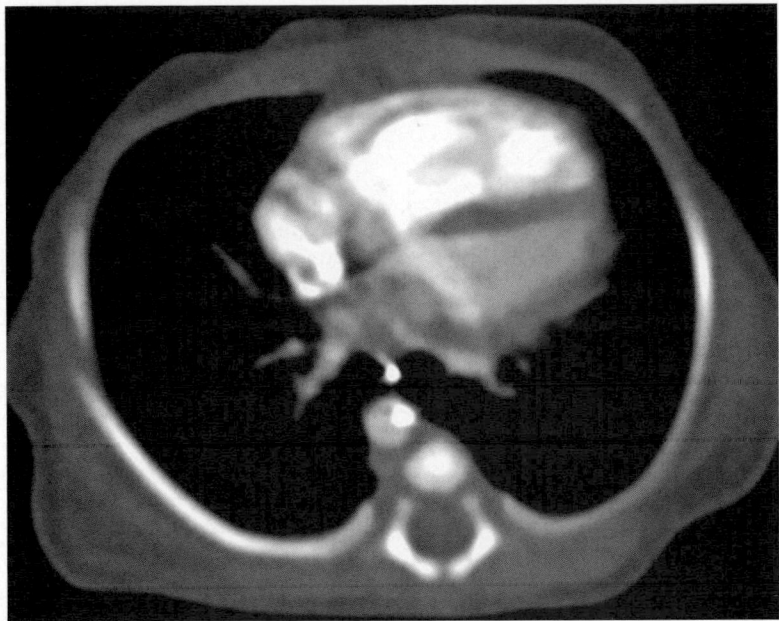

**Fig. 52.1**

| Total mAs 197 | Total DLP 6 mGycm | | | | | | |
|---|---|---|---|---|---|---|---|
| | Scan | KV | mAs / ref. | CTDIvol*<br>mGy | DLP<br>mGycm | TI<br>s | cSL<br>mm |
| Patient Position H-SP | | | | | | | |
| Topogram | 1 | 80 | 35 mA | 0.03 L | 0.4 | 1.3 | 0.6 |
| Ped CTA Chest | 2D | 70 | 32 /358 | 0.31 L | 5.1 | 0.28 | 0.6 |

**Fig. 52.2**

**HISTORY:** Pediatric patient ordered for a computed tomography (CT) scan

1. Radiation dose from medical imaging today makes up about how much of the total average radiation dose per citizen in the United States?
   A. 1/5
   B. 1/4
   C. 1/3
   D. 1/2

2. Which statement about the biologic effects of radiation is false?
   A. Biologic effects can be divided into stochastic and deterministic effects.
   B. Compton scatter, coherent scatter, and the photoelectric effect result in transfer of energy to electrons.
   C. Free radicals, formed via ionization from electrons, can cause DNA damage.
   D. The severity of stochastic effects is independent of dose.

3. Using computed tomography dose index $(CTDL)_{vol}$ and Dose Length Product (DLP) to estimate dose in pediatric patients may underestimate the dose by what percentage?
   A. 25% to 50%
   B. 50% to 75%
   C. 75% to 100%
   D. 100% to 200%

4. Which option is not a useful consideration in reducing the dosage to pediatric patients during CT scans?
   A. Tailor the protocol based on the age and weight of the patient.
   B. Reduce the peak kilovoltage (kVp) and milliampere-seconds (mAs) as much as possible.
   C. A single phase is often enough.
   D. Scan only the indicated area.

## CASE 52

### Radiation Exposure

1. D
2. B
3. D
4. A

### *Comment*

Radiation exposure from medical imaging now makes up about 50% of the total average radiation exposure in the United States, up from about 15% in the 1980s. Computed tomography (CT) scans and nuclear medicine procedures account for most of the medical radiation exposure. Approximately 80 million CT examinations are performed annually in the United States, and about 7 million of these are performed on children. Biologic effects from radiation can be deterministic (nonstochastic), for example, resulting in skin erythema, lens cataracts, or sterility. For these effects, there is a threshold dose above which the effect will occur, and the severity depends on the dose. Biologic effects from radiation can be also probabilistic (stochastic), for example, resulting in cancer. For stochastic effects, there is no defined lower threshold, and the severity of the effect is independent of the dose. The likelihood of the effect, however, does increase with higher dose. In the pediatric population in particular, stochastic effects from radiation are important to consider given the longer expected life span. Radiation-induced leukemia typically has a short latency period of about 5 years, but radiation-induced solid cancers can have latency periods of several decades.

X-rays interacting with matter can form free electrons through Compton scatter or the photoelectric effect (but not through coherent scatter, which results in no net transfer of energy), which in turn can form free radicals through ionization. Free radicals can, in turn, cause DNA damage, which may lead to development of cancer. Radiation dose during CT scanning should be decreased as much as reasonably achievable, by reducing peak kilovoltage (kVp) and milliampere-seconds (mAs) as much as possible, using a single phase if possible, and scanning only the indicated area. It is better to tailor the protocol (especially mAs) based on the size of the patient, rather than the age and weight. $CTDI_{vol}$ can underestimate the actual dose to a small pediatric patient by two- to threefold, because the energy is imparted on a smaller volume. Size-specific dose estimate (SSDE) tables have been created to better estimate dose based on the actual patient size.

### References

Alliance for radiation safety in pediatric imaging: image gently. <www.imagegently.org/>;Accessed 20.10.16.

Mettler Jr FA, Wiest PW, Locken JA, Kelsey CA. CT scanning: patterns of use and dose. *J Radiol Prot*. 2000;20(4):353–359.

### Cross-reference

Walters MM, Robertson RL. *Pediatric Radiology: The Requisites*. 4th ed. Philadelphia: Elsevier; 2017:1–2.

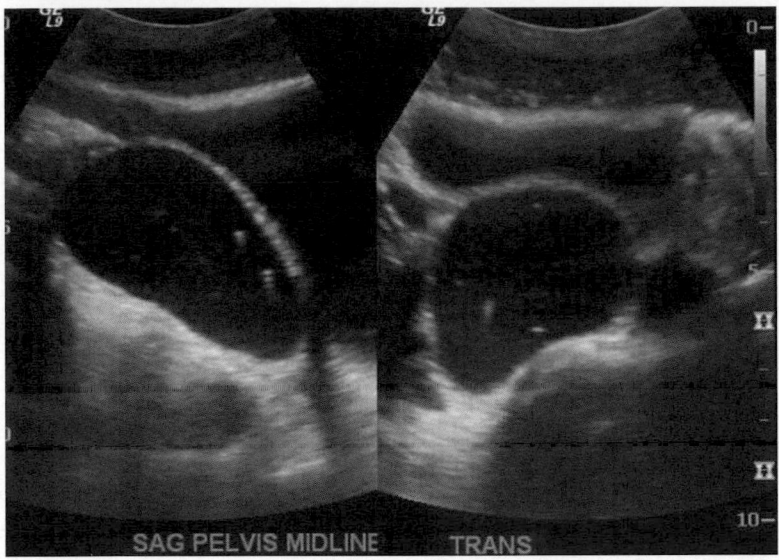

**Fig. 53.1**

**HISTORY:** 12-year-old female presenting with right lower quadrant pain

1. What is the most likely diagnosis?
   A. Ovarian cyst
   B. Lymphatic malformation
   C. Hydrometrocolpos
   D. Gastrointestinal (GI) duplication cyst

2. True or false?
   A. Eighty percent of duplication cysts contain gastric or pancreatic tissue.
   B. The most common location of GI duplication cysts is the esophagus.

3. Which statement is accurate?
   A. A duplication cyst may retain communication with the parent bowel.
   B. Perforation and hemorrhage are common complications.
   C. Fifty percent to 60% of duplication cysts contain gastric or pancreatic tissue.
   D. None of the above.

4. Which option describes the best imaging feature for duplication cysts?
   A. Bowel signature on ultrasound: echogenic inner mucosal layer, hypoechoic muscular layer, and echogenic outer serosal layer
   B. Bowel signature on ultrasound: hypoechoic inner mucosal layer, hypoechoic muscular layer, and echogenic outer serosal layer
   C. A signal drop in out-of-phase and in-phase imaging on magnetic resonance imaging (MRI)
   D. Restricted diffusion on diffusion weighted imaging (DWI)

## CASE 53

### Small Bowel Duplication Cyst

1. D

2. (A) False, (B) False

3. A

4. A

### *Comment*

Gastrointestinal (GI) duplication cysts can be seen along any part of the alimentary tract; the most common location is in the jejunum/ileum (~50%), followed by the esophagus (~20%). These are congenital cysts with three characteristic features: they are attached or were attached to some part of the GI tract, they have well-developed smooth muscle, and they have an epithelial lining representative of some part of the GI tract. They can be asymptomatic or result in intussusception. The imaging workup should start with ultrasound, which reveals the characteristic bowel wall signature, echogenic inner mucosal layer, hypoechoic muscular layer, and echogenic outer serosal layer. When a duplication cyst communicates with the bowel lumen, air or bowel content can be seen in the cysts, as demonstrated in this case. Treatment involves surgical resection.

### Reference

Tong SC, Pitman M, Anupindi SA. Best cases from the AFIP. Ileocecal enteric duplication cyst: radiologic-pathologic correlation. *Radiographics*. 2002;22(5):1217–1222.

### Cross-reference

Walters MM, Robertson RL. *Pediatric Radiology: The Requisites*. 4th ed. Philadelphia: Elsevier; 2017:113–114.

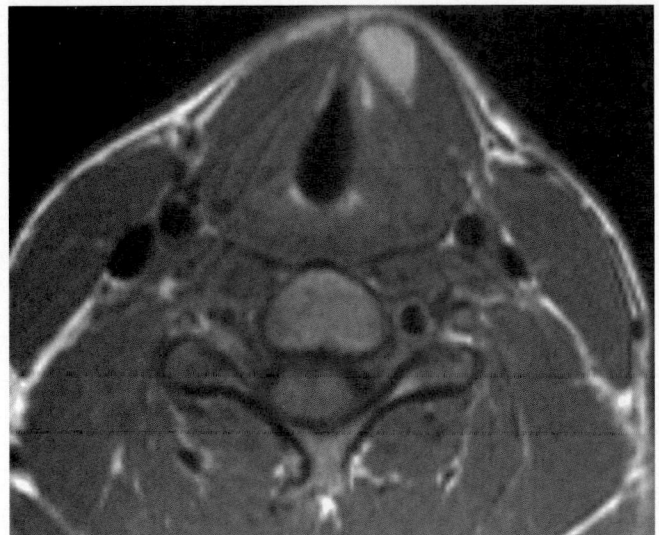

**Fig. 54.1**

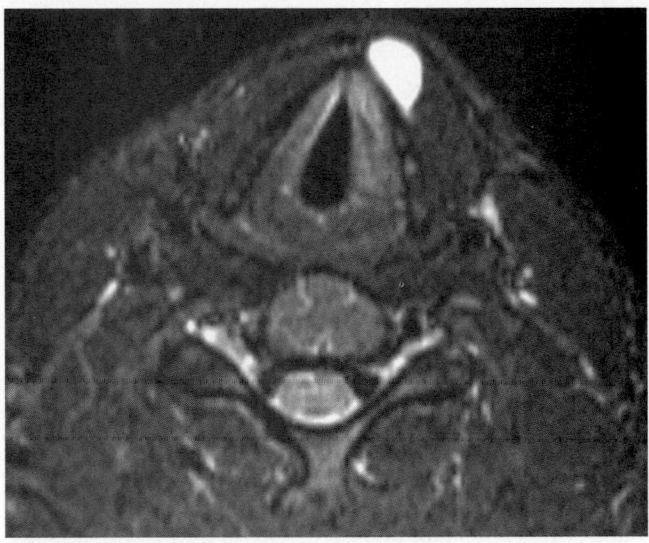

**Fig. 54.2**

**HISTORY:** 17-year-old female presenting with paramedian, compressible, painless neck mass

1. Which of the following should be included in the differential diagnosis for this lesion? (Choose all that apply.)
   A. Dermoid/epidermoid
   B. Thyroglossal duct cyst
   C. Suppurative lymph node
   D. Lymphatic malformation

2. Which feature is most specific for thyroglossal duct cysts?
   A. Embedded in the strap musculature
   B. T1 hyperintensity
   C. Location at the level of the hyoid bone
   D. Midline location

3. Which statement about thyroglossal duct cysts is *not* true?
   A. They are located at the midline above the hyoid bone and at the midline or paramidline below the hyoid bone.
   B. They may be associated with an ectopic thyroid.
   C. They can occur anywhere from the foramen cecum to the native thyroid gland location.
   D. Because they are benign, treatment is conservative with observation.

4. What is the name of the surgical procedure used to remove thyroglossal duct cysts?
   A. Sistrunk procedure
   B. Caldwell-Luc procedure
   C. Darrach procedure
   D. Frey procedure

## CASE 54

### Thyroglossal Duct Cyst

1. B, A, D

2. A

3. D

4. A

### *Comment*

In the infrahyoid neck, a cystic mass off midline embedded in the strap musculature is characteristic of a thyroglossal duct cyst. Most thyroglossal duct cysts present at the level of or below the hyoid bone. Above the hyoid, these lesions are typically at the midline. They can occur anywhere along the course of the thyroglossal duct, from the foramen cecum to the native thyroid gland location. Although these cysts are almost always benign, there is a small risk of cancer development (almost always papillary thyroid carcinoma). Treatment is surgical with the Sistrunk procedure, in which the cyst, tract to the foramen cecum, and midline portion of the hyoid may have to be removed. Before surgical removal, it is important to ascertain that the thyroid gland is orthotopic in location. Ectopic thyroid tissue may be located in the sublingual space in 10% of patients and at the base of the tongue (lingual thyroid) in 90% of patients. In 75% of patients, the ectopic tissue is the only functioning thyroid tissue. Neck ultrasound and nuclear scintigraphy may be helpful if ectopic thyroid tissue is suspected. On imaging, these are unilocular cysts, oftentimes diagnosed based on the location. Preferred imaging evaluation involves ultrasonography and magnetic resonance imaging (MRI). The echogenicity and signal characteristics may be variable depending on the degree of inflammation.

### Reference

Oomen KP, Modi VK, Maddalozzo J. Thyroglossal duct cyst and ectopic thyroid: surgical management. *Otolaryngol Clin N Am.* 2015;48(1):15–27.

### Cross-reference

Walters MM, Robertson RL. *Pediatric Radiology: The Requisites.* 4th ed. Philadelphia: Elsevier; 2017:370.

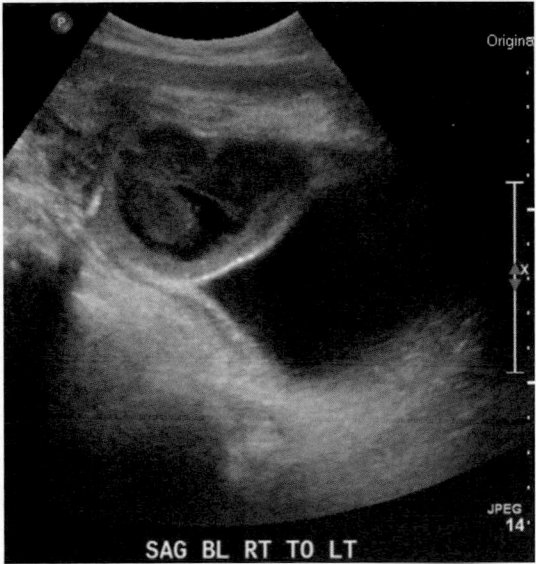

Fig. 55.1

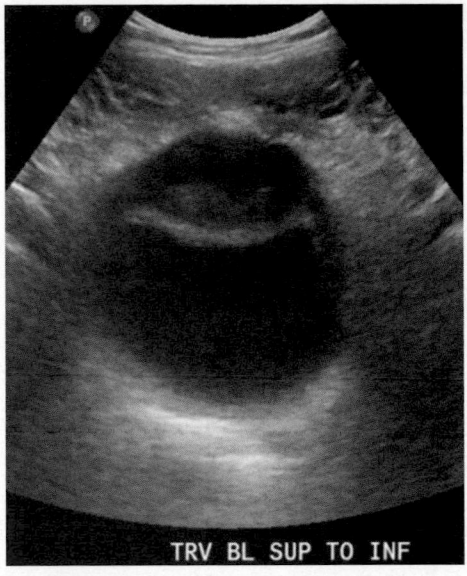

Fig. 55.2

**HISTORY:** 14-year-old male presenting with fever and periumbilical pain

1. What is the most likely diagnosis?
   A. Umbilical hernia
   B. Classic urinary tract infection with debris in the bladder
   C. Granulation tissue at the umbilical stump
   D. Urachal cyst, most likely infected

2. What is the most helpful diagnostic imaging clue for urachal cyst?
   A. Midline location between the dome of the bladder and the umbilicus
   B. Persistent and patent communication between the bladder and umbilicus
   C. Vascular solid mass attached to the naval
   D. None of the above

3. True or false?
   A. Developmental urachal abnormalities are more common in boys.
   B. Patent urachus is often diagnosed in late childhood to adolescence with irritative voiding system and fever as presented in this case.

4. What is the best diagnostic study for urachal abnormalities?
   A. Voiding cystourethrogram
   B. Plain radiography
   C. Ultrasonography
   D. A and C

## CASE 55

### Urachal Cyst

1. D

2. A

3. (A) True, (B) False

4. D

### Comment

Congenital urachal abnormalities encompass persistence of all or a portion of the connection between the dome of the bladder and the umbilicus, which is a remnant of the allantoic stalk. The spectrum of urachal abnormalities includes patent urachus (or urachal fistula), which represents an open channel from the bladder to the umbilicus; a urachal sinus, which represents persistence of the superficial segment of the channel opening to the skin surface (but sealed off on the bladder dome); a urachal diverticulum, which represents the persistence of the deep segment of the urachal channel creating a point or diverticulum off the anterosuperior segment of the bladder dome; and a urachal cyst, which represents the persistence of the intermediary segment connecting to the umbilicus and bladder dome with fibrous attachments. The presented case is a urachal cyst that demonstrates increased wall thickness and internal debris, secondary to infectious changes. Voiding cystourethrogram is best in demonstrating the patency of the urachus; however, infectious inflammatory changes can block the passage of contrast.

Patent urachus is diagnosed early on in neonates with leakage of urine from the umbilicus. A urachal diverticulum can remain silent, and urachal cysts are usually diagnosed in late childhood to adolescence, as seen in this case. To optimize ultrasonography, a relatively full bladder is helpful. Associations with omphalocele, cloacal anomalies, urogenital sinus malformation, meningomyelocele, kidney anomalies, and vaginal atresia have been reported. A urachal channel may remain patent as a response to bladder outlet obstruction, which resolves after treatment for obstruction. Surgical treatment should involve resection of the entire tract. Prognosis is excellent after resection. Risk of malignancy is considered if not resected, and the most common histopathologic types are adenocarcinoma, mucinous cystadenocarcinoma, and villous adenocarcinoma, which typically present in men 40 to 70 years of age.

### Reference

Yu JS, Kim KW, Lee HJ, Lee YJ, Yoon CS, Kim MJ. Urachal remnant diseases: spectrum of CT and US findings. *Radiographics*. 2001;21(2):451–461.

### Cross-reference

Walters MM, Robertson RL. *Pediatric Radiology: The Requisites*. 4th ed. Philadelphia: Elsevier; 2017:154.

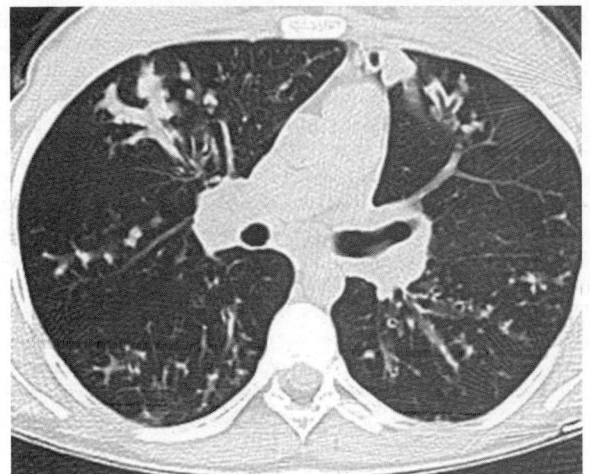

Fig. 56.1

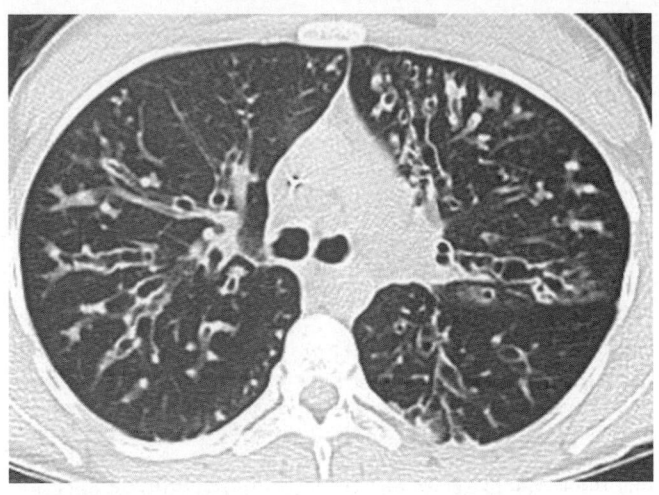

Fig. 56.2

**HISTORY:** 16-year-old presenting with cough

1. Given the imaging findings, which of the following would you include in your differential diagnosis? (Choose all that apply.)
   A. Allergic bronchopulmonary aspergillosis (ABPA)
   B. Cystic fibrosis (CF)
   C. Tuberculosis (TB)
   D. Sarcoidosis

2. What is typically the first lobe to be affected in CF?
   A. Left lower lobe
   B. Right upper lobe
   C. Right lower lobe
   D. Left upper lobe

3. Which option is *not* a common finding in patients with CF?
   A. Pancreatic insufficiency
   B. Meconium ileus in the newborn
   C. Dural venous thromboses
   D. Small opacified paranasal sinuses

4. Which finding on CT is the most specific in the setting of an acute exacerbation of CF?
   A. Mucous plugging
   B. Peribronchial thickening
   C. Air-fluid levels
   D. Centrilobular nodules

## CASE 56

### Cystic Fibrosis

1. A, B, C
2. B
3. C
4. C

### Comment

Cystic fibrosis (CF) is an inherited autosomal recessive disorder caused by defects in the gene for cystic fibrosis transmembrane conductance regulator (CFTR) located on the long arm of chromosome 17, resulting in abnormal chloride transport across cell membranes. Ultimately, this results in abnormal thick mucus secretions, predisposing to chronic infection and inflammation. In the lungs, this initially manifests on plain radiographs as an increase in lung volumes due to obstruction of small airways. Impaction of mucus in small airways results in small nodular or reticular opacities in the periphery of the lungs. More centrally, one may see linear opacities due to bronchial wall thickening or bronchiectasis. The earliest affected lobe is the right upper lobe. In older children and adults, more advanced findings include central mucoid impaction ("finger in glove" appearance), cysts and ring shadows in the upper lungs (from bronchiectasis, healed abscesses, or bullae), atelectasis, and hilar enlargement from adenopathy and/or pulmonary artery enlargement. On computed tomography (CT), early findings include tree-in-bud opacities and bronchial wall thickening (especially initially the right upper lobe bronchus), as well as mosaic perfusion and air trapping on expiratory views. Upper lobe predominance is due to the greater excursion of the lower lobes, which assists in clearing of airway secretions. Air-fluid levels are the most specific finding for an acute exacerbation. Allergic bronchopulmonary aspergillosis (ABPA) can develop in 10% of patients with CF. Tuberculosis (TB) may present with upper lobe–predominant bronchiectasis, consolidations, and cavities. In the absence of any other clinical information, TB should be ruled out. Sarcoidosis typically presents in patients in the third or fourth decade of life, and bronchiectasis is typically not a dominant finding.

### Reference

Shah RM, Sexauer W, Ostrum BJ, Fiel SB, Friedman AC. High-resolution CT in the acute exacerbation of cystic fibrosis: evaluation of acute findings, reversibility of those findings, and clinical correlation. *AJR Am J Roentgenol.* 1997;169:375–380.

### Cross-reference

Walters MM, Robertson RL. *Pediatric Radiology: The Requisites.* 4th ed. Philadelphia: Elsevier; 2017:40–41.

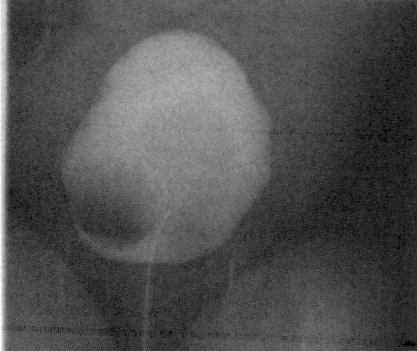

Fig. 57.1

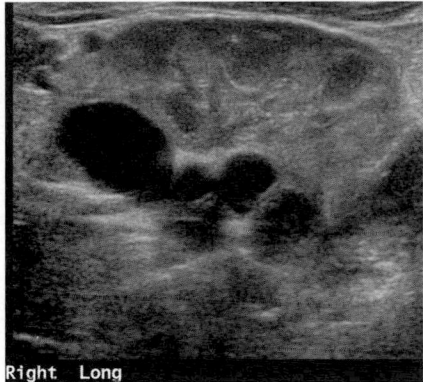

Fig. 57.2

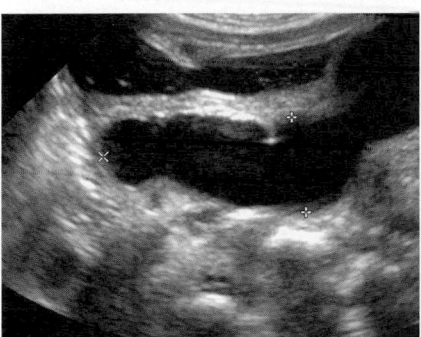

Fig. 57.3

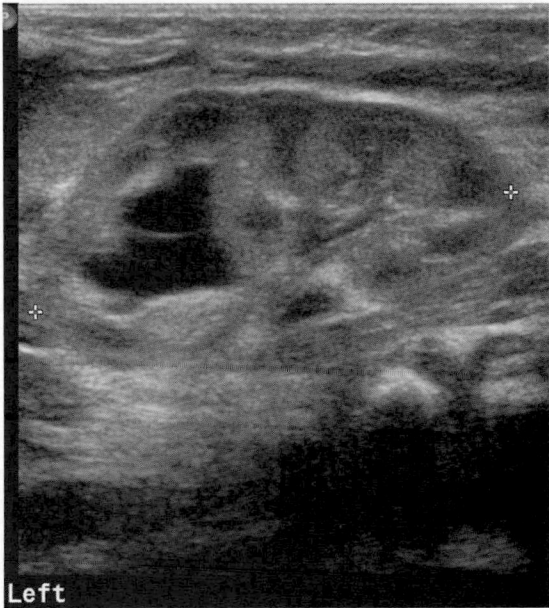

Fig. 57.4

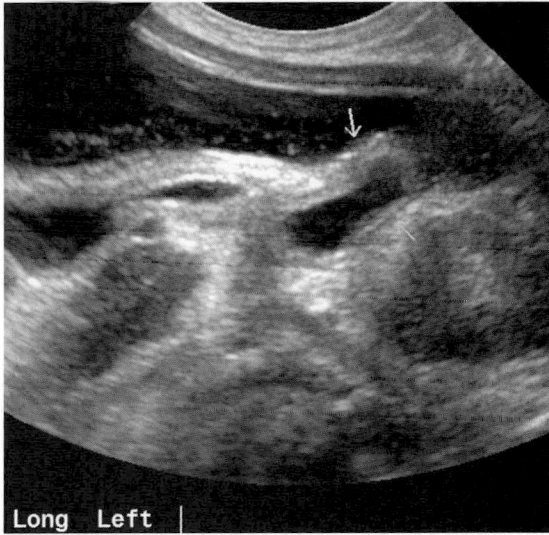

Fig. 57.5

**HISTORY:** Urinary tract infection in a 9-month-old baby girl

1. What is the most likely diagnosis?
   A. Rhabdomyosarcoma
   B. Ureterocele
   C. Mass effect on the bladder from the adjacent colon
   D. Hutch diverticulum

2. True or false?
   A. Ureteroceles can be seen with a single collecting system or in partial duplex systems.
   B. Ureteroceles can be intravesical or extravesical.

3. Which imaging recommendation is best in children with a suspected ureterocele?
   A. Although it may require anesthesia, magnetic resonance (MR) imaging provides the best anatomical detail, and thus the best diagnosis.
   B. Intravenous pyelogram (IVP) is the initial modality of choice.

C. Voiding cystourethrogram (VCUG) is the initial and best imaging modality.
D. Ultrasound is sufficient for diagnosis and has the advantage of avoiding radiation.

4. Which statement about ureteroceles is accurate?
   A. Ureteroceles are more likely to occur in complete duplication systems than in partial duplication systems.
   B. Females are more commonly affected than males.
   C. The ectopic, extravesical variety is more common than the orthotopic, intravesical variety.
   D. All of the above.

## Ureterocele

1. B

2. (A) False, (B) True

3. C

4. D

## *Comment*

A ureterocele is a congenital cystic dilation of the distal submucosal portion of the ureter. The ureterocele can be intravesical or partially extravesical extending into the urethra, bladder neck, or perineum. If the orifice of the ureterocele is located anywhere other than the bladder trigone, it is called an ectopic ureterocele. Duplex system ureteroceles are associated with complete duplication of the collecting system with two ureters. The Weigert-Meyer rule states that the ureter from the upper moiety of a duplicated kidney inserts inferomedially to the normal insertion site of the lower pole moiety. The upper pole moiety may be obstructed by the ureterocele and the lower pole moiety may have vesicoureteral reflux.

Ureteroceles may reflux, prolapse, or evert. A voiding cystourethrogram (VCUG) is the initial and best imaging modality. It is important to pay close attention to the bladder during the filling phase before intravesical pressure may compress the ureterocele. Females are more commonly affected than males (4 to 7:1) and the extravesical variety is more common than the simple intravesical variety. Prognosis is excellent if the ureterocele is nonobstructed and nonrefluxing.

This case shows bilateral ureteroceles, both partially extravesical. The VCUG shows two large filling defects representing the ureteroceles. On the ultrasound, note the asymmetrically smaller size of the left-sided ureterocele due to decompression. Dilation in the upper poles is secondary to obstruction.

### Reference

Berrocal T, López-Pereira P, Arjonilla A, Gutiérrez J. Anomalies of the distal ureter, bladder, and urethra in children: embryologic, radiologic, and pathologic features. *Radiographics*. 2002;22(5):1139–1164. [review].

### Cross-reference

Walters MM, Robertson RL. *Pediatric Radiology: The Requisites*. 4th ed. Philadelphia: Elsevier; 2017:144, 153.

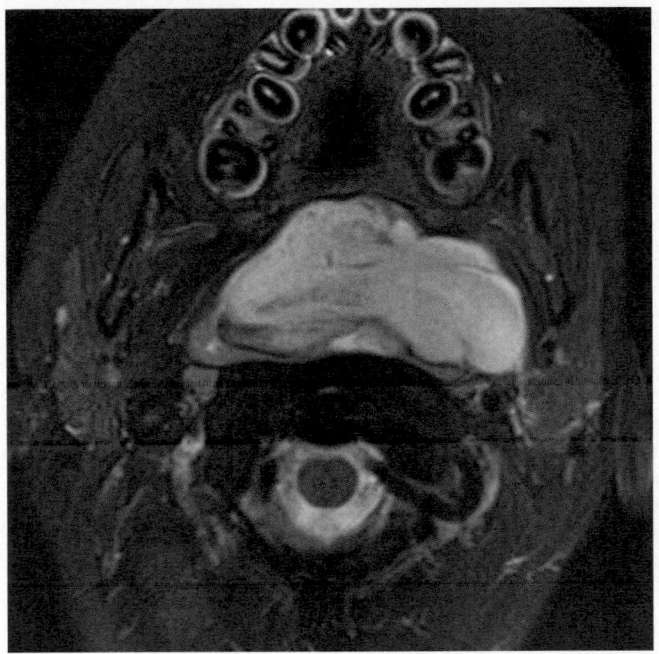

**Fig. 58.1**

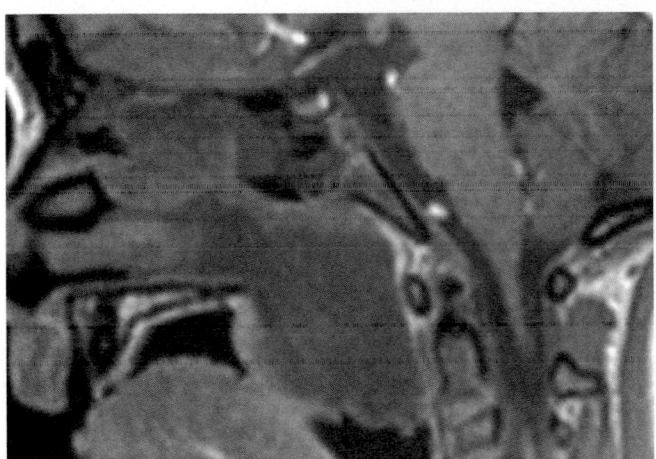

**Fig. 58.2**

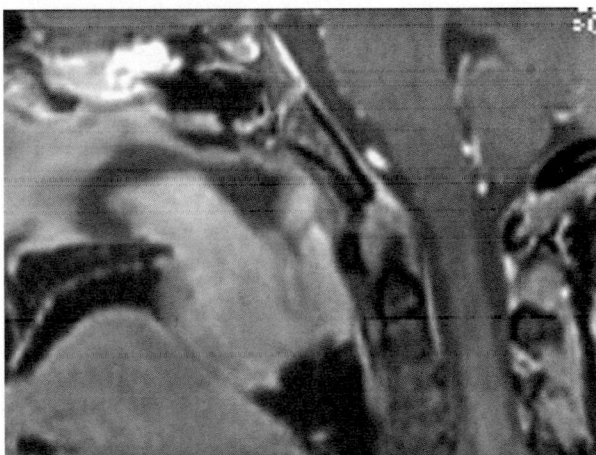

**Fig. 58.3**

**HISTORY:** 5-year-old boy presenting with progressive proptosis

1. Which of the following should be included in the differential diagnosis? (Choose all that apply.)
   A. Ewing sarcoma
   B. Rhabdomyosarcoma
   C. Venous malformation
   D. Lymphoma

2. In which anatomical region is rhabdomyosarcoma *least* common?
   A. Head and neck region
   B. Genitourinary tract
   C. Extremities
   D. Retroperitoneum

3. What is the age range for the peak incidence of rhabdomyosarcoma?
   A. 2 to 6 years
   B. 6 to 9 years
   C. 9 to 12 years
   D. 12 to 15 years

4. True or false, rhabdomyosarcoma is the most common soft tissue malignancy in children?

## CASE 58

### Rhabdomyosarcoma

1. A, B

2. D

3. A

4. True

## Comment

Rhabdomyosarcoma is the most common soft tissue malignancy in childhood. It can occur anywhere in the body, but does not arise primarily in bone. The most common sites are the head and neck (28%), extremities (24%), and genitourinary tract (18%). The major histologic subtypes are embryonal, botryoid (variant of embryonal), alveolar, and undifferentiated. The embryonal subtype is the most common and accounts for >50% of all rhabdomyosarcomas (as shown in this case), 70% to 90% of which occur in the head and neck or genitourinary regions. The botryoid variant arises in mucosal cavities such as the bladder, vagina, nasopharynx, and middle ear, is typically seen in children 2 to 6 years old, and has cysts filled with mucosanguinous fluid, giving it an appearance that has been compared to a bunch of grapes. Lesions in the extremities are most likely to have an alveolar type of histology, and these tend to occur in older children and young adults 15 to 25 years old.

Although ultrasound can be the first line of imaging, magnetic resonance imaging (MRI) is the modality of choice for lesion characterization. On T2-weighted imaging, these lesions typically appear as somewhat hyperintense to normal skeletal muscle and may show heterogeneous signals due to areas of hemorrhage and necrosis. Postcontrast enhancement is heterogeneous in most cases. There can be perilesional edema and enhancement. Treatment is with surgical debulking and adjuvant chemotherapy with or without radiation therapy.

### Reference

Stein-Wexler R. Pediatric soft tissue sarcomas. *Semin Ultrasound CT MR*. 2011;32(5):470–488.

### Cross-reference

Walters MM, Robertson RL. *Pediatric Radiology: The Requisites*. 4th ed. Philadelphia: Elsevier; 2017:166, 181, 241, 395, 396.

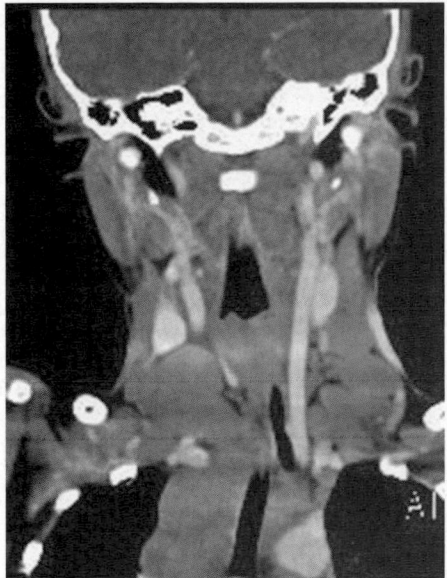

Fig. 59.1

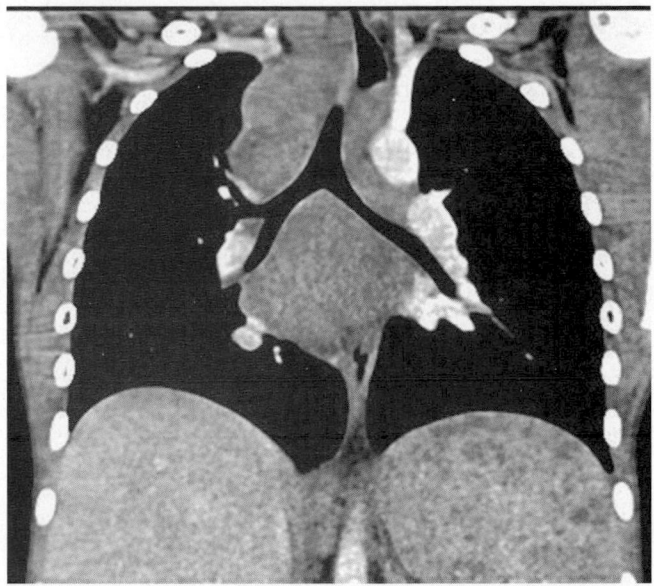

Fig. 59.2

**HISTORY:** Fatigue and night sweats.

1. What is your diagnosis in this teenage boy?
   A. Mediastinal teratoma
   B. Tuberculosis
   C. Thymoma
   D. Hodgkin lymphoma (HL)

2. What is the Ann Arbor staging for this patient with spleno-megaly and bone marrow disease documented on magnetic resonance imaging (MRI)?
   A. Stage I
   B. Stage II
   C. Stage III
   D. Stage IV

3. Which imaging modality offers the best diagnosis and stag-ing options for this patient?
   A. Contrast-enhanced MRI of the chest, abdomen, and pelvis
   B. Contrast-enhanced computed tomography (CT) of the chest
   C. Positron emission tomography-computed tomography (PET-CT) of the chest, abdomen, and pelvis
   D. Chest radiography

4. Which statement about HL is *not* true?
   A. It is associated with Epstein-Barr virus (EBV) in 90% of the cases.
   B. In cases with mediastinal lymphadenopathy, 50% reduc-tion in diameter trachea associated with respiratory fail-ure during induction of anesthesia.
   C. The 5-year survival exceeds 90%.
   D. Reed-Sternberg cells are pathognomonic for classic type HL.

## CASE 59

### Hodgkin Lymphoma

1. D
2. D
3. C
4. A

### Comment

Lymphoma is the third most common malignancy in children. The anterior mediastinum is the most common location for Hodgkin lymphoma (HL) and non-Hodgkin lymphoma. The World Health Organization (WHO) classifies HL as classic (90% to 95% of all HL) (nodular sclerosis 75%; mixed cellularity, lymphocyte rich, and lymphocyte depleted), and nodular lymphocyte-predominant HL. In classic HL, Reed-Sternberg cells are the pathologic hallmark. Approximately 50% of HL cases are associated with Epstein-Barr virus (EBV). HL is most commonly seen between 15 and 35 years of age, with a second peak after 55 years of age. HL is most commonly staged using the Ann Arbor classification. Stage I involves a single lymph node group, Stage II involves two lymph node groups on the same side of the diaphragm, Stage III includes nodes on both sides of the diaphragm, and Stage IV involves extranodal sites. In addition, the presence or absence of constitutional symptoms is designated as Stage A, asymptomatic, and Stage B, symptomatic with (20%) fever, night sweats, and >10% weight loss. More than 50% of the cases present with respiratory symptoms. Computed tomography (CT) shows a large, nodular, lobulated neck and anterior mediastinal mass (75% of the cases) with irregular borders and heterogeneous enhancement. Other sites of involvement are the hila, lungs (5% to 15%), pleura, and pericardium in the chest. Lymphoma distorts, displaces, and compresses adjacent structures. Calcifications are rare in untreated disease. Positron emission tomography with CT (PET-CT) has the highest sensitivity (96.5%) and specificity (100%) for diagnosis and follow-up. Active disease typically demonstrates increased radiolabeled [18F]-2-fluoro-2-deoxy-D-glucose (FDG) uptake. Differential diagnosis includes germ cell tumors (which would demonstrate the presence of fat, calcification, and mixed solid/cystic changes) or thymoma (rare in children, may show calcification). Survival has improved over time with 5-year survival now reaching 91%.

### Reference

Mauz-Körholz C, Metzger ML, Kelly KM, et al. Pediatric Hodgkin lymphoma. *J Clin Oncol.* 2015;33(27):2975–2985.

### Cross-reference

Walters MM, Robertson RL. *Pediatric Radiology: The Requisites.* 4th ed. Philadelphia: Elsevier; 2017:43.

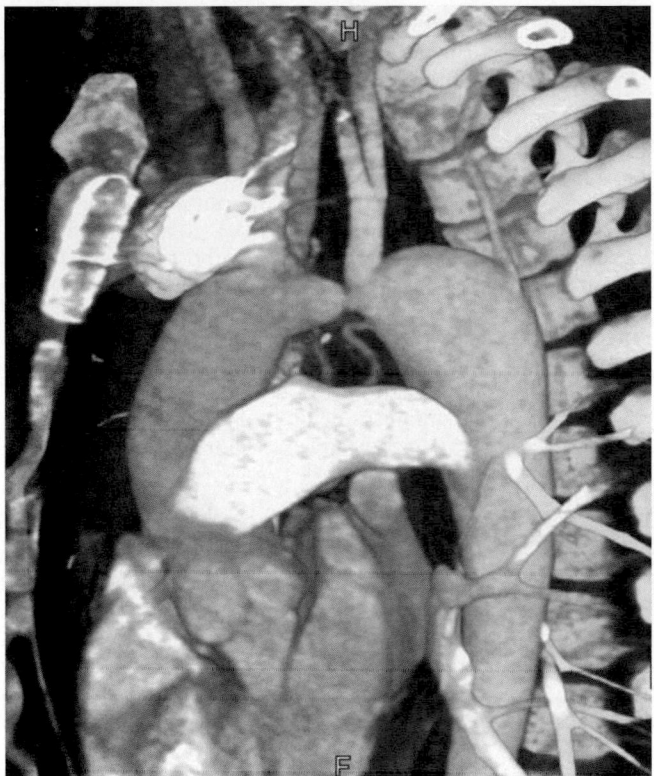

Fig. 60.1

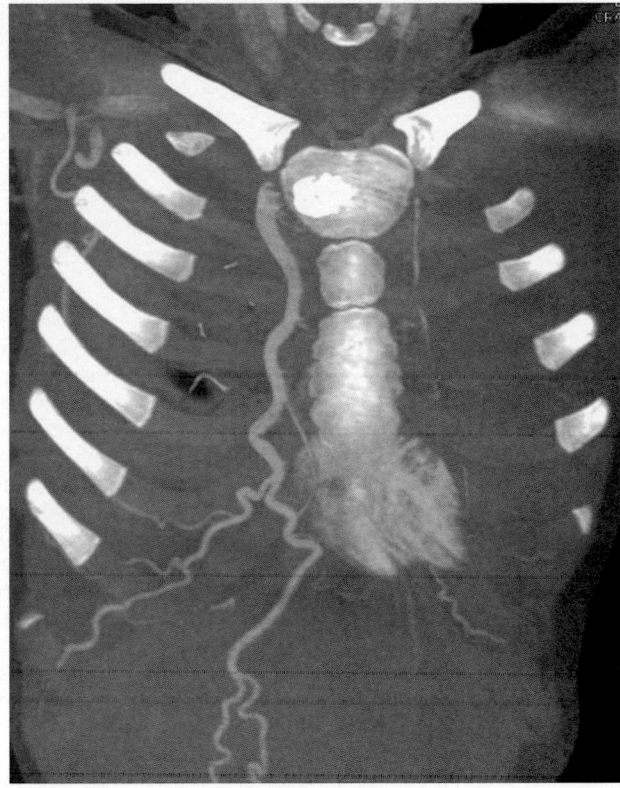

Fig. 60.2

**HISTORY:** 12-year-old boy with decreased left upper and lower extremity pulses

1. Based on the imaging findings, which option(s) would you include in your differential diagnosis? (Choose all that apply.)
   A. Aneurysm of the descending thoracic aorta
   B. Coarctation of the aorta
   C. Pseudoaneurysm of the aorta
   D. Pseudocoarctation

2. What is the most common cardiac anomaly associated with coarctation of the aorta?
   A. Atrial septal defect
   B. Bicuspid aortic valve
   C. Patent ductus arteriosus
   D. Ventricular septal defect

3. Infants with symptomatic coarctation are most likely to present with which of the following?
   A. Cyanosis
   B. Intracranial hemorrhage
   C. Heart failure
   D. Subclavian steal

4. Which statement regarding coarctation of the aorta is *not* true?
   A. Treatment in infants usually involves surgical correction.
   B. Treatment in children and young adults is typically with balloon angioplasty and then stenting in the setting of recoarctation.
   C. Rib notching can be seen in children and young adults and is due to collateral antegrade flow through intercostal arteries.
   D. The figure of three sign is a classic associated radiographic finding.

## CASE 60

### Coarctation of the Aorta

1. B
2. B
3. C
4. C

### Comment

Coarctation of the aorta represents a congenital narrowing of the aorta and can be classified in relation to the ductus arteriosus: preductal, ductal, and postductal types. Age at presentation is related to the degree of narrowing and the presence or absence of associated abnormalities. Simple coarctation is most commonly localized just beyond the origin of the left subclavian artery (postductal) and can present in children and young adults with leg claudication, hypertension, and its sequelae including intracranial aneurysms and chronic heart failure. Complex coarctation occurs in the presence of other intracardiac anomalies, tends to manifest in infancy, and is often preductal in location. It typically presents with acyanotic heart failure, similar to other causes of anatomical left-sided obstruction, including aortic stenosis, hypoplastic left heart, mitral stenosis, cor triatriatum, and pulmonary venous atresia. Unlike coarctation, pseudocoarctation presents in older individuals with elongation and kinking of the aorta without hemodynamically significant stenosis or collateral formation. Bicuspid aortic valve is the most common cardiac anomaly associated with aortic coarctation (>50%). Turner and Shone syndromes have a high association with coarctation of the aorta. Shone syndrome is comprised of four left-sided defects: aortic coarctation, subaortic stenosis, parachute mitral valve, and supravalvular mitral membrane. Treatment in infants is typically with surgical repair. In older children and young adults, treatment is commonly first with balloon angioplasty and stenting is reserved for recoarctation. The most common collateral arterial pathway is through the subclavian to the internal mammary arteries and then to the intercostal arteries (see second image provided in this case), which feed the poststenotic descending thoracic aorta via retrograde flow and may result in inferior rib notching. Magnetic resonance imaging (MRI) is useful in presurgical planning and can be used to assess pressure gradients across the stenosis and the degree of collateral flow in the descending thoracic aorta.

### References

Karaosmanoglu AD, Khawaja RD, Onur MR, Kalra MK. CT and MRI of aortic coarctation: pre- and postsurgical findings. *AJR Am J Roentgenol*. 2015;204(3):W224–W233.

Singh S, Hakim FA, Sharma A, et al. Hypoplasia, pseudocoarctation and coarctation of the aorta—a systematic review. *Heart Lung Circ*. 2015;24(2):110–118.

### Cross-reference

Walters MM, Robertson RL. *Pediatric Radiology: The Requisites*. 4th ed. Philadelphia: Elsevier; 2017:82–83.

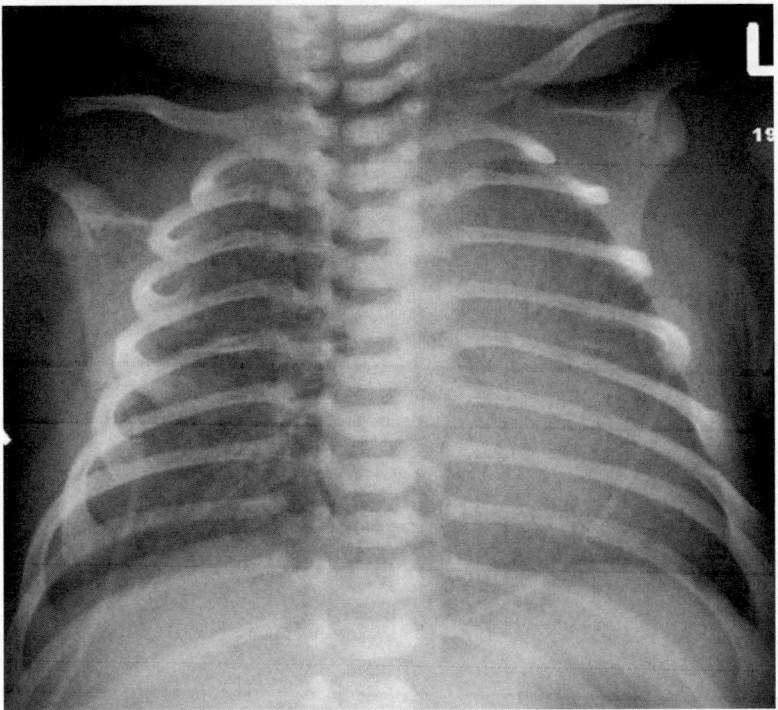

**Fig. 61.1**

**HISTORY:** Newborn full-term infant presenting with respiratory distress

1. Which of the following should be included in the differential diagnosis? (Choose all that apply.)
   A. Meconium aspiration
   B. Transient tachypnea of the newborn (TTN)
   C. Neonatal pneumonia
   D. Congenital heart disease

2. The imaging appearance in TTN is best explained by which of the following?
   A. Pulmonary venous congestion
   B. Retained fetal lung fluid
   C. Surfactant deficiency
   D. Shunt vascularity

3. Which statement about TTN is *not* correct?
   A. TTN is more common in infants born by cesarean section.
   B. TTN has a benign course and treatment is conservative.
   C. Respiratory symptoms peak after 2 to 3 days and are resolved within 1 week.
   D. TTN is more common in a setting of maternal diabetes, maternal sedation, and prolonged labor.

4. True or false?
   A. TTN is most common in premature infants.

## CASE 61

### Transient Tachypnea of the Newborn

1. A, B, C
2. B
3. C
4. False

### Comment

TTN, also known as wet lung disease, is caused by retention of fetal lung fluid after birth. Patients typically present with tachypnea and little to no oxygen requirement. Symptoms peak during day 1 and usually resolve within 2 to 3 days. TTN is a diagnosis of exclusion, and the main differential diagnoses that must be considered are meconium aspiration and neonatal infection. It is typically seen in full-term infants born via cesarean section, and it is believed that this mode of delivery prevents the usual physiologic external compression of the thorax that promotes clearing of fetal lung fluid during vaginal delivery. Additional risk factors include maternal diabetes, maternal sedation, and prolonged labor. The imaging appearance is that of fetal pulmonary edema related to the retained fetal lung fluid, and can range from mild to severe. Findings include pleural effusions, fluid in the fissures, septal interstitial markings, airspace opacities, and prominent but indistinct pulmonary vasculature.

### Reference

Pramanik AK, Rangaswamy N, Gates T. Neonatal respiratory distress: a practical approach to its diagnosis and management. *Pediatr Clin N Am.* 2015;62(2):453–469.

### Cross-reference

Walters MM, Robertson RL. *Pediatric Radiology: The Requisites.* 4th ed. Philadelphia: Elsevier; 2017:56.

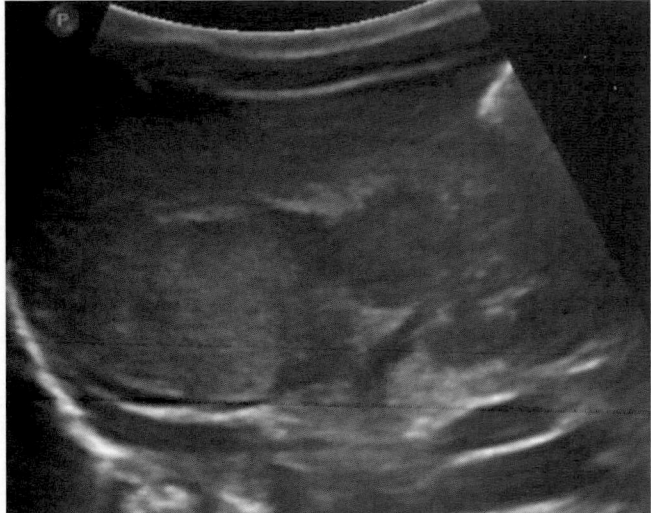

Fig. 62.1

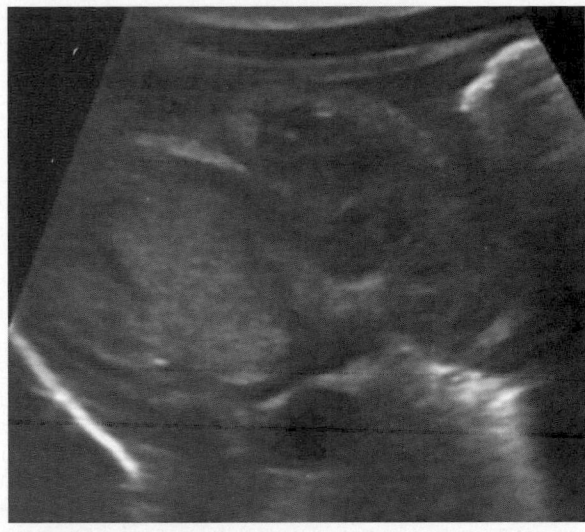

Fig. 62.2

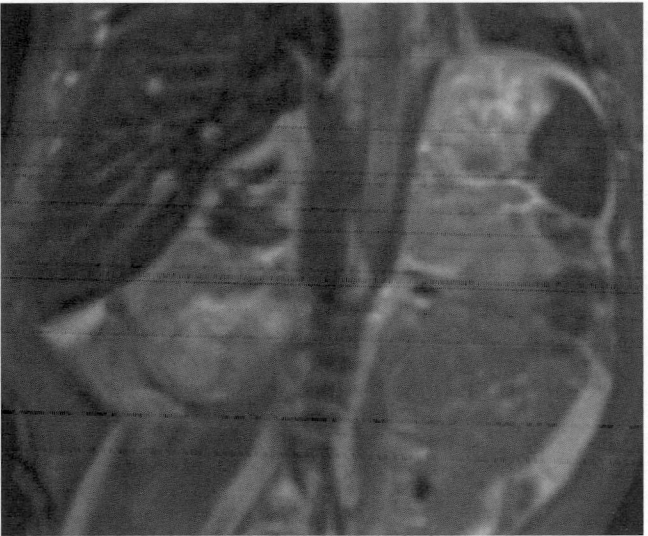

Fig. 62.3

**HISTORY:** Newborn ordered an abdominal ultrasound for history of prenatal mild hydronephrosis.

1. What is the most likely diagnosis in this newborn infant?
   A. Neuroblastoma
   B. Congenital adrenal hyperplasia
   C. Adrenal hemorrhage
   D. Subdiaphragmatic pulmonary sequestration

2. Which statement is accurate for this entity?
   A. It usually happens in full-term infants and babies who are large for their gestational age.
   B. Clinical presentation may include anemia, jaundice, or adrenal insufficiency, or the patient may be asymptomatic.
   C. Complications may involve cyst formation, calcification, and, rarely, fatal adrenal insufficiency.
   D. All of the above.

3. Which statement best describes the expected imaging findings in newborn adrenal hemorrhage?
   A. No internal blood flow is detected in Doppler ultrasonography (US).
   B. It is usually a well-circumscribed, heterogeneous mass with cystic components, although echogenicity of the mass would change depending on the stage.
   C. It involutes over time.
   D. All of the above.

4. Which option offers the best follow-up imaging option for this case?
   A. Magnetic resonance imaging (MRI) with contrast in 2 days to confirm diagnosis
   B. Computed tomography (CT) without contrast in 1 week
   C. US in 2 weeks
   D. Plain radiography in 3 days

## CASE 62

### Neonatal Adrenal Hemorrhage

1. C
2. D
3. D
4. C

### Comment

The exact incidence of this condition is unknown because neonatal adrenal hemorrhage can be asymptomatic. Most hemorrhages are believed to occur perinatally. Neonatal adrenal hemorrhage may be associated with perinatal stressors such as sepsis, asphyxia, birth trauma, or coagulopathies. Imaging findings reflect the stage of hemorrhage, with heterogeneous echogenicity and cystic changes seen in subacute to chronic stages. Early on, the hemorrhage may have a solid appearance as shown in this case. Ultrasonography (US) is the modality of choice to see the hemorrhage resolve. Presence of calcification on the initial US along with liver lesions would favor a neonatal neuroblastoma diagnosis. Systemic vessel feeding into the mass would favor a subdiaphragmatic pulmonary sequestration. Calcifications or cystic changes may be seen over time. In cases where an alternative diagnosis is suspected, magnetic resonance imaging (MRI) can be useful in assessing the presence of blood products, as shown in this case. Note the heterogeneous/decreased T2 signal of the hemorrhage in the right adrenal region. The kidney is displaced inferiorly due to mass effect.

### Reference

Gyurkovits Z, Maróti Á, Rénes L, Németh G, Pál A, Orvos H. Adrenal haemorrhage in term neonates: a retrospective study from the period 2001-2013. *J Matern Fetal Neonatal Med*. 2015;28(17):2062-2065.

### Cross-reference

Walters MM, Robertson RL. *Pediatric Radiology: The Requisites*. 4th ed. Philadelphia: Elsevier; 2017:171-172.

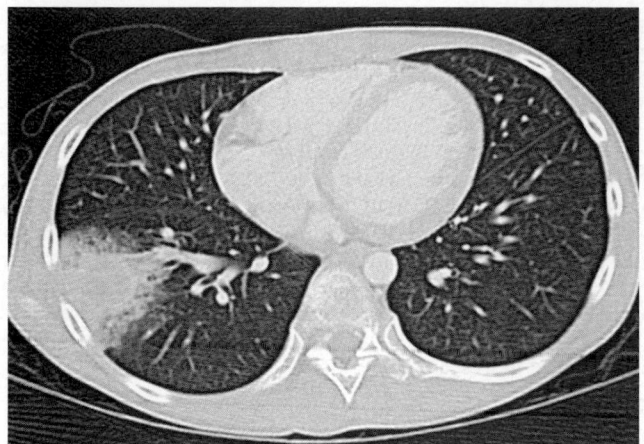

**Fig. 63.1**

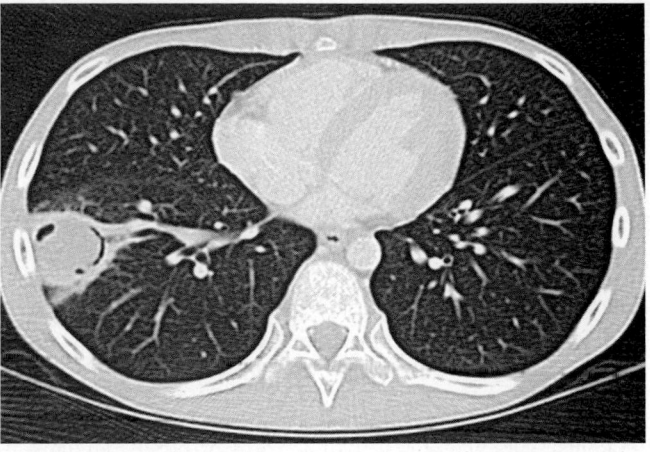

**Fig. 63.2**

**HISTORY:** 10-year-old female with aplastic anemia presenting with cough

1. Which of the following should be included in the differential diagnosis for the lesion seen on the second (right) computed tomography (CT) image? (Choose all that apply.)
   A. Invasive aspergillosis
   B. Mycetoma
   C. Echinococcus
   D. Kaposi sarcoma

2. What accounts for the imaging finding seen on the second CT image in the setting of invasive aspergillosis?
   A. Fistulous connection to the bronchial tree with air trapping related to a ball valve mechanism
   B. Cavitation with growth of a fungus ball
   C. Rupture between the outermost and inner layers of the fungal nodule with dissection of air between these layers.
   D. Lung necrosis with presence of a sequestrum of devitalized and necrotic lung occupying part of the cavity

3. What accounts for the imaging findings seen on the first CT image in the setting of invasive aspergillosis?
   A. Rim of hemorrhage surrounding a central fungal nodule
   B. Rim of edema surrounding a central fungal nodule
   C. Rim of fungal hyphae surrounding a central fungal nodule
   D. Rim of pus surrounding a central fungal nodule

4. True or false?
   A. The presence of the air crescent sign in the setting of angioinvasive aspergillosis indicates progression of disease.

## CASE 63

### Fungal Pneumonia

1. A, B, C

2. D

3. A

4. False

## Comment

Invasive aspergillosis is one of many infections to be on the lookout for in patients that are severely immunocompromised. Clinical scenarios that can lead to such an immunocompromised state include neutropenia in patients with acute leukemia, patients treated with steroids or other immunosuppressive agents (e.g., after organ transplant), and patients with malignancy. Other common infectious etiologies one might encounter in these patients include other fungal (e.g., mucormycosis) and mycobacterial infections, *Pneumocystis jiroveci* pneumonia (PCP), and viral pneumonia. Invasive aspergillosis is characterized by a nodule or nodules that, early on, show a rim of ground glass density that is due to a rim of hemorrhage secondary to invasion of fungal hyphae into capillaries. After about 2 weeks, nodules cavitate with formation of an air crescent sign, which is due to lung necrosis with the presence of a sequestrum or ball of necrotic lung occupying part of the cavity. Notably, cavitation in these patients is considered a good prognostic sign, because it is typically seen in patients with rising neutrophil counts. Other causes of the air crescent sign, whose clinical presentations are different, include mycetoma (fungus ball), seen in immunocompetent patients, and hydatid disease, seen in patients after ingestion of eggs of the echinococcal tape worm.

### Reference

Ketai L, Jordan K, Busby KH. Imaging infection. *Clin Chest Med*. 2015;36(2):197–217.

### Cross-reference

Walters MM, Robertson RL. *Pediatric Radiology: The Requisites*. 4th ed. Philadelphia: Elsevier; 2017:38–39.

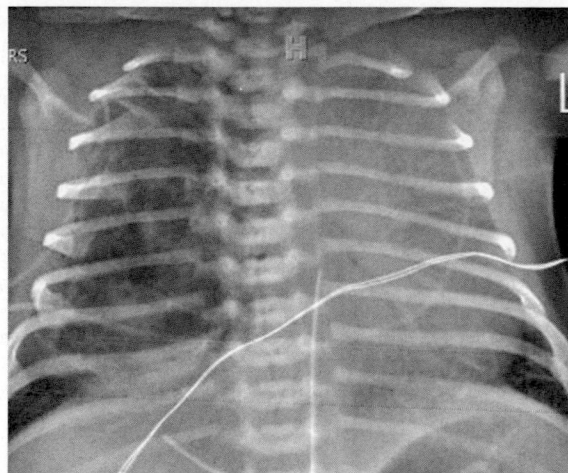

Fig. 64.1

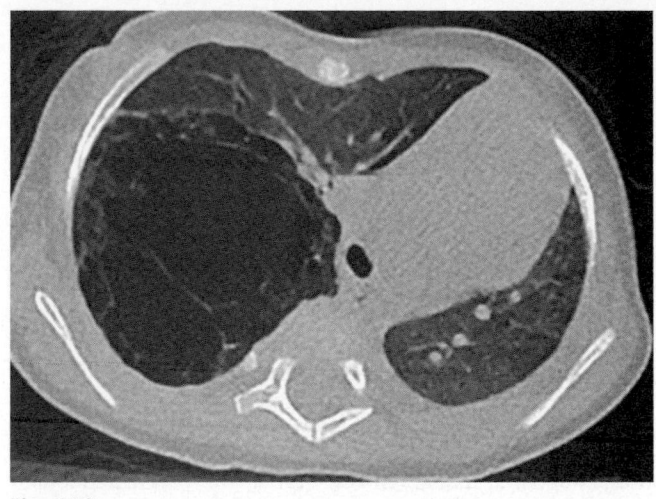

Fig. 64.2

**HISTORY:** Follow-up for prenatal diagnosis of lung mass

1. Based on the imaging findings, which of the following is most likely?
   A. Congenital pulmonary airway malformation (CPAM)
   B. Pulmonary sequestration
   C. Congenital diaphragmatic hernia
   D. Pleuropulmonary blastoma

2. Which CPAM subtype has a high association with other congenital abnormalities?
   A. Type 0
   B. Type 1
   C. Type 2
   D. Type 3

3. Which statement about CPAM is *not* true?
   A. It is often asymptomatic in the newborn period.
   B. It may show regression over time.
   C. It is most commonly found in the left lower lobe.
   D. Type 1 and type 4 CPAM present with large cysts and are difficult to reliably distinguish from type I pleuropulmonary blastoma.

4. True or false?
   A. The presence of a systemic arterial supply excludes the presence of CPAM.

## CASE 64

### Congenital Pulmonary Airway Malformation

1. A
2. C
3. C
4. False

## Comment

Congenital pulmonary airway malformation (CPAM) represents a heterogeneous group of cystic and noncystic lung lesions resulting from early airway maldevelopment. It is typically diagnosed on prenatal ultrasound as a lung mass and thus has a broad differential, including pulmonary sequestration, congenital diaphragmatic hernia, and pleuropulmonary blastoma. Type 2 CPAM (presence of numerous small cysts ranging in size between 0.5 and 1.5 cm) is associated with other congenital anomalies (renal, skeletal, intestinal, cardiac, other lung lesions) in about 50% of cases, which should be actively searched for. Type 1 and type 4 CPAM present with larger cysts and may not be reliably distinguished from one another or from type I pleuropulmonary blastoma by imaging. Type 3 CPAM has microcysts and appears almost solid by imaging. CPAM is often asymptomatic in the newborn period and may show regression over time. There is no lobar predilection. It sometimes presents in mixed form with pulmonary sequestration and thus can demonstrate the presence of a systemic arterial supply. Unlike in the setting of pulmonary sequestration, cysts in CPAM often contain air. Workup typically includes computed tomography angiography (CTA) to delineate the type of cysts (large, small, micro/solid) and presence/absence of arterial supply. Treatment of symptomatic CPAM involves surgical resection. Treatment in asymptomatic cases is more controversial, but surgery is sometimes advocated given the risk for infection and very low risk of malignancy.

### Reference

Fowler DJ, Gould SJ. The pathology of congenital lung lesions. *Semin Pediatr Surg.* 2015;24(4):176–182.

### Cross-reference

Walters MM, Robertson RL. *Pediatric Radiology: The Requisites.* 4th ed. Philadelphia: Elsevier; 2017:29–32.

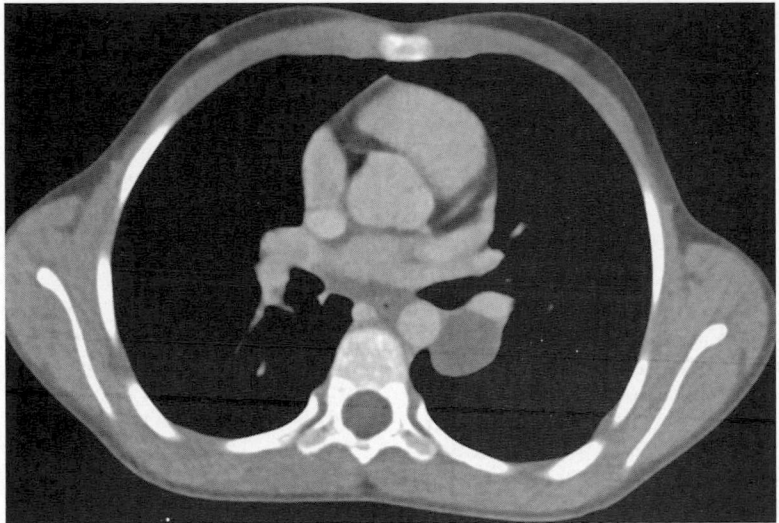

**Fig. 65.1**

**HISTORY:** 7-year-old presenting with chest pain

1. Given the imaging findings on the plain film, which of the following would you include in your differential diagnosis? (Choose all that apply.)
   A. Congenital pulmonary airway malformation (CPAM)
   B. Pulmonary sequestration
   C. Bronchogenic cyst
   D. Round pneumonia

2. What is the most common location of bronchogenic cysts?
   A. Pericardium
   B. Anterior mediastinum
   C. Middle mediastinum
   D. Medial one-third of the lung

3. The presence of air in a bronchogenic cyst may be normal in which of these locations?
   A. Neck
   B. Middle mediastinum
   C. Medial one-third of the lung
   D. Anterior mediastinum

4. Which statement about bronchogenic cysts is *not* true?
   A. They are almost always solitary.
   B. They are part of the family of foregut duplication cysts, which also includes pericardial cysts.
   C. They may compress the adjacent airway leading to downstream air trapping.
   D. Rare locations include the diaphragm, neck, and retroperitoneum.

### Bronchogenic Cyst

1. A, B, C, D
2. C
3. C
4. B

## Comment

Bronchogenic cysts are part of the family of foregut duplication cysts, which also includes enteric and neurenteric cysts (not pericardial cysts). On imaging, they appear as smooth, well-circumscribed, solid, dense masses and are most commonly found in the middle mediastinum (typically in the paratracheal, carinal, or hilar region), followed by the medial one-third of the lung parenchyma. Rarely, they are found in the diaphragm, neck, pericardium, or retroperitoneum. They are almost always solitary and typically do not communicate with the airway, and thus usually do not contain air. However, the parenchymal lesions are more likely to communicate with the airway than mediastinal lesions, and thus the presence of air in these lesions may be normal. In mediastinal bronchogenic cysts, the presence of air indicates infection. In the mediastinum, they may exert mass effect with compression of the adjacent airway or esophagus, resulting in air trapping or dysphagia, respectively. On cross-sectional imaging, they do not enhance centrally, but may have a thin and smooth enhancing rim. The presence of prominent wall enhancement suggests inflammation, and if the wall becomes thickened and irregular, concern for neoplasm should be raised. Principal differential considerations include congenital pulmonary airway malformation (CPAM), round pneumonia, and pulmonary sequestration. A CPAM commonly fills with air, is typically not unilocular, and does not involve the mediastinum. Patients with round pneumonia often present with fever, and imaging findings will resolve on follow-up evaluation. Pulmonary sequestration presents as an irregular enhancing mass and is a more heterogeneous mass than a bronchogenic cyst with a systemic arterial supply.

### Reference

Durell J, Lakhoo K. Congenital cystic lesions of the lung. *Early Hum Dev.* 2014;90(12):935–939.

### Cross-reference

Walters MM, Robertson RL. *Pediatric Radiology: The Requisites.* 4th ed. Philadelphia: Elsevier. 2017:28–30.

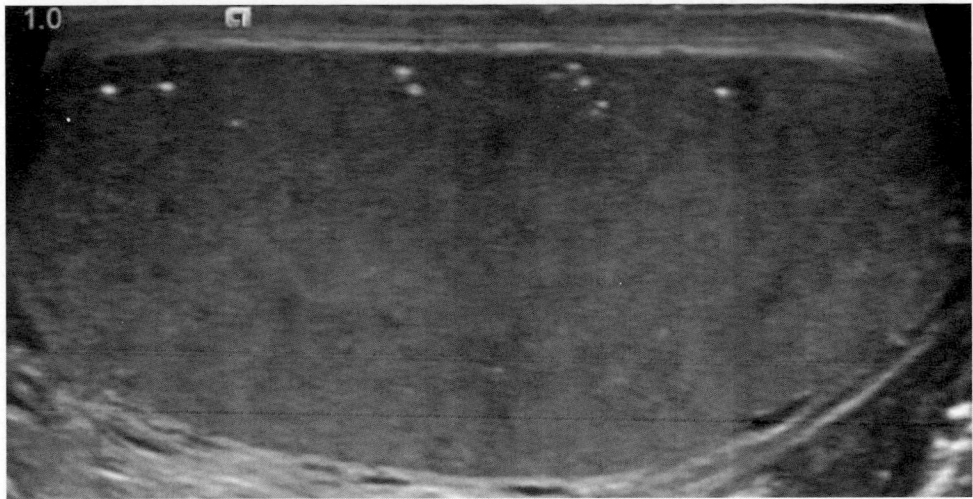

Fig. 66.1

**HISTORY:** 13-year-old male presenting with scrotal pain

1. Given the imaging findings, what is the best diagnosis?
   A. Multifocal germ cell tumor
   B. Microlithiasis
   C. Tuberculous orchitis
   D. Sarcoidosis

2. What is the standard definition of microlithiasis based on ultrasound findings?
   A. One to five echogenic foci per transducer field in one testicle
   B. Five or more echogenic foci per transducer field in one testicle
   C. 10 or more echogenic foci per transducer field in one testicle
   D. 20 or more echogenic foci per transducer field in one testicle

3. What is the approximate prevalence of microlithiasis in asymptomatic young males?
   A. About 1%
   B. About 12%
   C. About 5%
   D. About 8%

4. In an asymptomatic male with an incidental finding of microlithiasis on ultrasound, which option describes the best next course of action?
   A. Recommend referral for biopsy and/or testing for tumor markers (e.g., alpha-fetoprotein [AFP], human chorionic gonadotropin [hCG]).
   B. Recommend routine annual screening ultrasound.
   C. In the absence of any additional risk factors for developing germ cell tumors, recommend monthly scrotal self-examination only.
   D. Recommend further imaging with contrast-enhanced magnetic resonance imaging (MRI).

## CASE 66

### Testicular Microlithiasis

1. B
2. B
3. C
4. C

### Comment

Microlithiasis is typically defined as five or more nonshadowing discrete punctate echogenic foci per ultrasound transducer field in one testicle. About 5% of asymptomatic males between 17 and 35 have microlithiasis. Although the presence of microlithiasis confers an increased risk of developing a testicular germ cell tumor, the vast majority of patients with microlithiasis will not develop a testicular germ cell tumor. The presence of microlithiasis alone in the absence of other risk factors is therefore not an indication for regular scrotal ultrasound screening or biopsy. Risk factors include history of previous germ cell tumor, testicular maldescent, orchidopexy, testicular atrophy (<12 mL in volume), or history of germ cell tumor in a first-degree relative.

Annual screening ultrasound is advised for patients with microlithiasis and any of the previously described risk factors.

### Reference

Richenberg J, Belfield J, Ramchandani P, et al. Testicular microlithiasis imaging and follow-up: guidelines of the ESUR scrotal imaging subcommittee. *Eur Radiol*. 2015;25(2):323–330.

### Cross-reference

Walters MM, Robertson RL. *Pediatric Radiology: The Requisites*. 4th ed. Philadelphia: Elsevier; 2017:181.

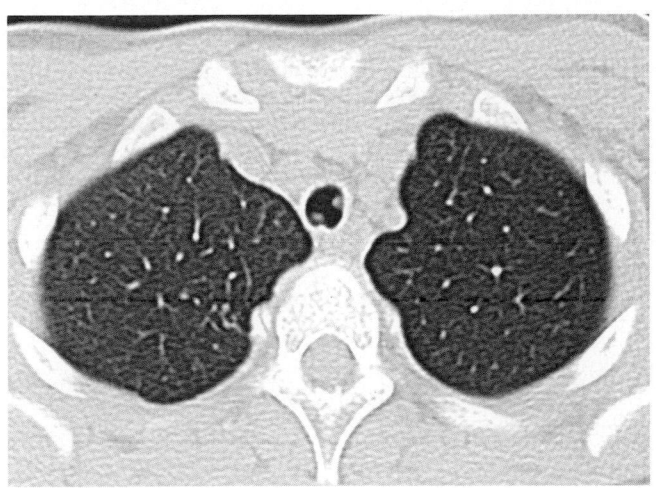

**Fig. 67.1**

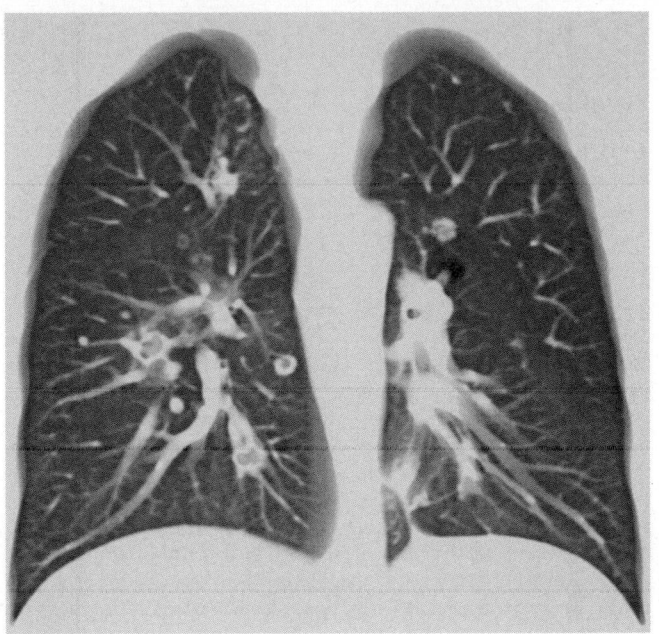

**Fig. 67.2**

**HISTORY:** 9-year-old girl presenting with cough

1. Based on the images provided, which of the following is the best diagnosis?
   A. Granulomatosis with polyangiitis (GPA; Wegener granulomatosis)
   B. Septic emboli
   C. Cavitary infection, e.g., tuberculosis (TB)
   D. Respiratory papillomatosis

2. What is the most common site involved by papillomatosis?
   A. Trachea
   B. Larynx
   C. Nasopharynx
   D. Peripheral airway/alveoli

3. What is the mean age at diagnosis in papillomatosis?
   A. Perinatal
   B. 4 years
   C. 10 years
   D. 14 years

4. True or false?
   A. Cavitary lung metastases are common in the pediatric age group.

## CASE 67

### Papillomatosis

1. D

2. B

3. B

4. False

### *Comment*

Papillomatosis is caused by infection with human papilloma virus (HPV) with development of benign tumors of the aerodigestive tract. Infection occurs through perinatal transmission of HPV from infected mother to child. Prolonged labor and vaginal delivery are risk factors. The most common site of infection is the larynx, and the mean age at presentation is 4 years. Patients typically present with hoarseness due to laryngeal involvement. Rarely, there is endotracheal spread to the lower trachea and central bronchi (11%), and even less commonly, there is spread to the peripheral airways and alveoli (3%). In the latter case, the imaging findings include multiple solid or cavitary lung nodules, as seen on the presented images. In addition, soft tissue nodules may be seen protruding into the airway lumen. Differential diagnosis for cavitary pulmonary lesions in a child include granulomatosis with polyangiitis (GPA), septic emboli, and cavitary infection (e.g., tuberculosis [TB]), but not metastatic disease, because cavitary lung metastases are very uncommon in the pediatric age group. Malignant degeneration of lung lesions to squamous cell carcinoma is a rare complication and presents with an enlarging heterogeneously enhancing lung mass and lymphadenopathy. In a child under 1 year of age presenting with a subglottic mass, the differential diagnosis should include infantile hemangioma in addition to papillomatosis.

### Reference

Shiau EL, Li MF, Hsu JH, Wu MT. Recurrent respiratory papillomatosis with lung involvement and malignant transformation. *Thorax*. 2014;69(3):302-303.

### Cross-reference

Walters MM, Robertson RL. *Pediatric Radiology: The Requisites*. 4th ed. Philadelphia: Elsevier; 2017:21-23.

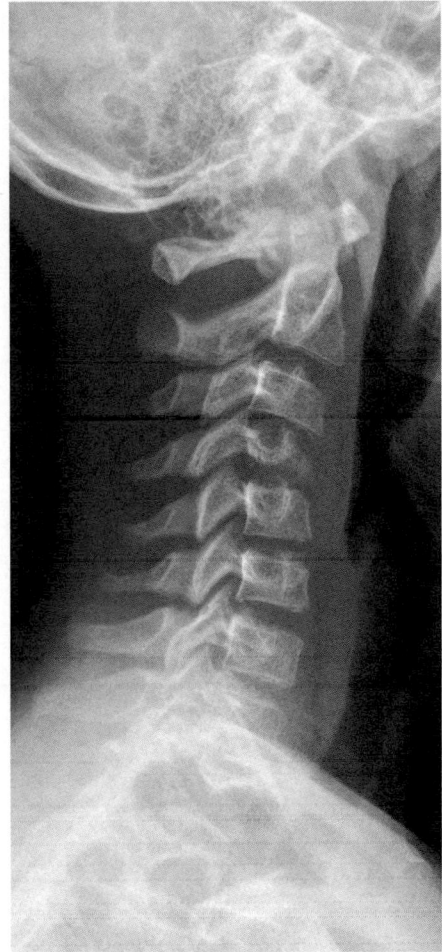

Fig. 68.1

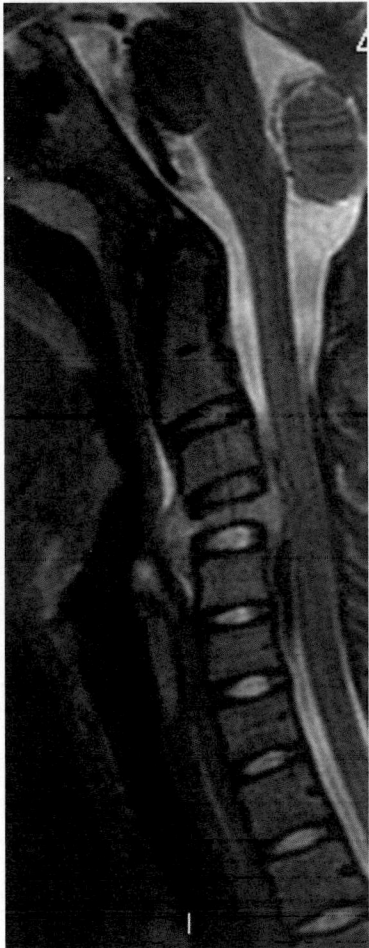

Fig. 68.2

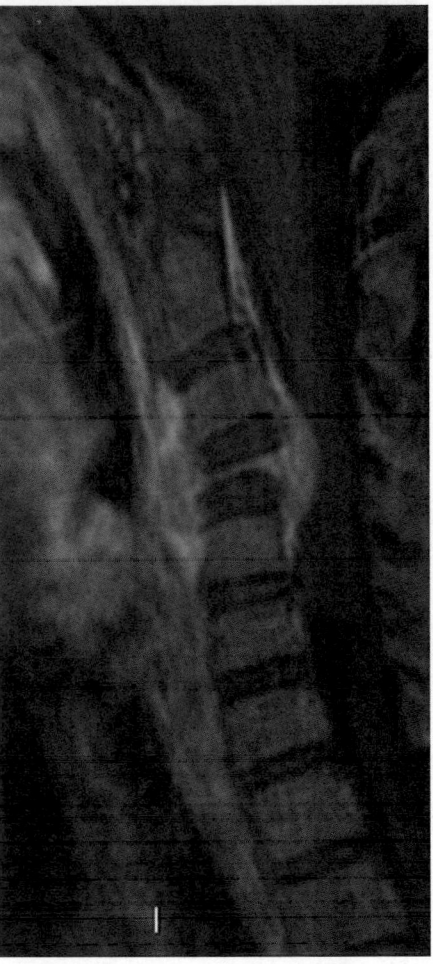

Fig. 68.3

**HISTORY:** Teenager presenting with neck pain after basketball tryouts

1. What is the most likely diagnosis?
   A. Compression fracture
   B. Osteomyelitis
   C. Langerhans cell histiocytosis
   D. Leukemia

2. What is the most likely imaging appearance in long-term follow-up?
   A. Vertebra plana
   B. Spontaneous complete recovery
   C. Short-term progression of disease in the entire spine
   D. None of the above

3. Which of the following is accurate regarding Langerhans cell histiocytosis?
   A. The best imaging tool is the radiograph and magnetic resonance imaging (MRI).
   B. A bone scan is the best imaging tool because all lesions demonstrate decreased tracer uptake.
   C. The most classic skull lesion is an ill-defined permeative lesion.
   D. None of the above.

4. True or false?
   A. The disease respects joint spaces.
   B. Girls are more commonly affected than boys.

## CASE 68

### Langerhans Cell Histiocytosis

1. C

2. A

3. A

4. (A) True, (B) False

## Comment

Langerhans cell histiocytosis (LCH) is a group of disorders involving abnormal proliferation of Langerhans cell histiocytes in organs of the reticuloendothelial system. Although the cause is debated between neoplastic or inflammatory processes, it is believed by most that this is a myeloid origin neoplastic disease. Letterer-Siwe is the acute disseminated form seen in 10% of the cases, usually in children less than 1 year of age; Hand-Schuller-Christian is the chronic disseminated form (20%); and eosinophilic granuloma is the form with isolated bone or lung involvement (70%).

Localized bone pain and tenderness is common. Patients may have fever, elevated sedimentation rate, and leukocytosis. LCH most commonly presents between 0 and 30 years of age (mean age of 5 to 10 years). Boys are 2 times more commonly affected than girls.

Plain radiography should be the first line of imaging because most lesions are visible on radiographs at the time of initial presentation. Classic imaging appearance is a well-defined lytic lesion without a sclerotic rim. A sclerotic rim appears during the healing phase. In the skull, the inner table of the calvarium is more commonly involved than the outer table, creating a "beveled edge." After the calvarium, the mandible is the second most commonly affected area in the head and neck. Alveolar bone destruction may result in the classic floating teeth. Soft tissue mass commonly accompanies the bone lesion in the acute phase of disease (as seen in this case as epidural enhancing mass). Spontaneous recovery can be seen, and partial or (less likely) complete improvement in vertebral body height can be seen.

Vertebra plana in children is most suggestive of LCH, unlike with adults, where metastasis is the leading differential. Other infiltrative processes like leukemia, metastatic neuroblastoma, lymphoma, and osteomyelitis can be considered in the differential diagnosis.

### References

Garg S, Mehta S, Dormans JP. Langerhans cell histiocytosis of the spine in children. Long-term follow-up. *J Bone Joint Surg Am.* 2004;86-A(8):1740–1750.

Monsereenusorn C, Rodriguez-Galindo C. Clinical characteristics and treatment of langerhans cell histiocytosis. *Hematol Oncol Clin N Am.* 2015;29(5):853–873.

### Cross-reference

Walters MM, Robertson RL. *Pediatric Radiology: The Requisites.* 4th ed. Philadelphia: Elsevier; 2017:229, 384, 395, 398.

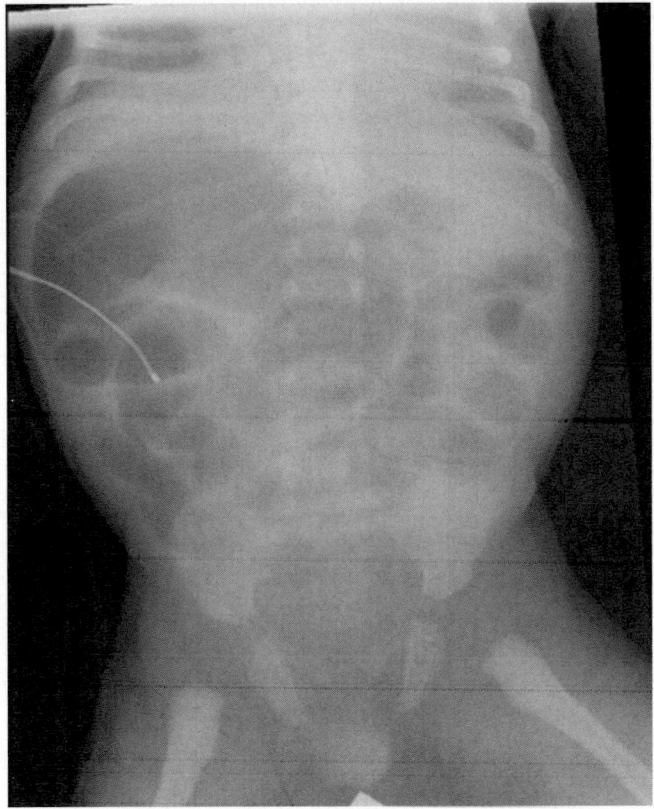

Fig. 69.1

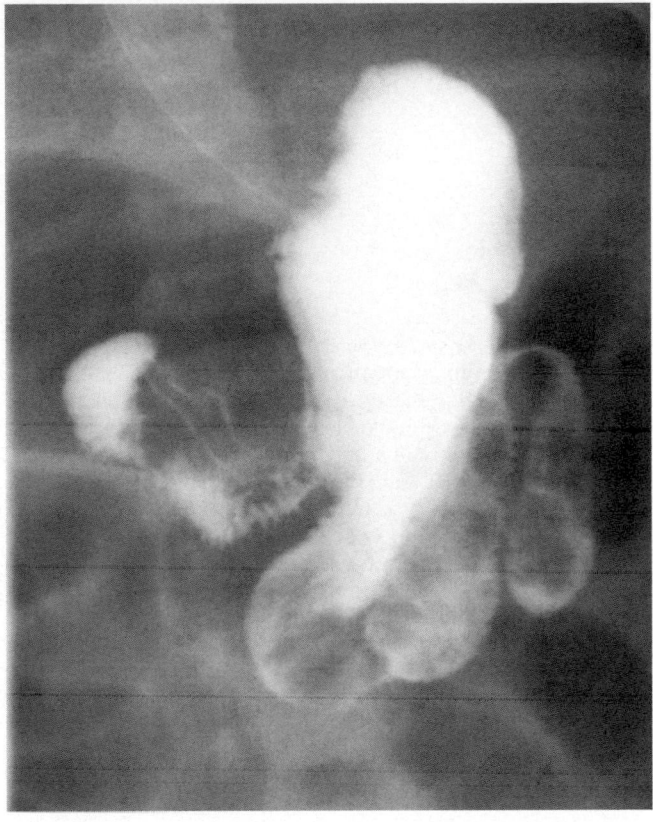

Fig. 69.2

**HISTORY:** Male 7-week-old neonate with acute onset of bilious emesis and "crampy" distended abdomen

1. Which signature pathological imaging finding do you see?
   A. Dilated bowel loops with multiple air-fluid levels
   B. Intramural air within multiple bowel loops
   C. Significantly thickened bowel wall
   D. Rigler sign

2. The difference in size and air distention of the bowel loops suggests which diagnosis?
   A. Duodenal atresia
   B. Jejunal atresia
   C. Midgut volvulus
   D. Sigmoid volvulus

3. What is the most frequent cause?
   A. Intestinal malrotation
   B. Meckel diverticula
   C. Heterotaxia
   D. Connective tissue disorder

4. Which statement is correct?
   A. Midgut volvulus results in a low intestinal obstruction.
   B. Midgut volvulus is a true pediatric emergency.
   C. The shorter the mesenteric root, the less likely it is that a midgut volvulus occurs.
   D. On cross-sectional imaging the superior mesenteric vein is typically seen to the right of the superior mesenteric artery.

## CASE 69

### Midgut Volvulus

1. A
2. C
3. A
4. B

### Comment

Midgut volvulus, or small bowel volvulus, is defined as a potentially life-threatening torsion or twisting of the small bowel around the superior mesenteric artery (SMA). Neonates and children with a congenital malrotation of the bowel are at high risk for a midgut volvulus. If the normal 270-degree counterclockwise rotation of the small bowel failed to occur during fetal life, the mesenteric root will be short and the duodenojejunal junction (DDJ) and cecum will be malpositioned. Acute or chronic twisting of the bowel loops around the mesenteric root may result in a critical perfusion of the bowel loops with resultant bowel ischemia or necrosis. Neonates with acute onset of bilious vomiting and high intestinal obstruction should be suspected of a midgut volvulus until proven otherwise. This entity represents a true acute radiologic and surgical emergency.

Ultrasound examination of the abdomen typically shows the switched position of the SMA and superior mesenteric vein (SMV) on axial imaging. Normally the SMA lies to the left of the SMV; in a midgut volvulus the SMA is seen to the right of the SMV. Computer tomography shows the same reversal of the normal vascular anatomy, and often a whirlpool of twisted, contrast-enhancing vessels is seen at the level of the mesenteric root. In addition to edematous, distended bowel loops with or without intramural air may be seen. Upper gastrointestinal fluoroscopic studies easily confirm the aberrant positioning of the DDJ, which failed to cross the midline to the left, and a characteristic corkscrew appearance of the proximal small bowel can be seen. If oral contrast passes the obstruction, the jejunum is seen within the right abdomen, and the misplaced cecum can be seen within the right or left upper quadrant.

In a high percentage of cases, associated anomalies are seen including congenital heart disease, duodenal webs, a preduodenal portal vein, and an annular pancreas.

### Reference

Lampl B, Levin TL, Berdon WE, Cowles RA. Malrotation and midgut volvulus: a historical review and current controversies in diagnosis and management. *Pediatr Radiol*. 2009;39:359–366.

### Cross-reference

Walters MM, Robertson RL. *Pediatric Radiology: The Requisites*. 4th ed. Philadelphia: Elsevier; 2017:99–102.

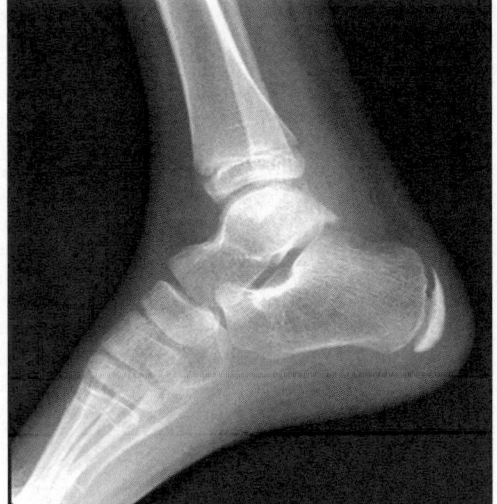

Fig. 70.1

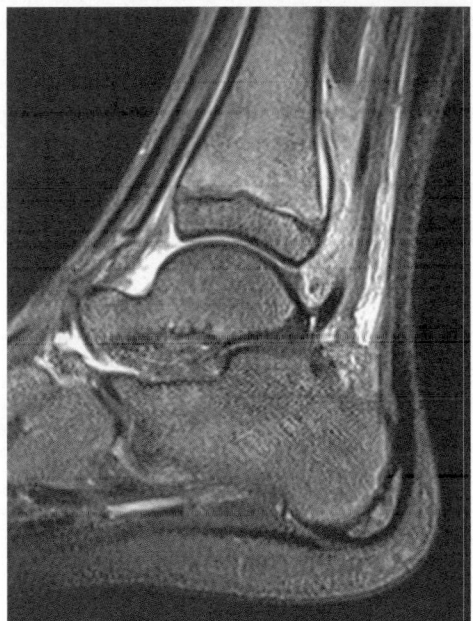

Fig. 70.2

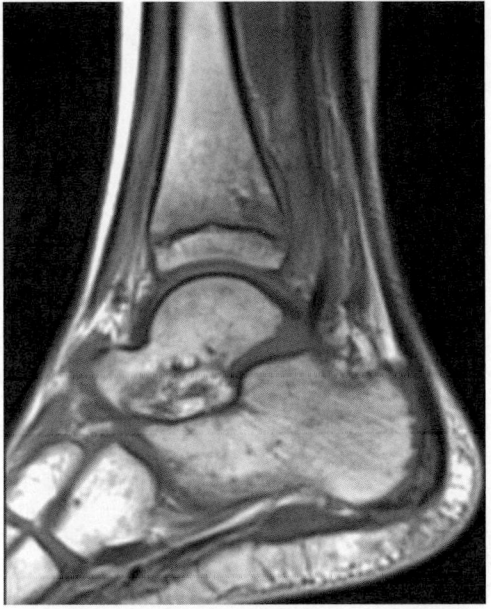

Fig. 70.3

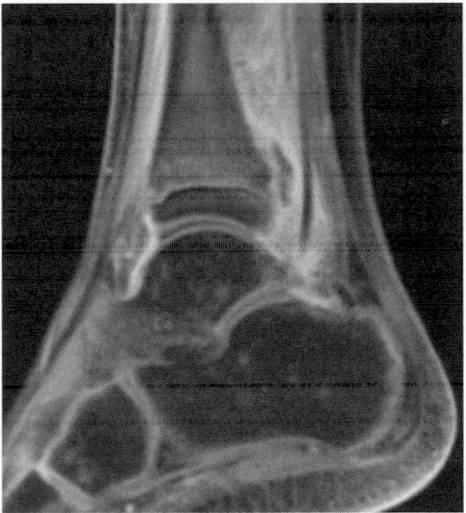

Fig. 70.4

**HISTORY:** 8-year-old male with pain in the lower leg

1. Based on the imaging findings, which of the following would you include in your differential diagnosis?
   A. Langerhans cell histiocytosis
   B. Neuroblastoma metastasis
   C. Leukemia
   D. Acute osteomyelitis

2. In infants (0–1 year), which option describes the most common location for acute osteomyelitis to develop?
   A. Diaphysis of long bone
   B. Metaphysis of long bone
   C. Physis and epiphysis of long bone
   D. Metaphyseal equivalent

3. In children (>1 year), which option describes the most common location for acute osteomyelitis to develop?
   A. Diaphysis of long bone
   B. Metaphysis of long bone
   C. Physis and epiphysis of long bone
   D. Metaphyseal equivalent

4. Which statement about acute osteomyelitis in children is *not* correct?
   A. Bony changes on a plain radiograph typically take more than 7 days to develop.
   B. About half of pediatric cases occur in children younger than 5 years.
   C. *Staphylococcus aureus* is the most common pathogen.
   D. An involucrum is an opening through the periosteum that permits pus from the infected bone to enter the surrounding soft tissue.

## CASE 70

### Acute Osteomyelitis

1. D
2. C
3. B
4. D

### Comment

Acute osteomyelitis in the pediatric population occurs most commonly in infants and young children, with one-third of cases occurring before 2 years of age, and one-half of cases occurring before 5 years of age. In infants (<1 year of age), metaphyseal vessels penetrate the growth plate and extend to the epiphysis. Consequently, infection in this age group primarily affects the epiphysis and growth plate. In children older than 1 year, metaphyseal vessels become terminal ramifications of nutrient arteries, with capillaries forming large slow-flow nutrient lakes in the metaphysis, which are common sites of osteomyelitis development. The earliest plain radiographic finding is nonspecific soft tissue swelling adjacent to the involved bone (as in the example provided in this case). Bony changes, including permeative bone lucency and periosteal reaction, are typically not seen until >7 days after onset of the infection. Magnetic resonance imaging (MRI) and radionuclide bone scan are more sensitive early on. On MRI, there is loss of the normal T1 bright marrow signal and replacement with T1-hypointense and T2-hyperintense signals. An adjacent soft tissue edema pattern (T2 bright) is usually moderate to marked. In infants and children, the periosteum is loosely adherent at the diaphysis and metaphysis, so transcortical spread of pus due to increased intramedullary pressure may cause marked elevation of the periosteum and formation of subperiosteal collections. Formation of an involucrum (envelope of thick, wavy periosteal reaction formed around the cortex of an infected tubular bone) is common in children and infants. A cloaca is an opening through the periosteum that permits pus from the infected bone to enter the soft tissue and may result in formation of a sinus tract to the skin surface. In the subacute and chronic setting, formation of a Brodie abscess in the pediatric age group is characteristic and consists of a well-circumscribed serpiginous or oval lytic defect on plain radiograph and an abscess on MRI, which is typically surrounded by a low T2 signal intensity rim of variable thickness representing fibrous tissue and reactive bone.

### References

Montgomery NI, Rosenfeld S. Pediatric osteoarticular infection update. *J Pediatr Orthop*. 2015;24(1):74–81.

Pugmire BS, Shailam R, Gee MS. Role of MRI in the diagnosis and treatment of osteomyelitis in pediatric patients. *World J Radiol*. 2014;6(8):530–537.

### Cross-reference

Walters MM, Robertson RL. *Pediatric Radiology: The Requisites*. 4th ed. Philadelphia: Elsevier; 2017:220–222.

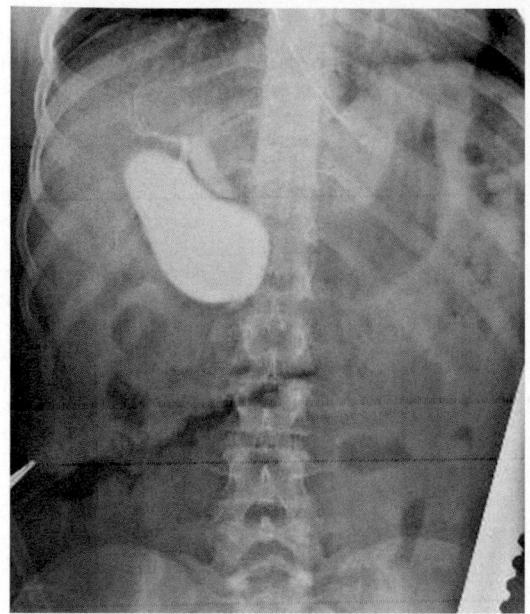

Fig. 71.1

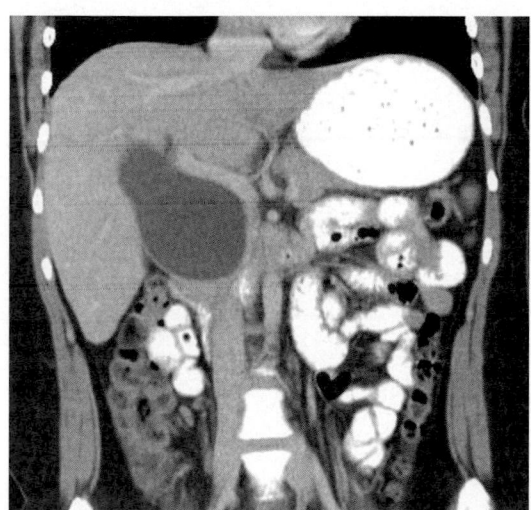

Fig. 71.2

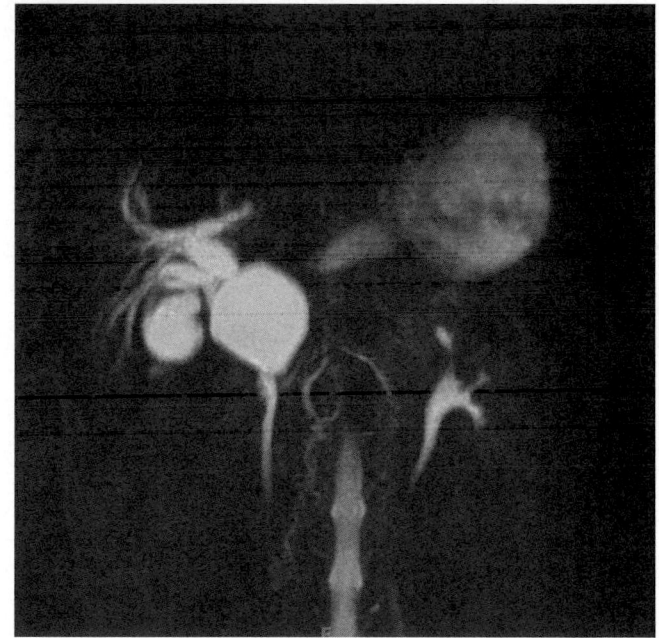

Fig. 71.3

See Supplemental Figures section for additional figures for this case.

**HISTORY:** 9-year-old boy with upper abdominal pain, intermittent jaundice, and a palpable upper abdominal mass

1. What is the most likely diagnosis based upon all available imaging studies?
   A. Gallbladder hydrops
   B. Duplication cyst of the duodenum
   C. Liver abscess
   D. Choledochal cyst

2. How would you classify this lesion?
   A. Todani type 1 choledochal cyst
   B. Todani type 2 choledochal cyst
   C. Todani type 3 choledochal cyst
   D. Todani type 4 choledochal cyst

3. Which condition may complicate biliary obstruction?
   A. Hepatic cirrhosis
   B. Portal hypertension
   C. Cholangitis/pancreatitis
   D. All of the above

4. Which statement is correct?
   A. Most choledochal malformations become apparent in the second decade of life.
   B. Caroli disease primarily affects the extrahepatic ducts.
   C. Choledochal cysts are associated with an increased risk for cholangiocarcinoma.
   D. Biliary atresia typically results from recurrent postnatal cholangitis.

## CASE 71

### Choledochal Cyst

1. D
2. A
3. D
4. C

### Comment

Choledochal cysts encompass a variety of congenital cystic malformations of the extra- and/or intrahepatic bile ducts. Neonates may present with prolonged neonatal jaundice or cholestasis prompting a diagnostic workup for biliary atresia. A palpable abdominal mass lesion is often noted. The clinical presentation in infants and older children is somewhat more variable and includes episodes of jaundice due to intermittent biliary obstruction as well as recurrent pancreatitis. Furthermore, acholic stool, hepatomegaly, and upper abdominal pain may be seen. Long-term sequelae include strictures of the bile ducts due to recurrent cholangitis, liver cirrhosis, and portal hypertension. The risk for cholangiocarcinoma is increased.

Ultrasound (US) is the primary imaging modality to examine choledochal cysts followed by magnetic resonance imaging (MRI) and magnetic resonance cholangiopancreatography (MRCP). Percutaneous cholangiography or endoscopic retrograde cholangiopancreatography are more invasive alternative tests. Computer tomography should be avoided in the pediatric population. The typical imaging findings include a focal or multifocal dilation of the involved segments of the biliary tree. Todani classified the malformation in five types. Type 1 is the most frequent form (75% to 85%) and is characterized by segmental or diffuse fusiform dilation of the common bile duct. Type 2 refers to a focal diverticulum of the choledochal duct, and type 3 is a choledochocele, which may protrude into the duodenum. Type 4 presents with multiple extrahepatic bile duct cysts, which may overlap the Caroli disease (type 5), which has multiple intrahepatic duct cysts.

On imaging, the relation to the pancreatic duct should always be carefully evaluated, in particular to guide the surgical planning. Occasionally stones may be seen within the choledochal cysts. Differential diagnosis includes secondary deformity of the hepatic ducts after recurrent cholangitis, or cholelithiasis. Furthermore, multifocal congenital or acquired liver cysts (e.g., after echinococcal disease) may mimic choledochal cysts.

Autosomal recessive polycystic kidney disease is often associated with Caroli syndrome. Choledochal malformations are rarely associated with autosomal dominant polycystic kidney disease.

### Reference

Chavhan GB, Babyn PS, Manson D, Vidarsson L. Pediatric MR cholangiopancreatography: principles, technique, and clinical applications. *Radiographics*. 2008;28:1951–1962.

### Cross-reference

Walters MM, Robertson RL. *Pediatric Radiology: The Requisites*. 4th ed. Philadelphia: Elsevier. 2017:119–121.

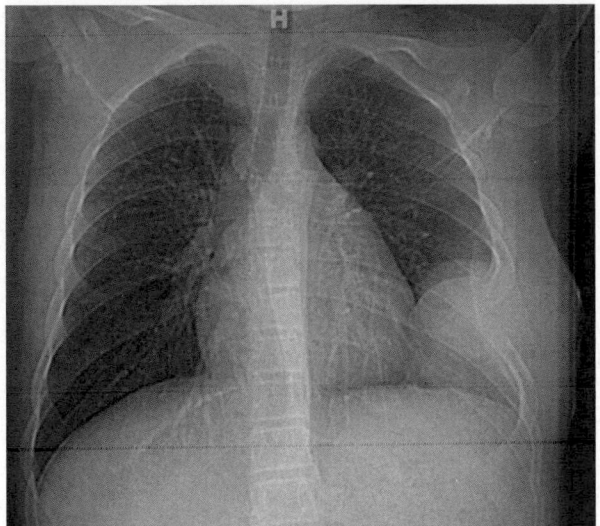

Fig. 72.1

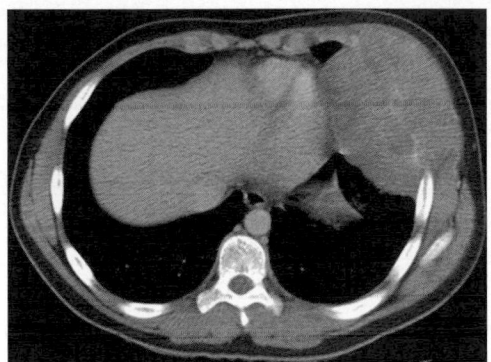

Fig. 72.2

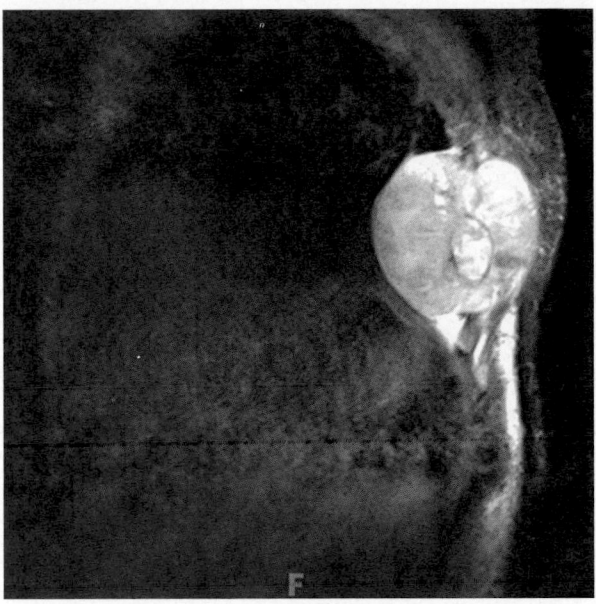

Fig. 72.3

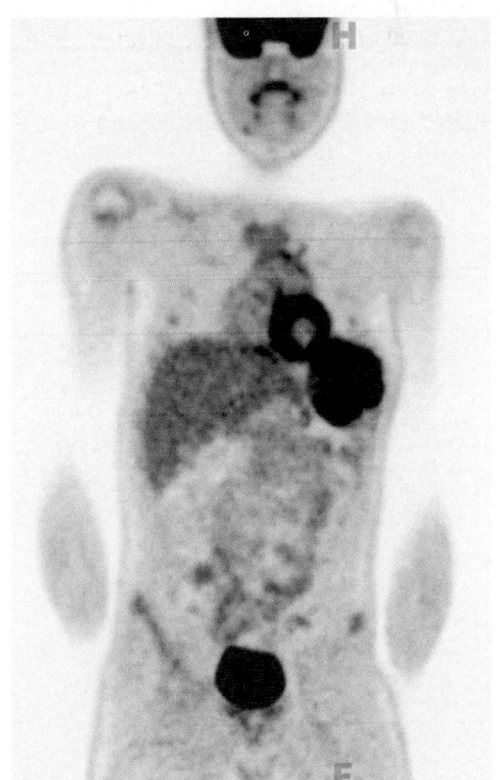

Fig. 72.4

**HISTORY:** 14-year-old boy with a newly discovered "bump" along the left lateral chest wall. Chest radiography, computed tomography (CT), and short tau inversion recovery (STIR) magnetic resonance (MR) images are available for analysis, along with a nuclear medicine study.

1. Which signature pathological imaging finding do you see?
   A. Focal mass lesion originating from the lung
   B. Focal mass lesion originating from the pleura
   C. Focal mass lesion originating from the ribs
   D. Focal mass lesion originating from the chest musculature

2. Based upon the CT, magnetic resonance imaging (MRI), and nuclear medicine study, which type of lesion is most likely?
   A. Benign
   B. Malignant
   C. Infectious
   D. Posttraumatic

3. What is the most likely diagnosis?
   A. Osteochondroma
   B. Osteosarcoma
   C. Ewing sarcoma
   D. Rhabdomyosarcoma

4. Which statement is correct?
   A. Ewing sarcoma rarely affects flat bones.
   B. Ewing sarcoma is typically seen within the first 5 years of life.
   C. Ewing sarcoma belongs to the group of small, round, blue cell tumors.
   D. Ewing sarcoma typically affects African American children.

## CASE 72

### Ewing Sarcoma

1. C
2. B
3. C
4. C

### Comment

Ewing sarcoma belongs to the group of aggressive, small, round blue cell tumors that may occur within the skeleton and in the soft tissues adjacent to the bones (extraosseous Ewing sarcoma). Ewing sarcoma is the second most common bone cancer in children, often diagnosed between the ages of 10 and 20 years. Clinically, children present with a focal swelling and/or localized pain. Ewing sarcomas may affect nearly any bone of the axial (spinal column, pelvis, ribs) and appendicular skeleton (long tubular bones). However, if a flat bone like the scapula or pelvis is affected, it is more likely a Ewing sarcoma than an osteosarcoma. If a tubular bone is affected, the metaphysis or diaphysis is mostly involved.

The first imaging usually involves radiography of the involved bone. Care should be taken to image the entire bone including the adjacent joints. The radiographic features follow the typical characteristics of an aggressive osseous lesion with various combinations of a permeative or moth-eaten focal destruction of the cortical bone and bone marrow, aggressive periosteal changes (Codman triangle, sunburst sign, onionskin appearance), adjacent sclerosis, and occasional pathologic fractures.

Computed tomography (CT) and magnetic resonance imaging (MRI) allow correct staging of the lesion with exact definition of tumor extension and identification of involved critical neurovascular structures. The osseous destruction, periosteal reaction, and intralesional calcifications are best seen on CT. In addition, lung CT should be performed to rule out metastatic pulmonary lesions. MRI allows study of the exact bony and soft tissue infiltration. Ewing sarcomas typically replace the T1-hyperintense fatty bone marrow and often show a heterogeneous contrast enhancement. On T2-weighted imaging the tumor is usually hyperintense. Nuclear medicine studies including positron emission tomography with CT (PET-CT) are characterized by an intense tumor radiotracer uptake.

Differential diagnosis includes primarily osteomyelitis and osteosarcoma.

### Reference

Kaste SC. Imaging pediatric bone sarcomas. *Radiol Clin North Am.* 2011;49:749–765.

### Cross-reference

Walters MM, Robertson RL. *Pediatric Radiology: The Requisites.* 4th ed. Philadelphia: Elsevier; 2017:238–240.

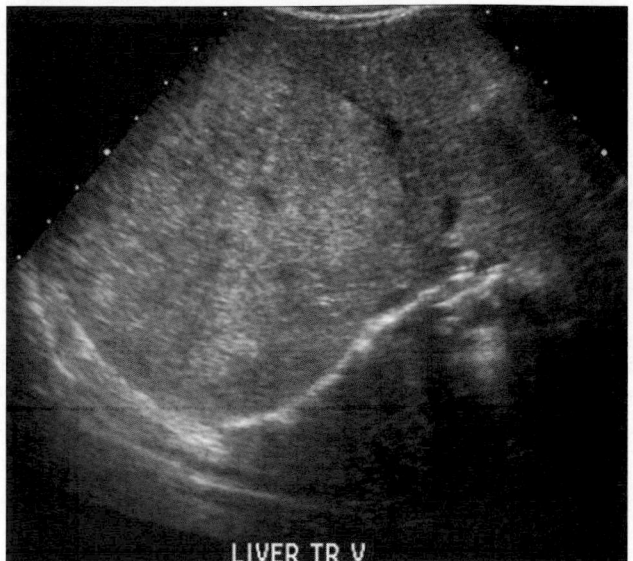

Fig. 73.1

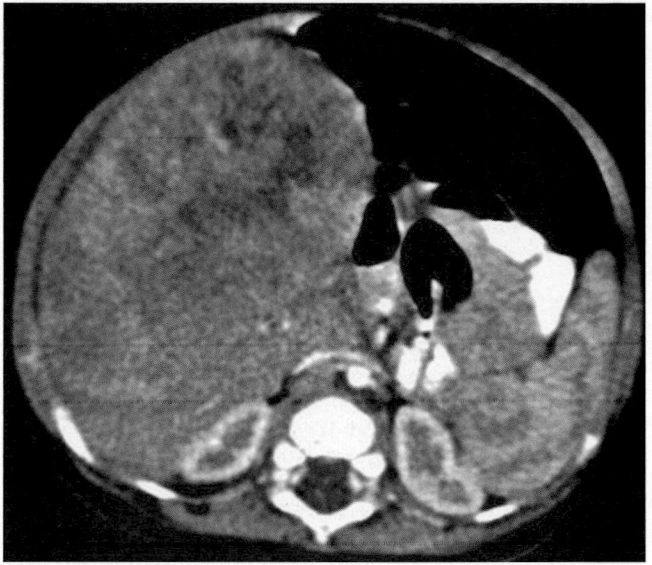

Fig. 73.2

**HISTORY:** 4-month-old male patient presenting with abdominal distension and poor oral intake

1. What is the most likely diagnosis?
   A. Hepatocarcinoma
   B. Cholangiocarcinoma
   C. Hemangioma
   D. Hepatoblastoma

2. What is the best treatment option?
   A. Tumor resection
   B. Tumor resection and radiation
   C. Tumor resection and chemotherapy
   D. Palliative care

3. Which statement is true regarding clinical presentation of hepatoblastoma?
   A. It is much rarer in preterm infants, especially those with very low birth weight.
   B. It typically presents with elevated alpha-fetoprotein levels.
   C. It is the most common malignant tumor in children 6 years of age or older.
   D. High alpha protein levels and thrombocytopenia are a classic presentation.

4. True or false?
   A. Tumor rupture and peritonitis are an unfavorable presentation for outcome.
   B. Only tumors that involve two segments of the liver are eligible for surgical resection.

## CASE 73

### Hepatoblastoma

1. D

2. C

3. B

4. A) True, B) False

## Comment

Hepatoblastoma is the most common primary malignant liver tumor in children and is usually diagnosed within the first 3 years of life. Most cases are sporadic; however, association with parental smoking, Beckwith-Wiedemann syndrome, familial polyposis, or deletion of chromosome 11 has been suggested. Typically, they are well-demarcated, solid, large (>5 cm) mass lesions at the time of diagnosis. Computed tomography (CT) or magnetic resonance imaging (MRI) is often performed to better delineate the anatomical involvement within the liver parenchyma and the relationship of the tumor to hepatic veins, inferior vena cava, and portal veins, which is crucial for preoperative planning. The tumor typically presents with heterogeneous density or signal intensity depending on the degree of intratumoral necrosis and hemorrhage. Contrast enhancement is less than that of liver parenchyma and is heterogeneous. Approximately 50% of these tumors demonstrate calcification on imaging. Serum alpha protein is the most important clinical marker and remains the clinical marker of malignant change, response to treatment, and relapse. Treatment options include complete surgical resection and chemotherapy. Patients with a single large localized tumor involving at most three segments of the liver can undergo complete surgical resection. Liver transplantation is an option when safe surgical resection is not possible. Differential diagnosis is guided by the clinical presentation and age of the child combined with the imaging findings. In children 4 years and older, hepatocarcinoma should be ruled out.

### References

Emre S, Umman V, Rodriguez-Davalos M. Current concepts in pediatric liver tumors. *Pediatr Transplant*. 2012;16(6):549-563.

Hiyama E. Pediatric hepatoblastoma: diagnosis and treatment. *Transl Pediatr*. 2014;3(4):293-299.

### Cross-reference

Walters MM, Robertson RL. *Pediatric Radiology: The Requisites*. 4th ed. Philadelphia: Elsevier; 2017:128-129.

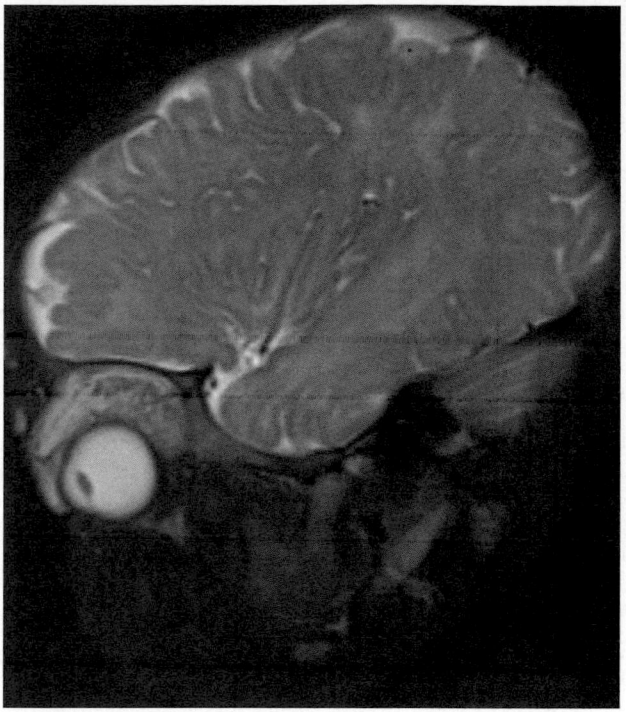

**Fig. 74.1**

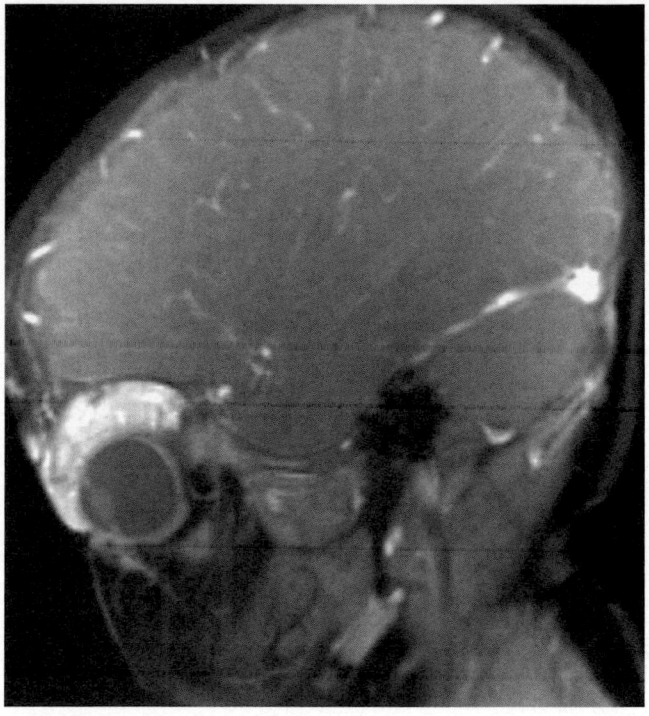

**Fig. 74.2**

1. What is the most likely diagnosis?
   A. Rhabdomyosarcoma
   B. Kaposiform hemangioendothelioma
   C. Infantile hemangioma
   D. Venous malformation

2. Which statement is accurate for clinical presentation of hemangiomas?
   A. Infantile hemangiomas are clinically recognizable as a palpable mass at the time of birth.
   B. Infantile hemangiomas are more commonly seen in males.
   C. Infantile hemangiomas are more commonly seen in low-birth-weight premature infants.
   D. Congenital hemangiomas have a predictable clinical course with proliferative, plateau, and involuted phases.

3. Choose the correct statement.
   A. Infantile hemangiomas typically do involute on their own.
   B. Infantile hemangiomas do not benefit from medical treatment with propranolol.
   C. Chemoembolization is helpful in 50% of infantile hemangiomas.
   D. None of the above.

4. What is the most commonly accepted classification system for vascular tumors and vascular malformations?
   A. International Society for the Study of Vascular Anomalies (ISSVA)
   B. World Health Organization (WHO)
   C. American College of Radiology (ACR)
   D. Radiological Society of North America (RSNA)

## CASE 74

### Infantile Hemangioma

1. C
2. C
3. A
4. A

## Comment

Infantile hemangiomas (IHs) are the most common benign tumor of infancy and the most common vascular tumor. Most IHs are diagnosed based on history and physical exam, and only a small portion of IH are referred for imaging. A higher incidence is noted among females and white Caucasians. Low-birth-weight prematurity is the single most important risk factor for developing an IH. The head and neck are the most common body parts involved, similar to other vascular anomalies (VAs). IH is characterized by a unique tripartite growth cycle of proliferation, plateau, and involution. The rapid phase of proliferation is complete by 8 weeks of life, most reach 80% of maximum size between 3 and 5 months of life, and almost all cases complete proliferation by 12 months of age. The most comprehensive and commonly used classification system is set forth by the International Society for the Study of Vascular Anomalies (ISSVA). Imaging findings vary with the stage of the IH. Most children are referred for imaging during the proliferative phase. Ultrasound (US) shows a highly vascular soft tissue mass with an arterial feeder. Magnetic resonance imaging (MRI) shows a T2 bright, avidly enhancing mass. The arterial feeder can be seen on T2-weighted imaging as a serpiginous flow void. Dynamic contrast-enhanced MRI can be very useful because it clearly demonstrates the arterial feeder and the venous drainage of the solid vascular mass. Large and segmental hemangiomas in the head and neck region raise suspicion for PHACES (Posterior fossa malformations, hemangiomas, arterial anomalies, cardiac defects, eye abnormalities, sternal cleft, and supraumbilical raphe) syndrome, and its lower body correlate is LUMBAR (Lower body hemangioma and other cutaneous defects, urogenital anomalies, ulceration myelopathy, bony deformities, anorectal malformations, arterial anomalies, renal anomalies) syndrome. IH is not visible at the time of birth, but becomes recognizable between 2 and 4 weeks of life. Unlike other VAs (including congenital hemangiomas and all vascular malformations), only IH stains positive for glucose transporter 1 (GLUT-1), an important pathologic marker. Most cases involute spontaneously. However those that ulcerate, compromise airways or other vital organs, or present with cardiac failure can be medically treated. The most widely used medication is a nonselective beta blocker, propranolol. Among all VAs, only IH responds to propranolol. Differentiation from congenital hemangiomas is mostly on a clinical basis; congenital hemangiomas are present at the time of birth, and whether or not they involute over time helps in the subclassification of congenital hemangiomas.

### Reference

Tekes A, Koshy J, Kalayci TO, et al. S.E. Mitchell Vascular Anomalies Flow Chart (SEMVAFC): a visual pathway combining clinical and imaging findings for classification of soft-tissue vascular anomalies. *Clin Radiol*. 2014;69(5):443–457.

### Cross-reference

Walters MM, Robertson RL. *Pediatric Radiology: The Requisites*. 4th ed. Philadelphia: Elsevier; 2017:390–391.

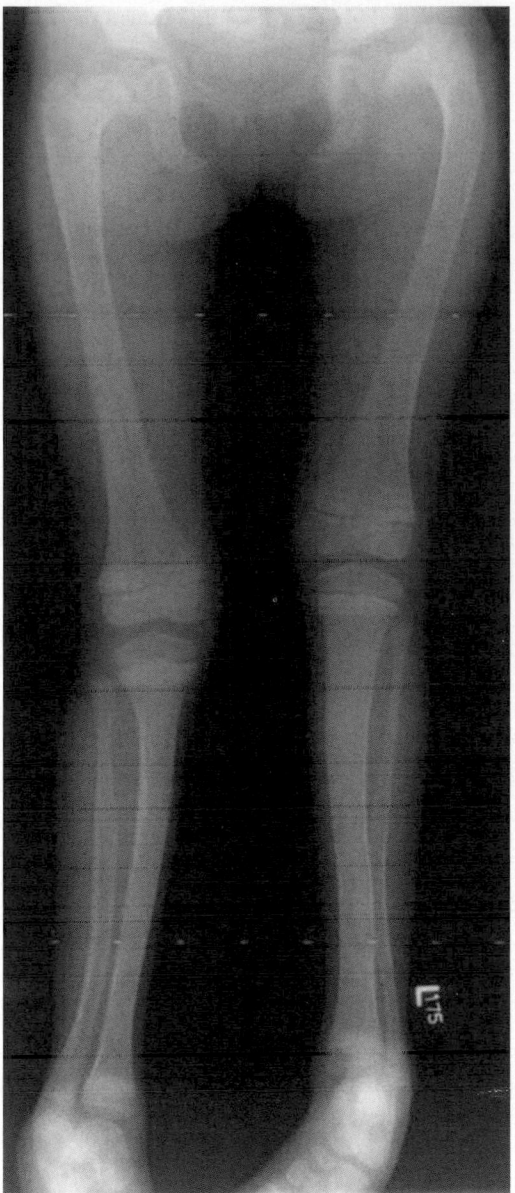

**Fig. 75.1**

**HISTORY:** 5-year-old girl presenting with leg length discrepancy and a limp

1. Based on the imaging findings, which is the best diagnosis?
   A. Langerhans cell histiocytosis (LCH)
   B. Chronic osteomyelitis
   C. Ewing's sarcoma
   D. Fibrous dysplasia (FD)

2. What percentage of cases of FD are monostotic?
   A. 10% to 20%
   B. 30% to 40%
   C. 50% to 60%
   D. 70% to 80%

3. Which statement about FD is *not* correct?
   A. Polyostotic FD typically presents before age 10.
   B. Monostotic FD typically presents after age 30.
   C. Polyostotic FD more commonly affects the skull base and facial bones than the monostotic form.
   D. McCune-Albright syndrome is associated with polyostotic FD and endocrine abnormalities including diabetes mellitus and acromegaly.

4. Which statement about FD is true?
   A. Malignant degeneration to sarcoma is rare and occurs in about 3% of cases.
   B. The monostotic form may progress to the polyostotic form.
   C. Mazabraud syndrome is characterized by polyostotic FD and multiple myxomatous soft tissue tumors.
   D. Treatment is typically with curettage and bone grafting.

## CASE 75

### Fibrous Dysplasia

1. D
2. D
3. B
4. D

## Comment

Fibrous dysplasia (FD) is a congenital disorder characterized by a defect in osteoblastic differentiation and maturation, with bony lesions caused by replacement of the normal marrow space with abnormal fibro-osseous tissue. Most cases (70% to 80%) are monostotic, and most of these patients present before the age of 30. Patients with the polyostotic form typically present before 10 years of age. On plain radiographs, lesions typically demonstrate loss of normal trabecular pattern and presence of ground glass opacity and/or lytic lucencies of the bony matrix. Long-segment involvement is typical, and the cortex is often diffusely thinned. The lesions remain diaphyseal and metaphyseal, stopping at the growth plate. Bowing of the proximal femur gives rise to the characteristic shepherd's crook deformity. The polyostotic form affects the skull and face more commonly than the monostotic form (about 50% vs. 25%, respectively). McCune-Albright syndrome is characterized by cutaneous hyperpigmentation, polyostotic FD, and polyendocrinopathy, including acromegaly, diabetes mellitus, hyperthyroidism, hyperparathyroidism, and sexual precocity. Patients with Mazabraud syndrome characteristically demonstrate polyostotic FD in combination with multiple myxomatous soft tissue tumors. Malignant degeneration of FD lesions is very rare, occurs in about 0.5% of cases, and the risk for malignant degeneration is significantly increased after irradiation of lesions. The monostotic form does not progress to the polyostotic form. Treatment is typically nonoperative and involves bisphosphonates and nonsteroidal antiinflammatory medications. Surgery is reserved for complications such as leg length discrepancies, vision loss, or severe calvarial deformities.

### Reference

Muthusamy S, Conway SA, Temple HT. Five polyostotic conditions that general orthopedic surgeons should recognize (or should not miss). *Orthop Clin North Am.* 2014;45(3):417–429.

### Cross-reference

Walters MM, Robertson RL. *Pediatric Radiology: The Requisites.* 4th ed. Philadelphia: Elsevier; 2017:227–229.

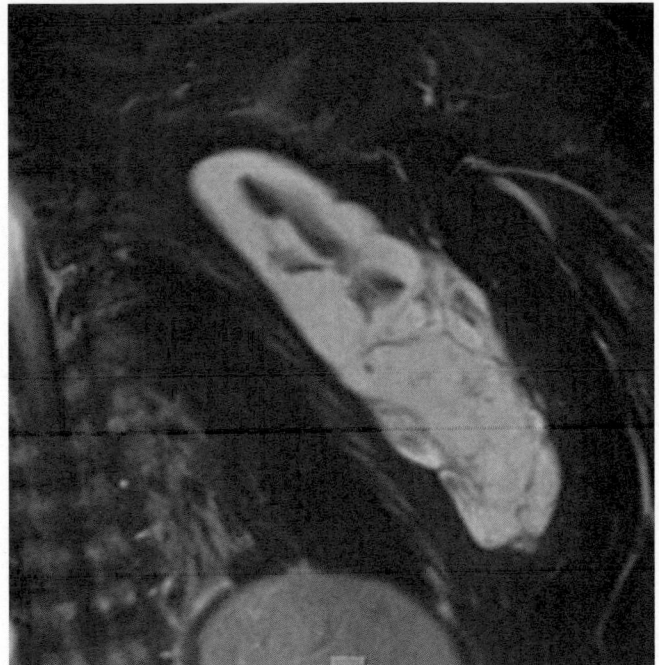

Fig. 76.1

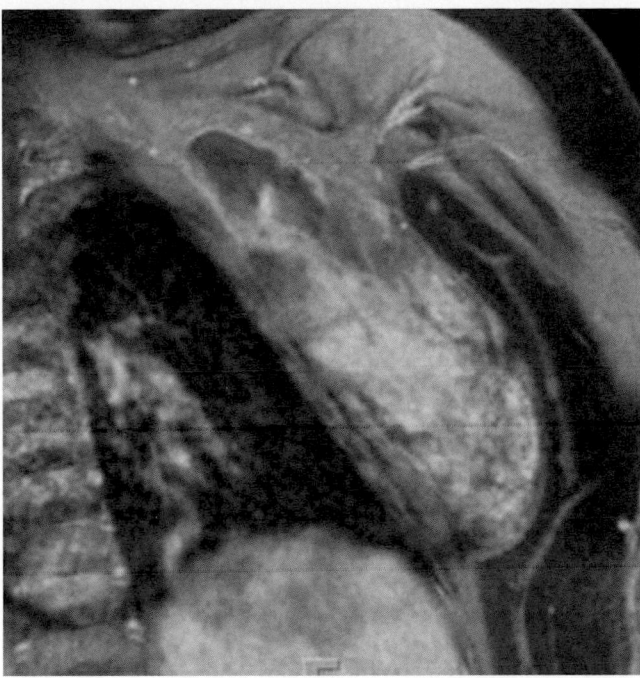

Fig. 76.2

**HISTORY:** Swelling, pain and bleeding in left lateral chest wall

1. What is the most common treatment for this lesion?
   A. Embolization
   B. Sclerotherapy
   C. Medical treatment with propranolol
   D. Surgery

2. What is a potential complication of the percutaneous embolization procedure?
   A. Skin necrosis
   B. Deep venous thrombosis
   C. Nerve damage
   D. All of the above

3. What is the most common vascular malformation?
   A. Solitary venous malformation
   B. Venolymphatic malformation
   C. Arteriovenous malformation
   D. Capillary malformation

4. Which option best describes magnetic resonance imaging (MRI) features of a venous malformation?
   A. Transspatial mass with phleboliths and a variable degree of contrast enhancement during the venous phase
   B. Transspatial multilocular mass without contrast enhancement
   C. Focal large solid mass with heterogeneous contrast enhancement
   D. None of the above

## CASE 76

### Venous Malformation

1. A
2. D
3. A
4. A

## Comment

The International Society for the Study for Vascular Anomalies classification (last updated in 2014) classifies vascular anomalies in two major groups: vascular tumors (VTs) and vascular malformations (VMs). The VMs are then subgrouped as simple, combined, and associated with syndromes. Simple venous malformations are the most common VM. Venous malformations most commonly present in the head and neck region followed by the extremities and trunk. There are some misnomers in the literature that confuse most practitioners: cavernous hemangiomas and intraosseous hemangiomas are in fact venous malformations. Clinically they may present with a palpable compressible painful mass, bluish skin discoloration, and disfigurement. Ultrasound (US) shows a heterogeneous/hypoechoic compressible mass with slow venous flow. Phleboliths may be seen with posterior acoustic shadowing. Magnetic resonance imaging (MRI) is the preferred imaging modality and gives superior detail for anatomical location, size, and proximity to vital structures such as major arteries, nerves, and veins. MRI demonstrates a T2 bright, focal, small to large transspatial mass with a variable degree of internal contrast enhancement. Phleboliths are best seen in T2-weighted imaging as T2 dark foci surrounded by a T2 bright signal. Dynamic contrast-enhanced magnetic resonance angiography (MRA) demonstrates progressive contrast enhancement only during the venous phase and can further detail the draining veins. Most cases are treated with percutaneous embolization. Alcohol and bleomycin are the commonly preferred agents. Pain killers and steroids can be used for pain and inflammation management. VMs do not respond to propranolol. Spontaneous resolution is unexpected. Klippel-Trenaunay, Maffucci, CLOVES (congenital lipomatous (fatty) overgrowth, vascular malformations, epidermal nevi, and scoliosis/skeletal/spinal anomalies), and Proteus syndromes are some of the syndromes with which VMs are associated.

### Reference

Higgins IJ, Koshy J, Mitchell SE, et al. Time-resolved contrast-enhanced MRA (TWIST) with gadofosveset trisodium in the classification of soft-tissue vascular anomalies in the head and neck in children following updated 2014 ISSVA classification: first report on systematic evaluation of MRI and TWIST in a cohort of 47 children. *Clin Radiol.* 2016;71(1):32–39.

### Cross-reference

Walters MM, Robertson RL. *Pediatric Radiology: The Requisites.* 4th ed. Philadelphia: Elsevier; 2017:370–373.

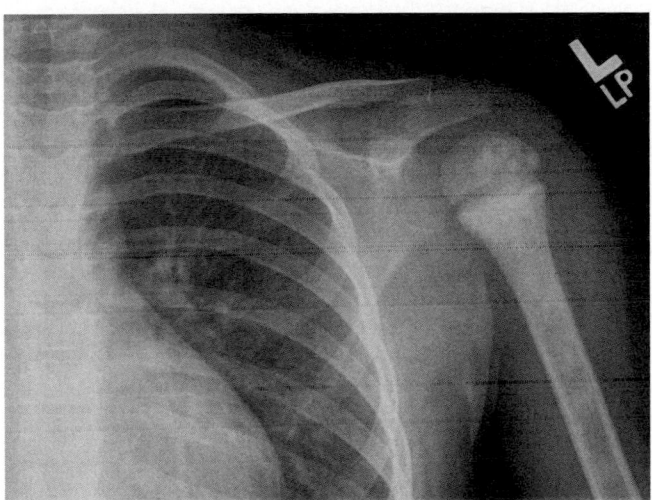

Fig. 77.1

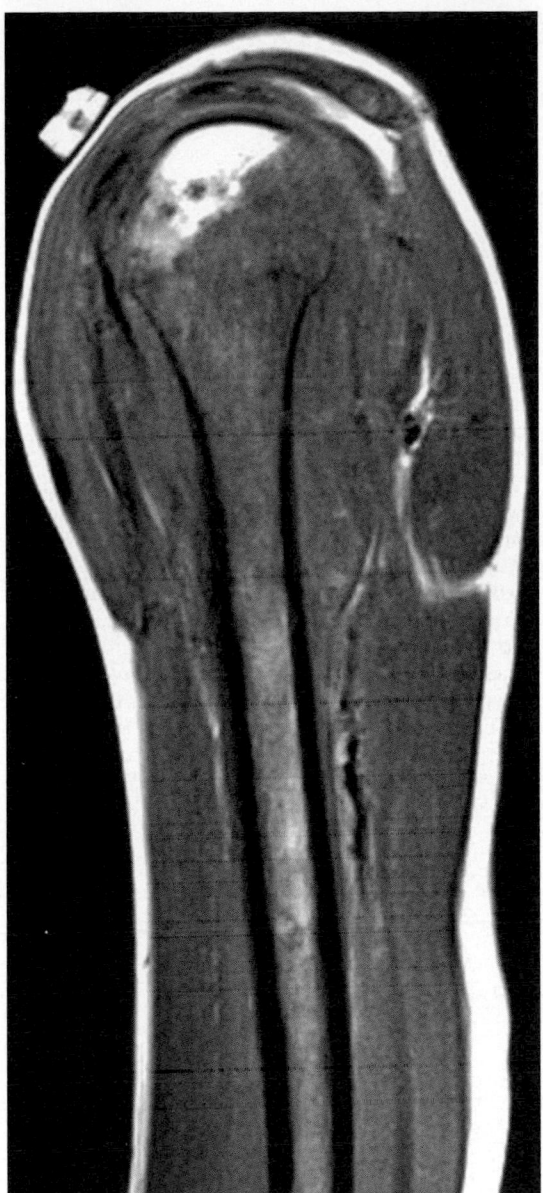

Fig. 77.2

**HISTORY:** 7-year-old girl presenting with shoulder pain

1. Given the imaging findings, which of the following would you include in your differential diagnosis? (Choose all that apply.)
   A. Ewing sarcoma
   B. Osteomyelitis
   C. Osteosarcoma
   D. Giant cell tumor
   E. Osteoblastoma

2. Which type of osteosarcoma has the best prognosis?
   A. Parosteal osteosarcoma
   B. Conventional osteosarcoma
   C. Periosteal osteosarcoma
   D. Telangiectatic osteosarcoma

3. Which type of osteosarcoma is least likely to involve the marrow cavity?
   A. Parosteal osteosarcoma
   B. Conventional osteosarcoma
   C. Periosteal osteosarcoma
   D. Telangiectatic osteosarcoma

4. Which statement about osteosarcoma is *not* true?
   A. Telangiectatic osteosarcomas cannot be reliably differentiated from aneurysmal bone cysts (ABCs) on imaging alone.
   B. Conventional osteosarcomas extend to the epiphysis in >75% of cases.
   C. The goal of neoadjuvant chemotherapy is >90% necrosis.
   D. Osteosarcomas are rarely entirely within soft tissues (extraskeletal osteosarcoma).

## CASE 77

### Osteosarcoma

1. A, C
2. A
3. C
4. A

### *Comment*

Osteosarcoma is the most common bone tumor in the pediatric age group. It typically presents between 10 and 30 years of age and most commonly affects the metaphysis of long bones, especially around the knee. Extension across the physis to involve the epiphysis is common (>75%) (as shown in this case), and along with skip lesions and joint space involvement. Osteosarcoma is best assessed on preoperative imaging for staging with magnetic resonance imaging (MRI). Ewing sarcoma is more commonly centered in the diaphysis, but may elicit prominent reactive bone proliferation and may thus overlap on imaging with osteosarcoma. Ewing sarcoma commonly has a large associated soft tissue mass, but unlike osteosarcoma, there is no mineralized matrix in the soft tissue mass. Osteomyelitis does not cause osteoid or bone production, although chronic osteomyelitis may present with mixed sclerotic and lucent regions. Giant cell tumor is centered in the epiphysis and osteoblastoma would typically be less aggressive in appearance, with less permeative osseous destructive change. Parosteal osteosarcoma is a type of surface osteosarcoma and has a better prognosis than periosteal (another type of surface osteosarcoma), conventional, and telangiectatic osteosarcomas. Periosteal osteosarcoma presents as a broadbased soft tissue mass that commonly causes thickening and scalloping of the outer margin of the cortex and typically has associated hair on end periosteal reaction. Marrow involvement in periosteal osteosarcoma is very rare. Telangiectatic osteosarcoma may appear largely lytic on plain radiographs and may have multiple fluid-fluid levels on cross-sectional imaging, thus mimicking an aneurysmal bone cyst (ABC). However, unlike ABCs these tumors typically have thick peripheral soft tissue enhancement around centrally necrotic regions, and on computed tomography (CT) often have an osteoid in the periphery. Osteosarcoma is rarely entirely within soft tissues (extraskeletal osteosarcoma). Treatment is with neoadjuvant chemotherapy with a goal of >90% necrosis followed by surgery and adjuvant chemotherapy.

### Reference

Moore DD, Luu HH. Osteosarcoma. *Cancer Treat Res.* 2014;162:65–92.

### Cross-reference

Walters MM, Robertson RL. *Pediatric Radiology: The Requisites.* 4th ed. Philadelphia: Elsevier; 2017:237–239.

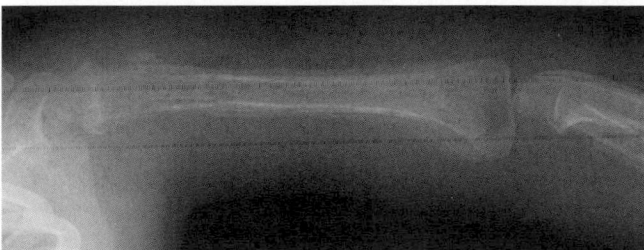

Fig. 89.1

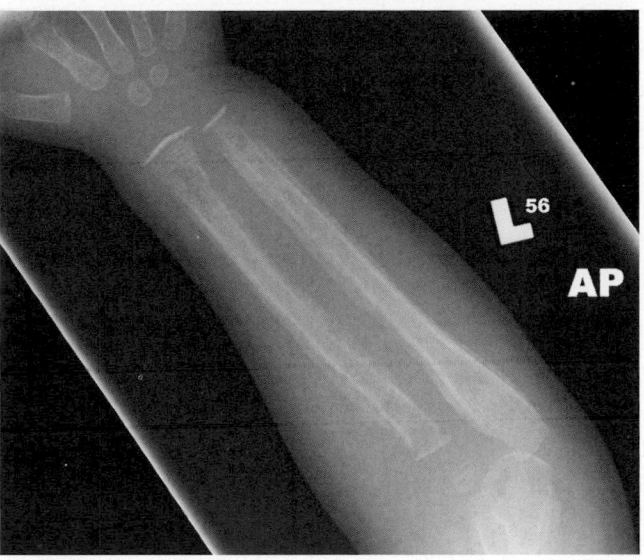

Fig. 89.2

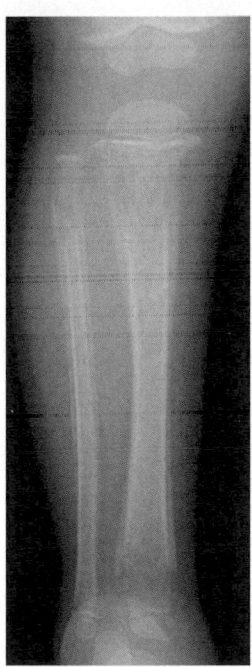

Fig. 89.3

**HISTORY:** 8-year-old male presenting with generalized bone pain

1. Which of the following should be included in the differential diagnosis for permeative lytic lesions in a child of this age? (Choose all that apply.)
   A. Ewing sarcoma
   B. Osteomyelitis
   C. Lymphoma/leukemia
   D. Neuroblastoma metastases

2. Given the imaging findings, what is the most likely diagnosis in this case?
   A. Ewing sarcoma
   B. Osteomyelitis
   C. Lymphoma/leukemia
   D. Neuroblastoma metastases

3. Which of the following should be included in the differential diagnosis for periostitis in a child? (Choose all that apply.)
   A. Osteomyelitis
   B. Stress fracture
   C. Leukemia
   D. Ewing sarcoma

4. True or false?
   A. Leukemia can present with pathologic fractures in the metaphyseal region and simulate nonaccidental trauma.

## CASE 89

### Leukemia

1. A, B, C
2. C
3. A, B, C, D
4. True

### Comment

Although radiographs are often normal in patients with leukemia, it is important to be aware of the imaging findings of leukemia so that diagnosis is not delayed. In the extremities, imaging findings consist of diffuse osteopenia, lucent metaphyseal bands ("leukemic lines"), periostitis, and lytic lesions ranging from geographic to permeative in appearance. Neuroblastoma metastases may also appear as lytic bony lesions, but this entity is rare in a child older than 5 years. Pathologic fractures can occur in patients with leukemia, are most common in the metaphyseal region, and may mimic nonaccidental trauma. In the spine, osteopenia and compression fractures can be seen. On magnetic resonance imaging (MRI), the typical imaging finding includes diffuse abnormal T1 hypointensity (relative to the intervertebral disc signal) due to replacement of the normal mixed fatty marrow by abnormal marrow proliferation of leukemic cells. The patient in this case had relapsed acute myeloid leukemia.

### Reference

Gallagher DJ, Phillips DJ, Heinrich SD. Orthopedic manifestations of acute pediatric leukemia. *Orthop Clin N Am*. 1996;27(3):635–644.

### Cross-reference

Walters MM, Robertson RL. *Pediatric Radiology: The Requisites*. 4th ed. Philadelphia: Elsevier; 2017:165.

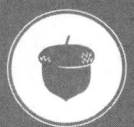

# Challenge

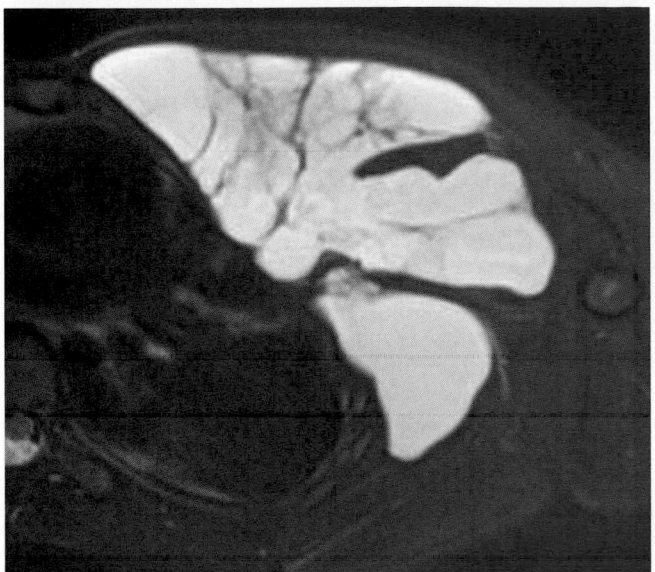

Fig. 90.1

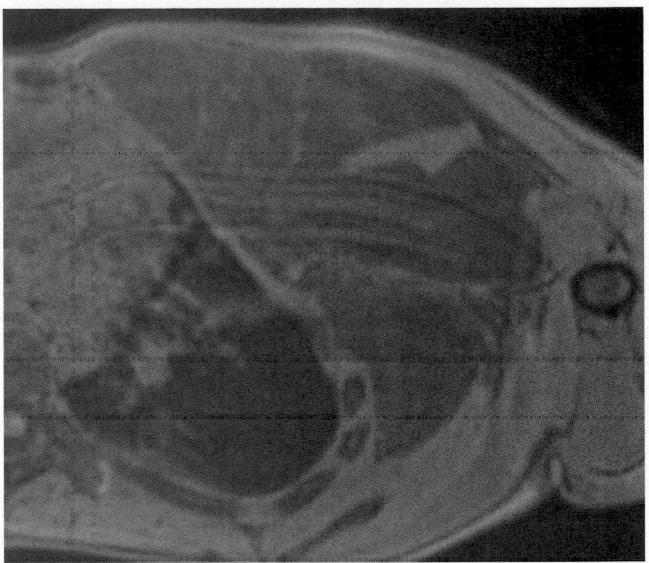

Fig. 90.2

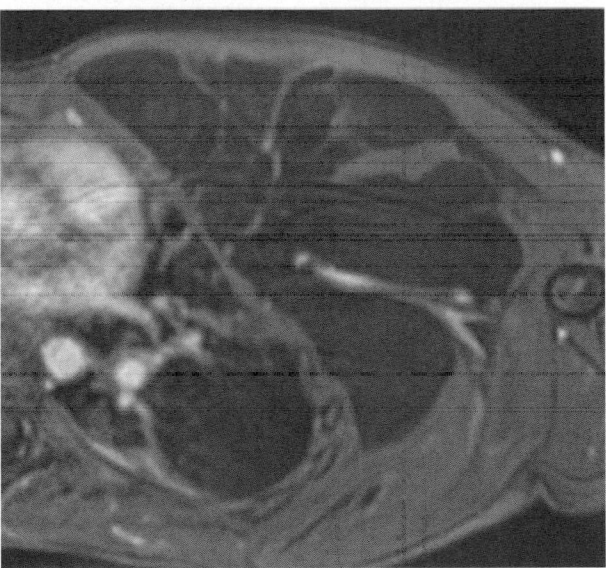

Fig. 90.3

1. What is the most likely treatment option for this case?
   A. Sclerotherapy
   B. Coil embolization
   C. Propranolol
   D. Surgery

2. Which statement is most accurate about lymphatic malformations (LMs)?
   A. Typically they are fast-flow vascular malformations.
   B. Phleboliths are pathognomonic for LMs.
   C. Avid enhancement of a solid mass during the arterial phase is a classic magnetic resonance imaging (MRI) finding.
   D. A transspatial cystic mass (either macro- or microcystic) without internal contrast enhancement.

3. Which of the following syndromes could be associated with LMs?
   A. Noonan syndrome
   B. Turner syndrome
   C. Klippel-Trenaunay syndrome
   D. All of the above

4. What is the most common location for vascular anomalies?
   A. Head and neck
   B. Trunk
   C. Upper extremity
   D. Lower extremity

## CASE 90

### Lymphatic Malformation

1. A

2. D

3. D

4. A

### Comment

Lymphatic malformations (LMs) are the second most common vascular malformation following venous malformations. The term lymphatic malformation should be preferred over lymphangioma; the suffix "oma" implies "tumor," but LMs are true vascular malformations resulting from morphological maldevelopment of the embryonic vascular system between the 4th and 10th gestational weeks. The head and neck are the most common areas of involvement, similar to the rest of the vascular anomalies. LMs can be macrocystic, microcystic, or mixed. It is important to define the nature of LMs because macrocystic LMs are most amenable to percutaneous sclerotherapy. Percutaneous sclerotherapy is the most common treatment method. The cyst walls or septa may enhance; however, the internal content of the cysts do not. Wall enhancement of the microcysts may mimic diffuse enhancement; however, careful evaluation of T2-weighted imaging along with pre- and postcontrast T1-weighted imaging is helpful in differentiating the microcystic lymphaic malformation from other solid mass lesions. On magnetic resonance imaging (MRI), a precontrast high/intermediate signal can be seen due to hemorrhages within the cyst. Dynamic contrast-enhanced magnetic resonance angiography (MRA) does not demonstrate any enhancement during the arterial or venous phase. Fluid-fluid levels can be seen due to internal hemorrhage or proteinaceous content. Although this has been initially described for LMs; it is not a specific finding for lymphatic malformations, rather a finding for slow-flow vascular malformations. LMs can be focal, multifocal and transspatial, but even with focal lesions, multicystic appearance is common. LMs can be associated with Noonan, Turner, Klippel-Trenaunay, CLOVES (congenital lipomatous overgrowth, vascular malformations, epidermal nevi, and scoliosis/skeletal/spinal anomalies), and Proteus syndromes.

### Reference

Thawait SK, Puttgen K, Carrino JA, et al. MR imaging characteristics of soft tissue vascular anomalies in children. *Eur J Pediatr*. 2013;172(5):591–600.

### Cross-reference

Walters MM, Robertson RL. *Pediatric Radiology: The Requisites*. 4th ed. Philadelphia: Elsevier; 2017:370–372.

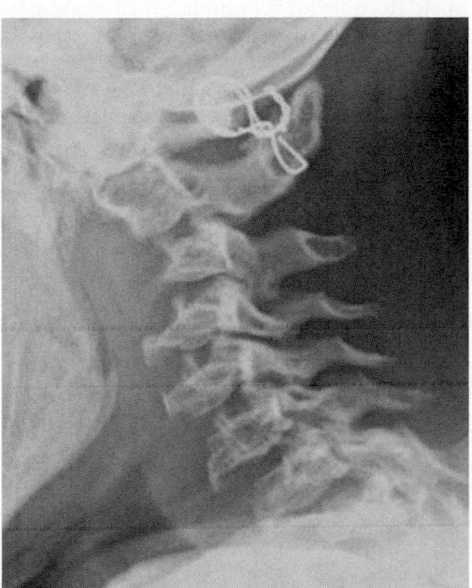

Fig. 91.1

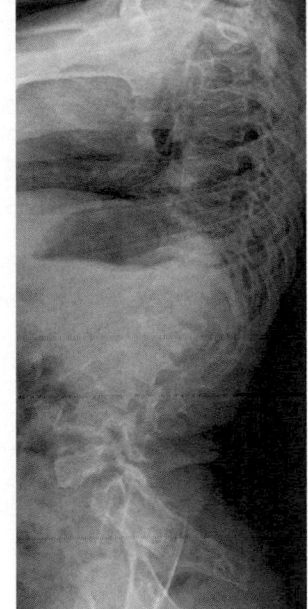

Fig. 91.2

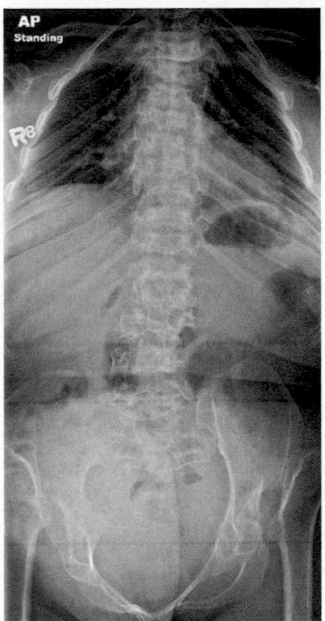

Fig. 91.3

**HISTORY:** 18 year old female with short stature, bell shaped chest, and widely spaced teeth.

1. Which of the following should be included in the differential diagnosis? (Choose all that apply.)
   A. Jeune syndrome
   B. Hurler syndrome
   C. Osteogenesis imperfecta, type I
   D. Morquio syndrome

2. Which statement about mucopolysaccharidoses is *not* true?
   A. They form a heterogeneous group of lysosomal storage diseases characterized by a deficiency of enzymes that degrade glycosaminoglycans.
   B. Dysostosis multiplex refers to a constellation of bony dysplasias seen variably in mucopolysaccharidoses.
   C. Testing the urine for glycosaminoglycans is a common screening test for mucopolysaccharidoses.

D. They are lysosomal storage disorders resulting in deposition of glucocerebroside in cells of the reticuloendothelial system, including bone marrow.

3. Which option is *not* a characteristic finding of dysostosis multiplex?
   A. Oval-shaped vertebral bodies with anterior beaking
   B. Thick, "canoe paddle" shaped ribs (thin proximally, wide distally)
   C. Wormian bones
   D. Metacarpals with proximal tapering

4. Which option is a characteristic finding in the spine in patients with mucopolysaccharidoses?
   A. S-shaped scoliosis
   B. Narrowed interpedicular distance
   C. Gibbus deformity
   D. Segmentation anomalies

## CASE 91

### Morquio Syndrome

1. B,D
2. D
3. C
4. C

### Comment

The images presented in this case are from a patient with Morquio syndrome, which is a member of the group of mucopolysaccharidoses, a heterogeneous group of lysosomal storage diseases characterized by a deficiency in enzymes that degrade glycosaminoglycans (also known as mucopolysaccharides). Other examples of syndromes in this group include Hunter, Hurler, Scheie, and Sanfilippo syndromes. Dysostosis multiplex refers to a constellation of skeletal findings that are variably seen in these patients, including oval vertebral bodies with anterior beaking, gibbus deformity of the spine, thick "canoe-paddle" ribs (thin proximally, wide distally), proximally tapered metacarpals, and short thick clavicles. In the pelvis, bony changes include flared iliac wings that are tapered inferiorly, shallow and steep acetabula, and coxa valga. Patients with Morquio syndrome have anterior beaking in the mid-anterior body, whereas patients with Hurler syndrome have anteroinferior beaking. Patients with Morquio syndrome are also at high risk of cervical myelopathy due to odontoid hypoplasia and ligamentous laxity leading to atlantoaxial subluxation.

### Reference

Solanki GA, Martin KW, Theroux, et al. Spinal involvement in mucopolysaccharidosis IVA (Morquio-Brailsford or Morquio A syndrome): presentation, diagnosis and management. *J Inherit Metab Dis*. 2013;36(2):339–355.

### Cross-reference

Walters MM, Robertson RL. *Pediatric Radiology: The Requisites*. 4th ed. Philadelphia: Elsevier; 2017:206–207.

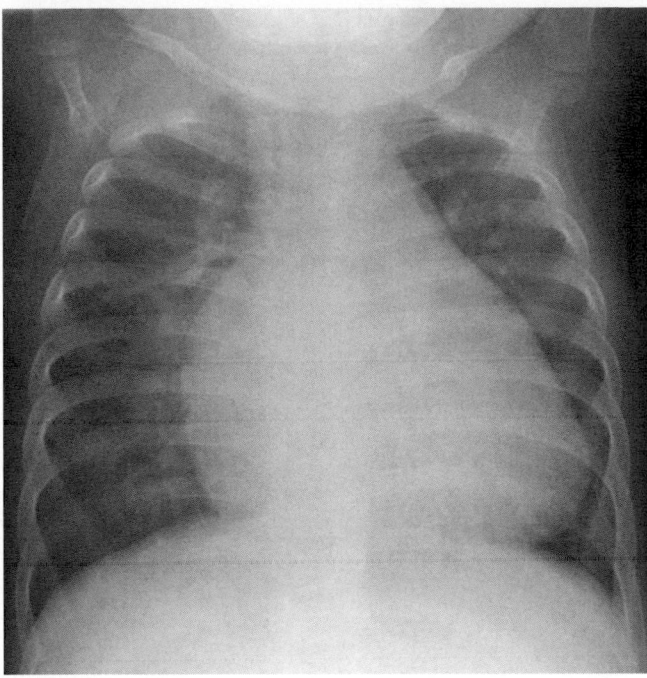

Fig. 92.1

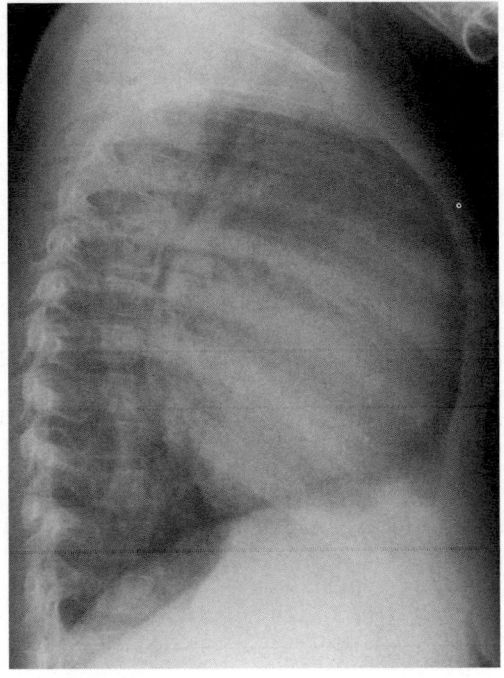

Fig. 92.2

**HISTORY:** 2-month-old child presenting with tachypnea

1. Based on the imaging findings, which of the following would you include in your differential diagnosis? (Choose all that apply.)
   A. Endocardial cushion defect
   B. Ventricular septal defect (VSD)
   C. Atrial septal defect (ASD)
   D. Patent ductus arteriosus

2. In endocardial cushion defect, which type of ASD is typically encountered?
   A. Ostium secundum
   B. Ostium primum
   C. Patent foramen ovale
   D. Sinus venosus

3. In endocardial cushion defect, which type of VSD is typically encountered?
   A. Membranous/perimembranous
   B. Muscular/trabecular
   C. Inlet/inflow
   D. Outlet/subarterial

4. Which statement about endocardial cushion defects is *not* true?
   A. Surgery is the definitive treatment modality.
   B. A complete atrioventricular (AV) canal is characterized by a common AV valve and large defects in the atrial and ventricular septa.
   C. They are associated with trisomy 21 in more than 40% of cases.
   D. They are present in the perinatal period with profound cyanosis, tachypnea, and tachycardia.

## CASE 92

### Endocardial Cushion Defect

1. A, B, C, D

2. B

3. C

4. D

## *Comment*

An endocardial cushion defect (also known as atrioventricular septal defect or atrioventricular canal defect) represents a broad spectrum of defects of the atrial septum (ostium primum type), ventricular septum (inflow type), and atrioventricular valves. It is a type of congenital left-to-right shunt that has a strong association with trisomy 21 (more than 40% of cases). It may be partial, with presence of mild defects in the atrial septum and atrioventricular valves; intermediate, with additional findings of a mild ventricular septal defect (VSD), or complete, with a common atrioventricular (AV) valve and large ASDs and VSDs. Other common causes of congenital left-to-right shunts include isolated ASDs, VSDs, and patent ductus arteriosus. Imaging findings in left-to-right shunts include an enlarged heart, prominent pulmonary arteries, and mild to moderate pulmonary edema (shunt vascularity). Because oxygenated blood is being shunted in these cases, cyanosis does not typically occur to any significant degree. In complete endocardial cushion defects, cyanosis may be encountered, but is typically mild and intermittent. Surgical correction is the definitive method of treatment.

### Reference

Jacobs JP, Jacobs ML, Mavroudis C, et al. Atrioventricular septal defects: lessons learned about patterns of practice and outcomes from the congenital heart surgery database of the Society of Thoracic Surgeons. *World J Pediatr Congenit Heart Surg*. 2010;1(1):68–77.

### Cross-reference

Walters MM, Robertson RL. *Pediatric Radiology: The Requisites*. 4th ed. Philadelphia: Elsevier; 2017:72.

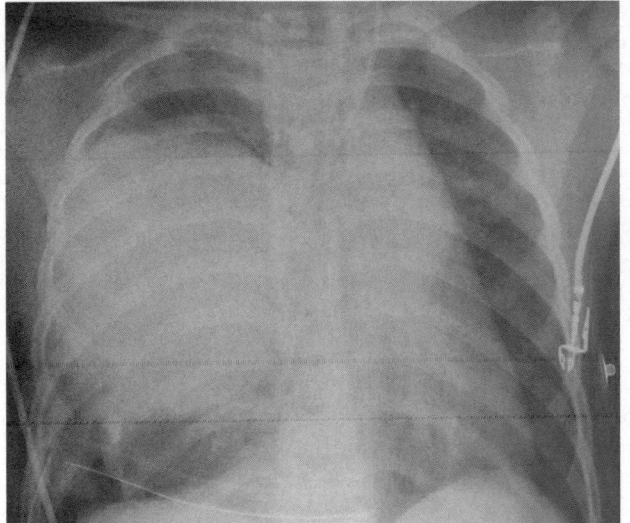

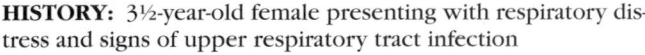

Fig. 93.1

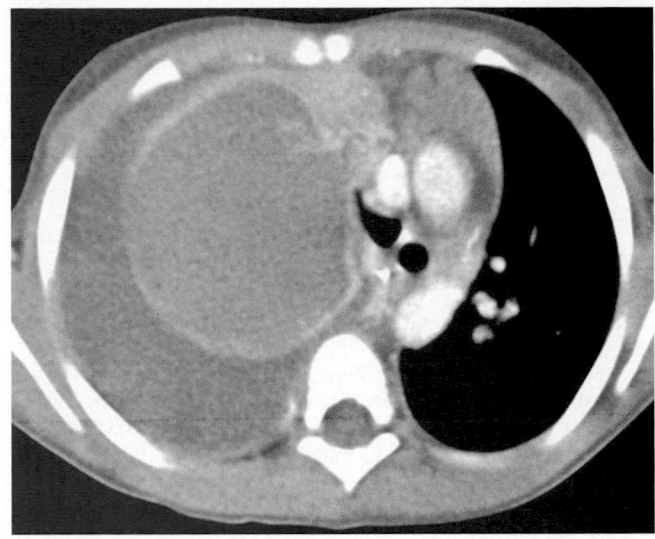

Fig. 93.2

**HISTORY:** 3½-year-old female presenting with respiratory distress and signs of upper respiratory tract infection

1. Based on the plain radiograph, which of the following should be included in the differential diagnosis? (Choose all that apply.)
   A. Congenital pulmonary airway malformation (CPAM)
   B. Congenital lobar emphysema/overinflation
   C. Pulmonary sequestration
   D. Pleuropulmonary blastoma

2. Which lesion has the best prognosis?
   A. Pleuropulmonary blastoma type 1
   B. Pleuropulmonary blastoma type 2
   C. Pleuropulmonary blastoma type 3
   D. Pleuropulmonary blastoma type 4

3. Which statement about pleuropulmonary blastoma is correct?
   A. It is histologically distinct from adult pulmonary blastoma, which has malignant epithelial and mesenchymal components.
   B. It is typically seen in children older than 6 years.
   C. Type 3 typically has the youngest age at presentation, followed by type 2, and then type 1.
   D. Type 3 occurs more frequently in males than in females.

4. True or false?
   A. Type 1 congenital cystic adenomatoid malformation and type 1 pleuropulmonary blastoma are indistinguishable.

### Pleuropulmonary Blastoma

1. A, C, D

2. A

3. A

4. True

## Comment

Pleuropulmonary blastoma (PPB) is a malignant embryonal mesenchymal neoplasm of the lung and pleura that arises during organ development, and most lesions present in children under 6 years of age. By imaging alone, it is often difficult to distinguish this lesion from congenital pulmonary airway malformation (CPAM), because both have cystic and solid subtypes. Cross-sectional imaging can help distinguish PPB from pulmonary sequestration (systemic circulation) and congenital lobar emphysema/overinflation (not a true cystic lesion). There are three PBB subtypes. Type 1 is purely cystic, has the best prognosis, and is indistinguishable from CPAM type 1. Type 2 (cystic and solid) and type 3 (purely solid) have a worse prognosis and typically present later in life than type 1. It is believed that there is a progression from type 1 to type 2 and then type 3.

### Reference

Odev K, Guler I, Altinok T, Pekcan S, Batur A, Ozbiner H. Cystic and cavitary lung lesions in children: radiologic findings with pathologic correlation. *J Clin Imaging Sci.* 2013;3:60.

### Cross-reference

Walters MM, Robertson RL. *Pediatric Radiology: The Requisites.* 4th ed. Philadelphia: Elsevier; 2017:48–51.

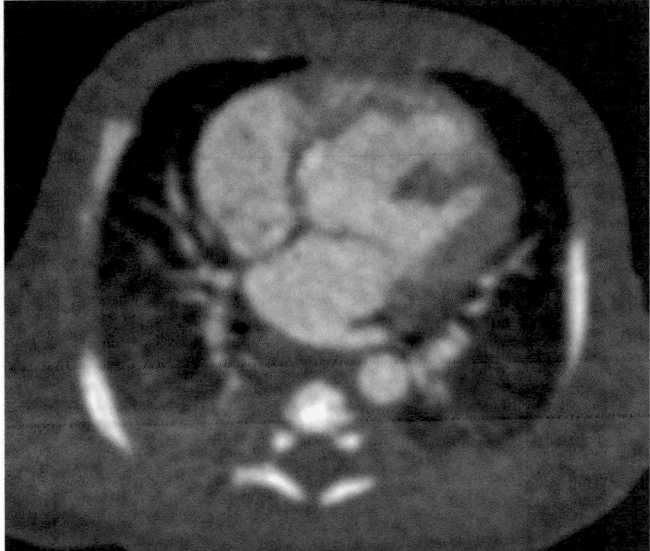

**Fig. 94.1**

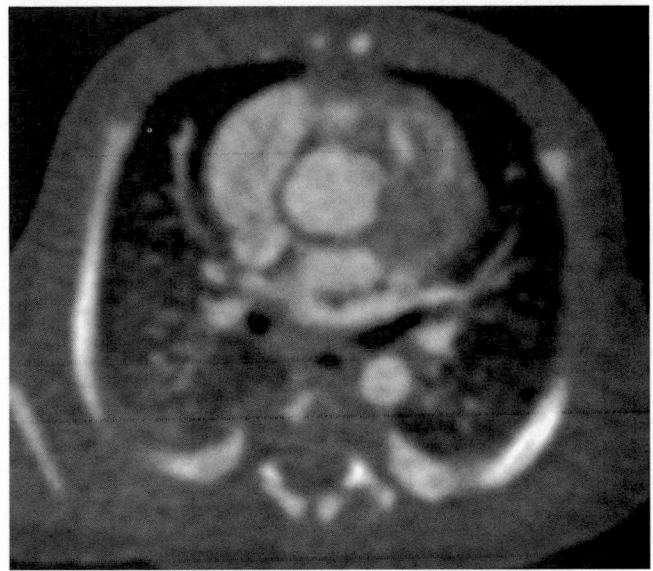

**Fig. 94.2**

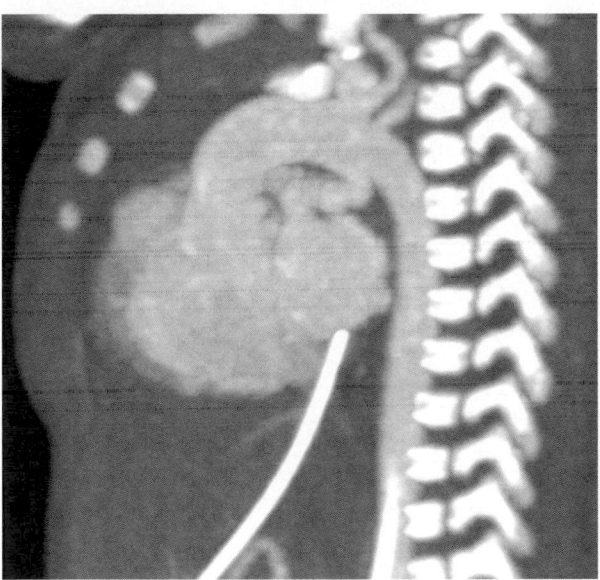

**Fig. 94.3**

**HISTORY:** 1-month-old infant presenting with cyanosis

1. Given the imaging findings and history of cyanosis, which of the following would you include in your differential diagnosis?
   A. D-transposition of the great vessels
   B. Ebstein anomaly
   C. Tetralogy of Fallot (TOF)
   D. Pulmonary atresia with intact ventricular septum

2. Which of the four classic components of TOF is believed to precede and be partially responsible for the other three?
   A. Ventricular septal defect
   B. Right ventricular outflow tract (RVOT) stenosis
   C. Right ventricular hypertrophy
   D. Overriding aorta

3. A right aortic arch is seen with TOF in what percentage of cases?
   A. 5%
   B. 15%
   C. 25%
   D. 45%

4. Which statement about TOF is *not* true?
   A. TOF is the most common congenital cyanotic heart disease.
   B. TOF typically presents by 3 months of age.
   C. 10% of patients have associated arteriovenous canal abnormalities.
   D. The mainstay of treatment consists of placing a shunt from the subclavian artery to the pulmonary artery (Blalock-Taussig shunt).

## CASE 94

### Tetralogy of Fallot

1. C

2. B

3. C

4. D

## Comment

Tetralogy of Fallot (TOF) is the most common type of cyanotic congenital heart disease in children. It is typically diagnosed by 3 months of age. Common associations include right-sided aortic arch (25%) and atrioventricular canal abnormalities (10%). Infundibular right ventricular outflow tract (RVOT) stenosis is believed to precede and result in the other three classic components. Decreased blood flow through the RVOT results in hypoplasia of the RVOT and malalignment of the membranous and muscular septa, leaving a ventricular septal defect. The aorta is drawn medially due to lack of supporting tissue and straddles the septum. The right ventricle hypertrophies because it is exposed to elevated systemic pressures and is forced to pump against a stenosed RVOT. Typical imaging findings include decreased pulmonary blood flow, a normal to slightly enlarged cardiac size, a "boot-shaped" heart due to an upturned cardiac apex (a result of right ventricular hypertrophy), and a concave main pulmonary artery segment. On computed tomography (CT) imaging, an overriding aorta, hypoplastic RVOT, and right ventricular enlargement are typically observed. Ebstein anomaly and pulmonary atresia with intact ventricular septum also present with cyanosis and decreased pulmonary blood flow, but in those cases, there is typically massive cardiomegaly. D-transposition of the great arteries also presents with cyanosis, but typically shows increased pulmonary blood flow. Treatment most commonly involves complete repair of the RVOT and closure of the ventricular septal defect. RVOT restenosis and pulmonary regurgitation are common complications after surgical repair.

### Reference

Puranik R, Mathurangu V, Celermajer DS, Taylor AM. Congenital heart disease and multi-modality imaging. *Heart Lung Circ.* 2010;19(3):133–144.

### Cross-reference

Walters MM, Robertson RL. *Pediatric Radiology: The Requisites*. 4th ed. Philadelphia: Elsevier; 2017:78–81.

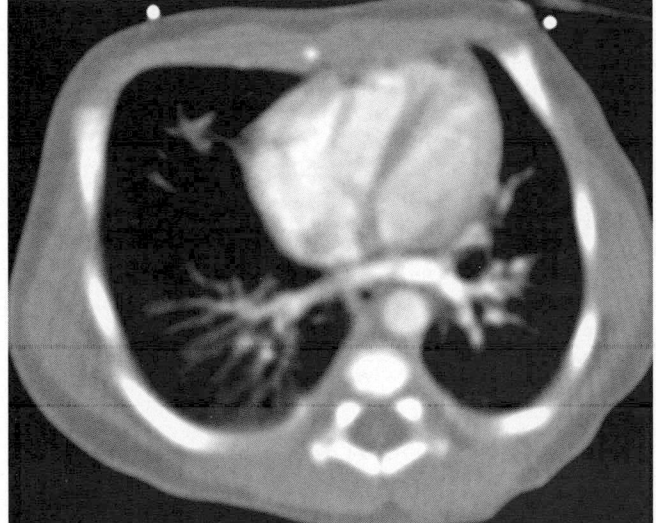

Fig. 95.1

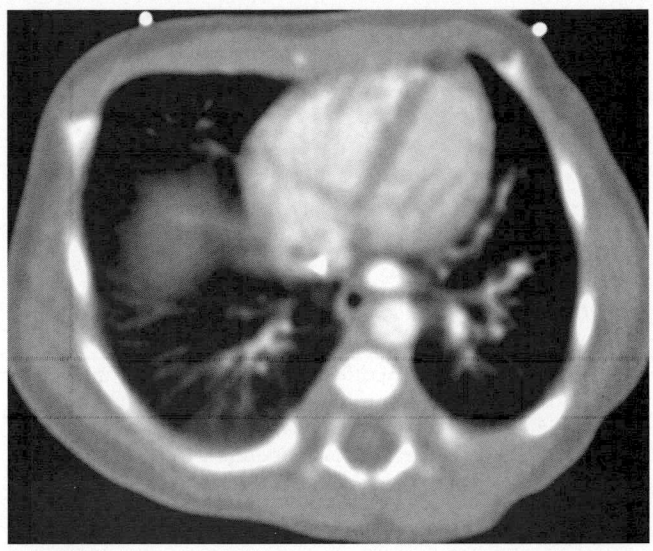

Fig. 95.2

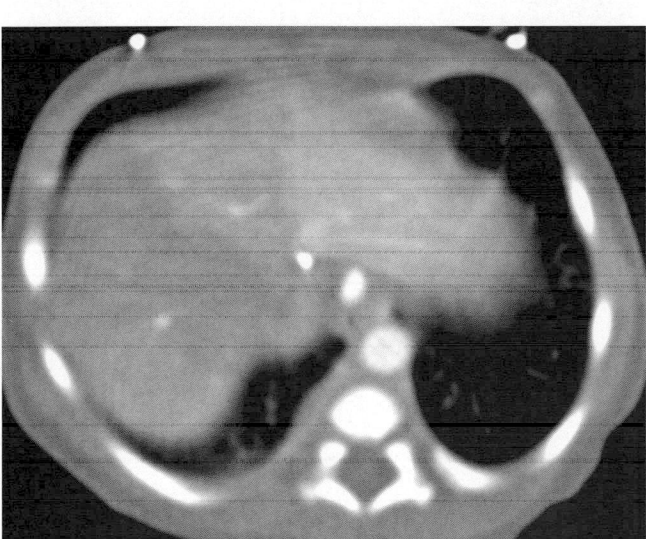

Fig. 95.3

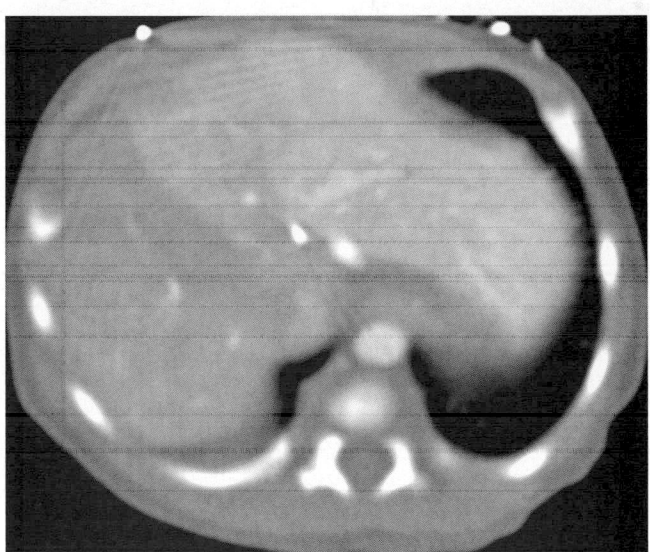

Fig. 95.4

**HISTORY:** Newborn infant presenting with cyanosis

1. Based on the imaging findings and clinical history, what is the best diagnosis?
   A. Truncus arteriosus
   B. Total anomalous pulmonary venous return (TAPVR)
   C. D-transposition of the great arteries
   D. Tetralogy of Fallot

2. Which type of TAPVR is most likely to present with pulmonary venous congestion?
   A. Type I: Supracardiac
   B. Type II: Cardiac
   C. Type III: Infracardiac
   D. Cannot tell, not enough information.

3. In type I TAPVR, the left superior aspect of the "snowman" appearance on the anteroposterior (AP) radiograph of the chest is due to which of the following?
   A. Dilation of the superior vena cava (SVC)
   B. Left vertical vein
   C. Duplicate SVC
   D. Reactive mediastinal adenopathy

4. Which type of TAPVR presents earliest and with the most severe cyanosis?
   A. Type I: Supracardiac
   B. Type II: Cardiac
   C. Type III: Infracardiac
   D. No significant difference between the different types

## CASE 95

### Total Anomalous Pulmonary Venous Return

1. B
2. C
3. B
4. C

### *Comment*

In total anomalous pulmonary venous return (TAPVR), the pulmonary veins are connected to systemic venous structures that drain into the right atrium, thus forming a left-to-right shunt resulting in hypoxemia. There are three TAPVR subtypes, supracardiac, cardiac, and infracardiac, depending on where the pulmonary veins connect to the systemic venous circulation. In the supracardiac type, the pulmonary veins converge to form a left vertical vein that drains into the left brachiocephalic vein. In the cardiac type, the pulmonary veins drain directly into the right atrium or coronary sinus. In the infracardiac type, the veins pass through the esophageal hiatus of the diaphragm to connect to the portal vein, ductus venosus, or inferior vena cava (IVC). These veins can be obstructed as they pass through the diaphragm, leading to venous congestion and pulmonary edema, which is why this type presents earliest and with the most severe cyanosis. In types I and II, there is no obstruction to flow and the imaging findings are those of a left-to-right shunt with shunt vascularity (e.g., prominent proximal pulmonary arteries), as can be seen, for example, with atrial septal defect (ASD). In type I, the "snowman" appearance is classic and is formed by the left vertical vein and superior vena cava (SVC) forming the left and right upper border of the snowman, respectively, and the heart forming the lower part of the snowman.

### Reference

Dyer KT, Hlavacek AM, Meinel FG, et al. Imaging in congenital pulmonary vein anomalies: the role of computed tomography. *Pediatr Radiol.* 2014;44(9):1158–1168.

### Cross-reference

Walters MM, Robertson RL. *Pediatric Radiology: The Requisites.* 4th ed. Philadelphia: Elsevier; 2017:78.

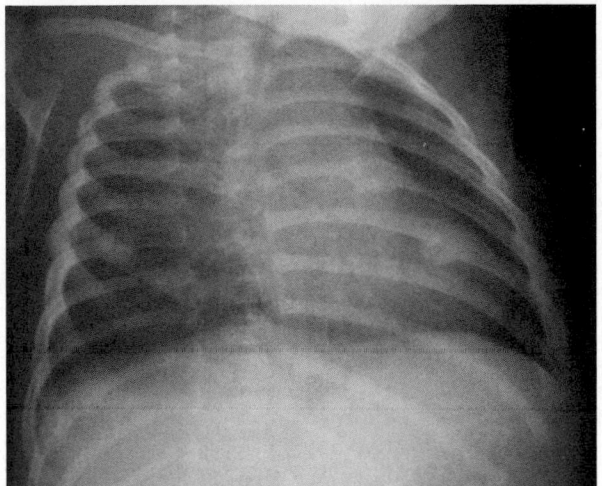

Fig. 96.1

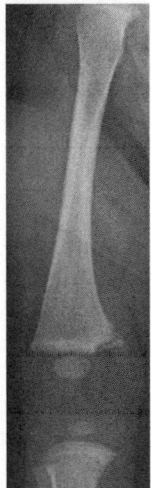

Fig. 96.2

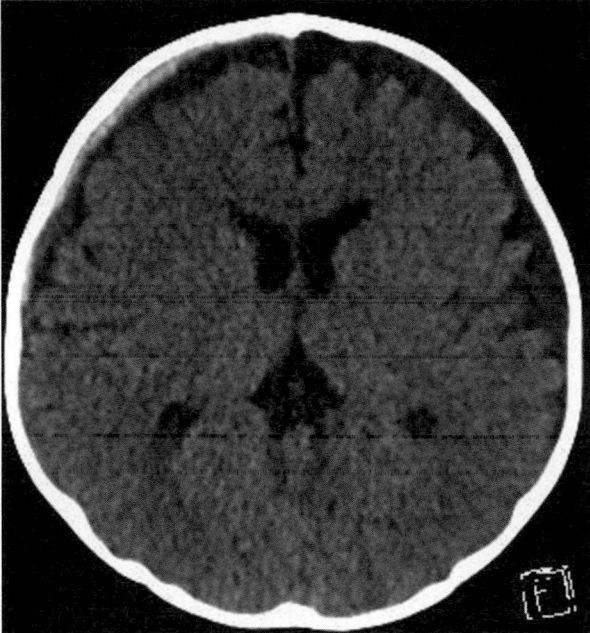

Fig. 96.3

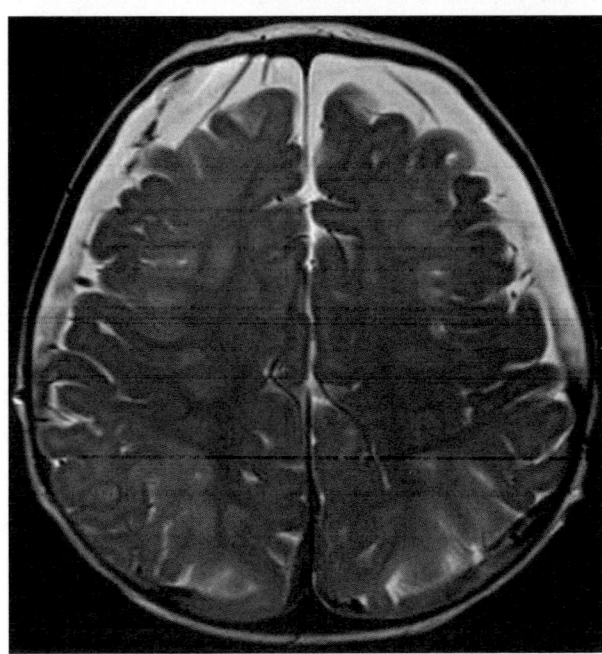

Fig. 96.4

**HISTORY:** 5-month-old male brought to the emergency department due to a fall from the couch 2 days ago

1. Based on the provided images, what is the most likely diagnosis?
   A. Abusive head trauma (AHT)
   B. Shaken baby syndrome
   C. Nonaccidental injury
   D. All of the above

2. Which of the following findings are present in the provided images?
   A. Thin supratentorial hemorrhage
   B. Metaphyseal corner fracture of the femur
   C. Bilateral multiple healing rib fractures
   D. Ischemic injury to bilateral brain parenchyma as evidenced by increased T2 signal and thrombosis in the right frontal bridging vein
   E. All of the above

3. Neuroimaging has become an important tool in court in cases with suspected AHT. Which statement is most accurate?

A. The presence of subdural and retinal hemorrhages is sufficient to make an AHT diagnosis.
B. Computed tomography (CT) of the head is accurate in determining the age of subdural and parenchymal hemorrhages.
C. Magnetic resonance imaging (MRI) is accurate in determining the age of subdural and epidural hemorrhages but not parenchymal hemorrhages.
D. The presence of extraaxial hemorrhages (most commonly subdural), parenchymal ischemic injuries, and retinal hemorrhages can be highly suggestive of AHT in the setting of a discordant clinical history.

4. Which of the following choices best describes the skeletal manifestations of nonaccidental injury?
   A. Multiple, especially posterior, rib fractures of different ages are common.
   B. Metaphyseal fractures in the lower extremities are common.
   C. Scapula and metatarsal fractures are highly suggestive.
   D. All of the above.

## CASE 96

### Child Abuse

1. D
2. E
3. D
4. D

### Comment

Abusive head trauma (AHT) is suspected if the caregiver denies a history of trauma or there is a discrepancy between the caregiver's explanation and the lesions. AHT is also suspected if there are injuries of different ages or multiple injuries, a change or inconsistency in history, delay in medical care, or overall poor care of the child. Although shaking an infant has the potential to cause neurologic injury, blunt impact or a combination of shaking and blunt impact can cause injury as well. The American Academy of Pediatrics recommends a less mechanistic term, AHT, when describing an inflicted injury to the head and its contents. In 2012, there were more than 678,000 confirmed cases of child abuse associated with 1640 fatalities in the United States. At least one-third of AHT cases are not identified upon initial presentation to the emergency department, which indicates that a careful history and physical exam are required, including a skeletal survey when abuse is suspected. AHT is the most common reason for traumatic death in children less than 1 year of age. AHT most commonly affects children younger than 6 months, and the median age is 2 to 4 months. Males are more commonly affected than females and the perpetrators are usually the father, the mother's boyfriend, or a female babysitter.

AHT includes any nonaccidental inflicted injury to a child's head and body. AHT, often characterized but not limited to repetitive acceleration-deceleration forces with or without blunt head impact, has a mortality rate of 30%, and 80% of survivors suffer permanent neurologic damage. Ocular manifestations of AHT are typically identified by dilated funduscopic ophthalmic exam showing retinal hemorrhages that are too numerous to count, multilayered, and extending to the periphery. Because almost 80% of AHT causes retinal abnormalities, a noninvasive imaging tool, ophthalmic ultrasound, is a potential screening tool.

Dating of skeletal fractures is challenging because although metaphyseal fractures become somewhat more prominent during their healing phase, they do not heal with typical callus formation. Metaphyseal fractures are usually seen within the first year of life. A bucket-handle fracture of the distal tibial metaphysis and corner fractures of the distal femur metaphysis are highly suggestive of nonaccidental injury. Tight gripping of the chest during inflicted injury is believed to result in posterior rib fractures.

Dating of intracranial hemorrhages is known to be inaccurate when based on computed tomography (CT) and magnetic resonance imaging (MRI), despite the use of advanced techniques. This is partly due to a mixture of cerebrospinal fluid (CSF) and blood products that creates heterogeneity. Thin subdural hemorrhages are common in the supratentorial brain, but can be seen infratentorially as well. White matter contusional tears (little hemorrhagic clefts in the subcortical and periventricular white matter) can be seen in infants younger than 4 to 6 months of age. Bridging vein thrombosis (as shown in this case) is another common finding. A variety of ischemic injuries, limited to a single lobe, single hemisphere, bilateral hemispheres, or diffuse anoxic ischemic injuries, can be seen. Skull fractures can be seen, most commonly affecting the parietal bone. Subdural and subarachnoid hemorrhages are more common in AHT than in accidental head trauma, but diffuse axonal injury and epidural hematoma are more common in accidental trauma. Parenchymal ischemia and laceration are more common in AHT.

Although a very serious health concern, there is no gold standard for diagnosis. Early suspicion is critical and detailed imaging data must be collected and interpreted to provide a clinical history with a multidisciplinary approach.

### References

Christian CW, Block R. Committee on Child Abuse and Neglect, American Academy of Pediatrics. Abusive head trauma in infants and children. *Pediatrics.* 2009;123(5):1409–1411.

Tung GA, Kumar M, Richardson RC, Jenny C, Brown WD. Comparison of accidental and nonaccidental traumatic head injury in children on non-contrast computed tomography. *Pediatrics.* 2006;118(2):626–633.

### Cross-reference

Walters MM, Robertson RL. *Pediatric Radiology: The Requisites.* 4th ed. Philadelphia: Elsevier. 2017;258–259:316–317.

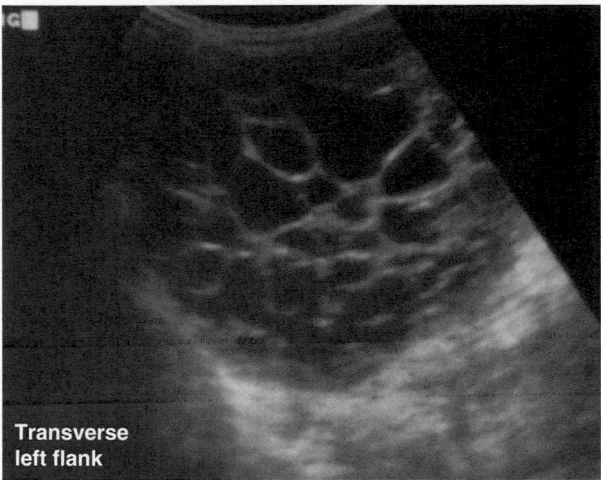

**Fig. 111.1**

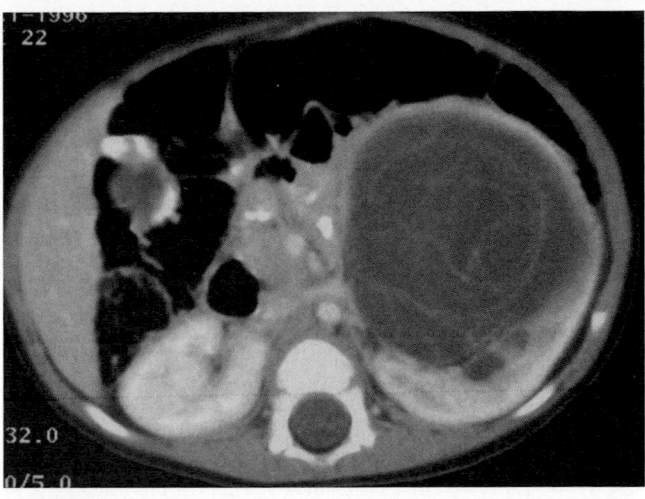

**Fig. 111.2**

**HISTORY:** Patient referred to imaging for evaluation of a painless abdominal mass

1. Based on the imaging findings, which of the following would you include in your differential diagnosis? (Choose all that apply.)
   A. Multicystic dysplastic kidney
   B. Cystic nephroma
   C. Cystic partially differentiated nephroblastoma (CPDN)
   D. Cystic Wilms tumor
   E. Cystic renal cell carcinoma

2. Which statement about multilocular cystic renal tumors (MCRTs) is *not* true?
   A. MCRTs may have small areas of nodular enhancement.
   B. There are two types of MCRT: cystic nephroma and CPDN.
   C. MCRTs are more common in males in the pediatric age group and more common in females in the adult age group.
   D. There is no contrast excretion into the cystic spaces.

3. Which statement about MCRTs is true?
   A. Cystic nephroma and CPDN can be reliably distinguished based on their imaging appearance.
   B. MCRT and cystic Wilms tumor can be reliably distinguished based on their imaging appearance.
   C. MCRT and multicystic dysplastic kidney can be reliably distinguished based on their imaging appearance.
   D. MCRT and cystic renal cell carcinoma can be reliably distinguished based on their imaging appearance.

4. Which option describes the typical management of MCRTs?
   A. Radiofrequency ablation
   B. Renal sonography for screening at 3-month intervals until 7 years of age
   C. Chemotherapy
   D. Partial or complete nephrectomy

## CASE 111

### Multilocular Cystic Renal Tumor

1. B, C, D, E
2. A
3. C
4. D

### *Comment*

There are two types of multilocular cystic renal tumors (MCRTs): cystic nephroma and cystic partially differentiated nephroblastoma (CPDN). Both are benign neoplasms containing multiple cysts without any solid tissue except for the thin septa separating the cysts and a surrounding fibrous capsule. These are typically not familial and are thus not present at birth. The difference on histology between these tumors is the presence of blastemal elements (nephrogenic rests) within the septa in CPDN. Neither metastasize, but the presence of blastemal elements in CPDN is associated with slightly more aggressive behavior of these tumors and a higher rate of recurrence. Nevertheless, prognosis is excellent with both tumors, and treatment is with resection. There is a bimodal age distribution. Children show male predominance, and presentation is between 3 months and 4 years of age. In adults, there is female predominance, and presentation is typically between 40 and 60 years of age. The two tumors cannot be distinguished by clinical or imaging criteria. Both appear as a well-circumscribed multicystic mass with thin septations and a surrounding fibrous capsule. The tumor may herniate into the renal sinus, and there is no excretion of contrast material into the cysts. In larger tumors, there is typically a "claw sign" of normal, compressed renal tissue at the periphery of the mass. In addition, imaging cannot reliably distinguish these tumors from a cystic Wilms tumor or cystic renal cell carcinoma, underscoring the importance of resection of these tumors. Multicystic dysplastic kidney, unlike MCRTs, is present in utero and at birth, and there is no normal renal parenchyma present.

### References

Grania MF, O'brien AT, Trujillo S, Mancera J, Aguirre DA. Multilocular cystic nephroma: a systematic literature review of the radiologic and clinical findings. *AJR Am J Roentgenol*. 2015;205(6):1188–1193.

Joshi VV, Beckwith JB. Multilocular cyst of the kidney (cystic nephroma) and cystic, partially differentiated nephroblastoma. Terminology and criteria for diagnosis. *Cancer*. 1989;64(2):466–479.

### Cross-reference

Walters MM, Robertson RL. *Pediatric Radiology: The Requisites*. 4th ed. Philadelphia: Elsevier; 2017:162.

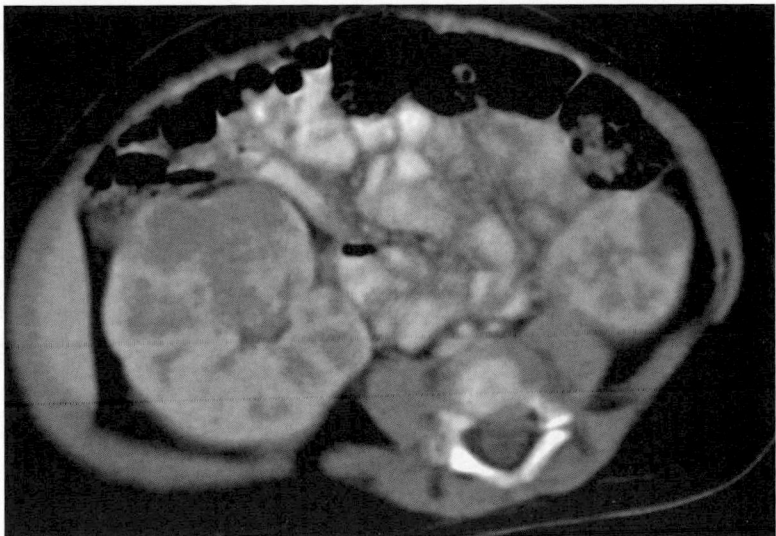

**Fig. 112.1**

**HISTORY:** 4-month-old infant with abdominal distention

1. Based on the imaging findings, which of the following would you include in your differential diagnosis? (Choose all that apply.)
   A. Pyelonephritis
   B. Wilms tumor
   C. Nephroblastomatosis
   D. Leukemia/lymphoma

2. Perilobar nephrogenic rests are associated with which syndromes? (Choose all that apply.)
   A. Beckwith-Wiedemann syndrome
   B. Hemihypertrophy syndrome
   C. Trisomy 18 syndrome
   D. Denys-Drash syndrome
   E. WAGR (Wilms tumor, aniridia, genitourinary anomalies, and intellectual disability [formerly referred to as mental retardation]) syndrome

3. Intralobar nephrogenic rests are associated with which syndromes? (Choose all that apply.)
   A. Beckwith-Wiedemann syndrome
   B. Hemihypertrophy syndrome
   C. Trisomy 18 syndrome
   D. Denys-Drash syndrome
   E. WAGR syndrome

4. Which statement about nephroblastomatosis is *not* true?
   A. Most cases show spontaneous regression.
   B. Syndromic Wilms tumors are more commonly associated with nephroblastomatosis than are sporadic cases of Wilms tumor.
   C. Screening for Wilms tumor in the setting of nephroblastomatosis is most commonly performed with ultrasound (US) and/or magnetic resonance imaging (MRI).
   D. Nephroblastomatosis may appear on imaging as homogeneous hyperenhancing subcapsular masses.

## CASE 112

### Nephroblastomatosis

1. B, C, D
2. A, B, C
3. D, E
4. D

### Comment

Nephroblastomatosis is characterized by the abnormal presence of diffuse or multifocal nephrogenic rests (persistent meta-nephric blastema) beyond 36 weeks' gestational age. The two pathologic subtypes are perilobar and intralobar nephrogenic rests. The perilobar subtype is found in the renal cortex or at the corticomedullary junction and is associated with a 1% to 2% risk of developing Wilms tumor. It is associated with Beckwith-Wiedemann syndrome, Perlman syndrome, hemihypertrophy, and trisomy 18. The intralobar subtype is found deeper in the renal parenchyma and is associated with a higher (4% to 5%) risk of developing Wilms tumor than is the perilobar type. It is associated with Denys-Drash and WAGR (Wilms tumor, aniridia, genitourinary anomalies, and intellectual disability [formerly referred to as mental retardation]) syndromes. In general, Wilms tumors associated with underlying syndromes are more commonly bilateral and found together with nephrogenic rests than is the case for sporadic Wilms tumors. Overall, only a small percentage of persistent nephrogenic rests develop into Wilms tumor, and most cases of nephroblastomatosis regress spontaneously. However, given the risk of developing Wilms tumor, especially in patients with underlying syndromes, short interval screening is performed with ultrasound (US) and/or magnetic resonance imaging (MRI). On imaging, nephro-blastomatosis may be diffuse or multifocal, and typical imaging appearance consists of homogeneous subcapsular oval or thick rind-like renal masses that enhance less than the rest of the renal parenchyma (the image provided demonstrates multiple perilobar nephrogenic rests in a patient with Beckwith-Wiedemann syndrome). On US, these masses are typically iso- to hypoechoic. On MRI, they demonstrate iso- to hypointensity on both T1- and T2-weighted images. Findings that suggest conversion to Wilms tumor include interval increase in size and/or increase in heterogeneity of the mass(es). Biopsy is often not helpful because microscopic patterns of nephrogenic rests and Wilms tumor can be similar.

### Reference

Heller MT, Haarer KA, Thomas E, Thaete FL. Neoplastic and proliferative disorders of the perinephric space. *Clin Radiol*. 2012;67(11): e31–e41.

### Cross-reference

Walters MM, Robertson RL. *Pediatric Radiology: The Requisites*. 4th ed. Philadelphia: Elsevier; 2017:164–165.

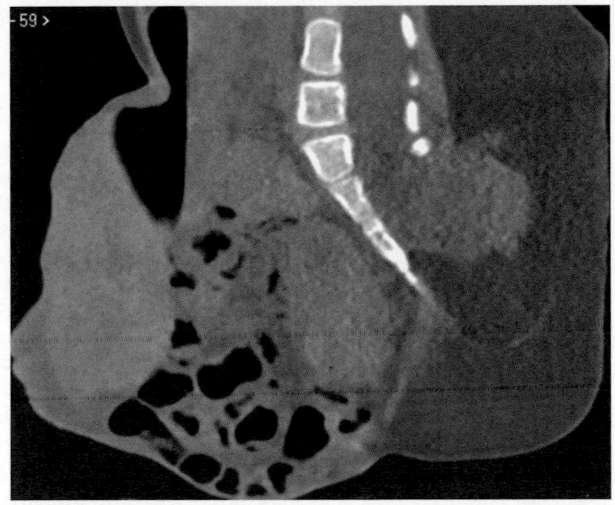

**Fig. 113.1**

See Supplemental Figures section for additional figures for this case.

**HISTORY:** History withheld

1. What is the most likely diagnosis?
   A. Caudal regression syndrome
   B. Vertebral defects, anal atresia, cardiac defects, tracheo-esophageal fistula, renal anomalies, and limb abnormalities (VACTERL)
   C. Gastroschisis
   D. Omphalocele, exstrophy, imperforate anus, spinal defects (OEIS)

2. Which of the following is most appropriate for genetic counseling?
   A. Autosomal dominant inheritance pattern, therefore a parental genetic workup is necessary
   B. Autosomal recessive inheritance pattern, therefore a parental genetic workup is necessary
   C. X-linked inheritance pattern, therefore only the father needs a genetic workup
   D. Sporadic but somewhat increased risk reported in the siblings

3. Which of the following embryonic structures is maldeveloped in OEIS?
   A. Vitelline duct
   B. Cloaca
   C. Mullerian duct
   D. Notochord

4. True or false?
   A. Classic bladder exstrophy is more common than epispadias.
   B. Pubic diastasis progressively worsens from classic bladder exstrophy to OEIS complex.
   C. Iliac osteotomy is helpful in reducing the pelvic tension and increasing the chances of successful primary closure of the exstrophy.

## CASE 113

### OEIS (Omphalocele, Exstrophy, Imperforate Anus, and Spinal Defects)

1. D

2. D

3. B

4. A) True, B) True, C) True

## Comment

Omphalocele, exstrophy, imperforate anus, and spinal defects (OEIS) is a rare complex and represents the most severe form of epispadias-exstrophy sequence, ranging from epispadias, pubic diastasis, classic bladder exstrophy (isolated), to cloacal exstrophy, that is, OEIS. OEIS occurs with an incidence of 1 in 200,000 to 400,000 live births. The occurrence of classic exstrophy of the bladder appears to be more common (1 in 30,000 to 40,000). The incidence of OEIS is probably higher because many cases are incorrectly diagnosed as omphalocele, which is the most prominent component of this malformation complex. In humans, the cloaca is a phylogenetic embryonic structure where the genital, urinary, and digestive organs have a common outlet. The normal development gives origin to the lower abdominal wall with the bladder, the intestine, the anus, the genital organs, part of the pelvic bones, and the lumbosacral spine. OEIS is considered to be a defect in blastogenesis, beginning in the first 4 weeks of human development. In patients with exstrophy the lower abdominal wall has a midline defect, through which the bladder plate is exposed. Pubic diastasis is the pelvic skeletal hallmark of the exstrophy, which progressively worsens toward the OEIS complex end of the spectrum. Additional pelvic bony abnormalities include widened iliac wing angles. The levator ani is flattened and the anus is anteriorly displaced in classic exstrophy patients, whereas atresia is seen in OEIS.

Differential diagnosis includes omphalocele or gastroschisis (isolated), classic bladder exstrophy, and limb-body wall complex. Associated cardiac and renal anomalies can also be seen. A multidisciplinary approach with collaboration among pediatric surgeons, urologists, orthopedic surgeons, neurosurgeons, gynecologists, and neonatologists is paramount in the management of children with OEIS syndrome. Initial management consists of identifying associated anomalies including renal, gastrointestinal, and spine anomalies. During the initial surgical management of the newborn, the omphalocele must be repaired and the fecal stream diverted due to anal atresia. Bladder exstrophy closure needs to be repaired either primarily or in stages.

This 2-year-old patient never had the omphalocele repaired. Note the herniation of the bowel loops. The surface-rendered 3D reconstructed image shows the marked pubic diastasis and formation/segmentation anomalies. Note the lipomyelomeningocele that is partially visualized.

### Reference

Allam ES, Shetty VS, Farmakis SG. Fetal and neonatal presentation of OEIS complex. *J Pediatr Surg*. 2015;50(12):2155–2158.

### Cross-reference

Walters MM, Robertson RL. *Pediatric Radiology: The Requisites*. 4th ed. Philadelphia: Elsevier; 2017:156, 328.

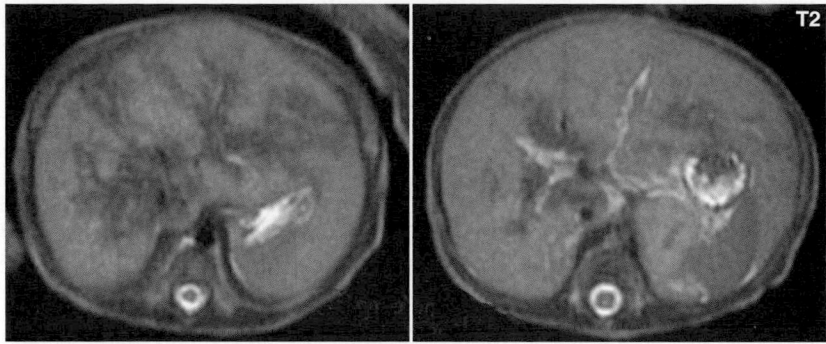

5-day-old neonate

**Fig. 114.1**

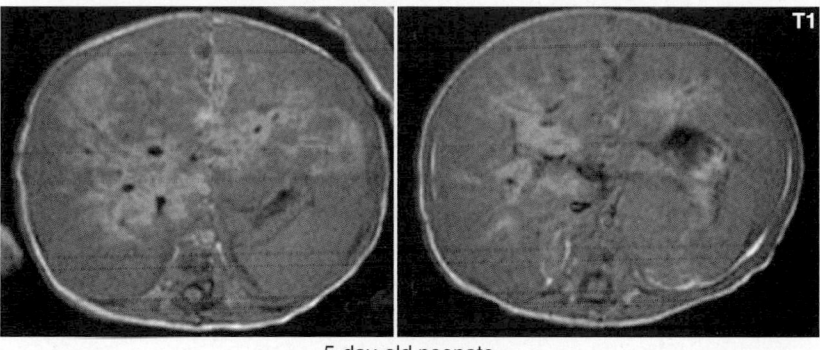

5-day-old neonate

**Fig. 114.2**

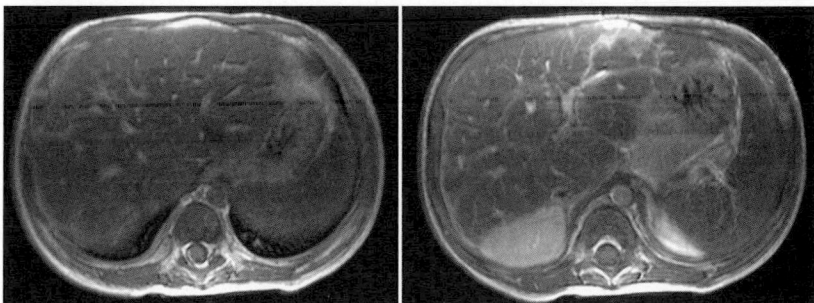

Follow-up at 10 months

**Fig. 114.3**

**HISTORY:** Initial T2- and T1-weighted magnetic resonance imaging (MRI) of a neonate with a protuberant abdomen and follow-up at 10 months without treatment

1. Which signature pathologic imaging finding do you see?
   A. Enlarged liver secondary to storage disease
   B. Enlarged liver secondary to portal vein thrombosis
   C. Enlarged liver secondary to congenital heart disease
   D. Enlarged liver due to diffuse metastatic disease

2. Is there an additional lesion that could be linked to the liver abnormality?
   A. Left paravertebral neurofibroma
   B. Left paravertebral Ewing sarcoma
   C. Left adrenal gland neuroblastoma
   D. Left adrenal gland hemorrhage

3. If no other lesions are present, what is the most likely diagnosis/staging?
   A. Neuroblastoma stage 1
   B. Neuroblastoma stage 2
   C. Neuroblastoma stage 3
   D. Neuroblastoma stage 4S

4. Which statement is correct?
   A. Neuroblastomas typically arise from the urogenital crest.
   B. Neuroblastoma stage 4S may have a spontaneous regression.
   C. Neuroblastoma typically has elevated serum levels of alpha-fetoprotein.
   D. Neuroblastoma may present with excessive hirsutism.

## CASE 114

### Neuroblastoma

1. D
2. C
3. D
4. B

## Comment

Neuroblastoma (NBL) is one of the most common solid malignancies in children originating from the neural crest cells of the sympathetic nervous system. There are increasing degrees of cellular differentiation/benignity along a spectrum: neuroblastoma (malignant), ganglioneuroblastoma (GNBL), and ganglioneuroma (GN, benign).

Neuroblastomas can be seen anywhere along the sympathetic chain reaching from the neck into the pelvis, usually in a paravertebral location. The adrenal glands are most often affected. Clinical presentation varies with the primary location. Neuroblastomas may be large with heterogeneous calcifications, displace solid organs, and wrap or engulf major vessels. Paravertebral neuroblastomas have a tendency to invade the spinal canal through widened neuroforamina. Epidural tumor extension with compression of the spinal cord can result in significant neurologic deficits. Diffuse metastatic disease may affect the liver, bone marrow, and skin. The characteristic raccoon eyes are a result of metastatic disease in the orbits and skull base. Nearly 90% of cases have elevated levels of catecholamines in the urine.

Neuroblastomas are classified in four stages. In stage 1, the tumor involves a single organ. Stages 2 and 3 show extension beyond the organ, crossing the midline or not crossing the midline, respectively. Stage 4 is characterized by metastatic disease. Stage 4S is a unique form in which children younger than 1 year of age have a localized tumor with metastatic dissemination limited to the liver, skin, or bone marrow. The survival rate of stage 4S is nearly 100%. This good prognosis relies on the unique feature that a spontaneous regression occurs with transformation of undifferentiated tumor cells into benign, well-differentiated cells.

Conventional radiography may show a nonspecific soft tissue mass with intralesional calcifications. Cross-sectional imaging is essential for tumor staging. The tumor is typically heterogeneous on ultrasound and computed tomography (CT), and dispersed calcifications are well seen on CT. Magnetic resonance imaging (MRI) is, however, the imaging modality of choice. The tumor is typically T2 hyperintense and T1 hypointense. Neuroblastomas show avid radiotracer uptake on metaiodobenzylguanidine (MIBG) scans.

### Reference

Irwin MS, Park JR. Neuroblastoma: paradigm for precision medicine. *Pediatr Clin North Am*. 2015;62:225-256.

### Cross-reference

Walters MM, Robertson RL. *Pediatric Radiology: The Requisites*. 4th ed. Philadelphia: Elsevier; 2017:350.

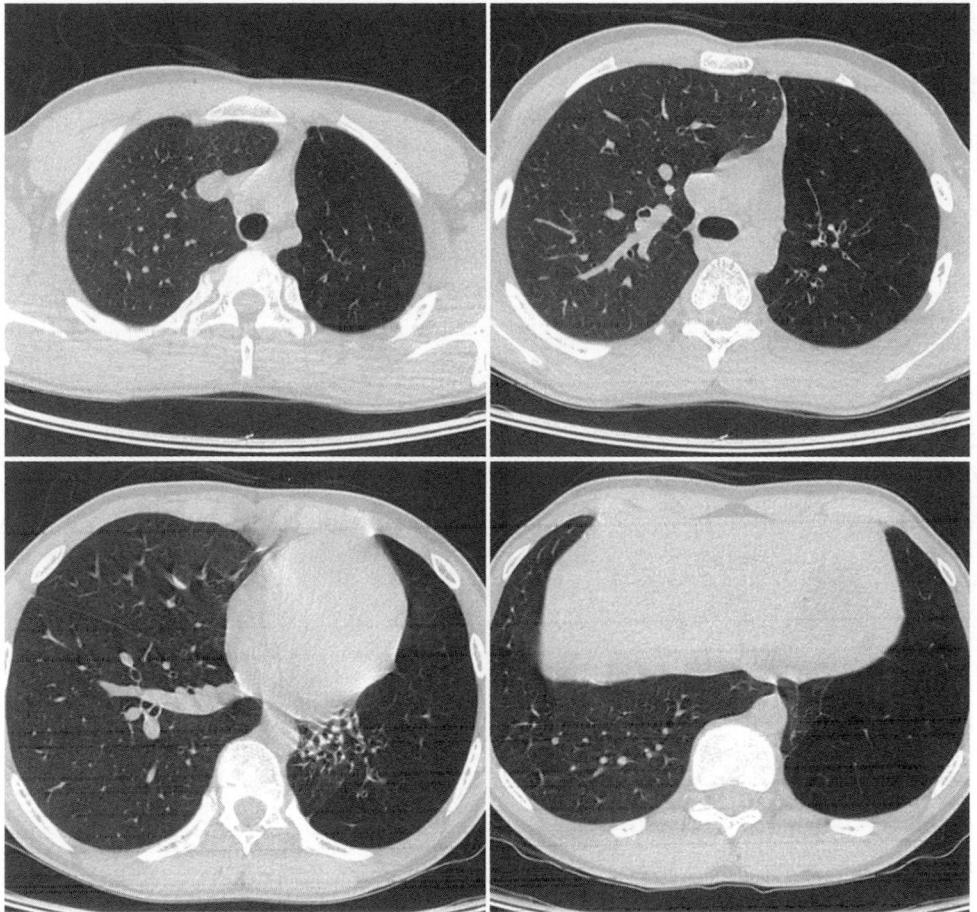

Fig. 115.1

**HISTORY:** Patient with history of recurrent pneumonia presenting with chronic cough and wheezing

1. Based on the imaging findings, which of the following is the best diagnosis?
   A. Poland syndrome
   B. Pneumothorax
   C. Swyer-James syndrome
   D. Proximal interruption of the pulmonary artery

2. What is believed to be the underlying etiology in Swyer-James syndrome?
   A. Congenital hypoplasia of a lobe or lung segment
   B. Congenital hypoplasia of the pulmonary artery
   C. Acquired pulmonary hypoplasia due to postinfectious bronchiolitis obliterans early in life (less than age 8)
   D. Congenital unilateral absence of the pectoralis musculature leading to a unilateral hyperlucent hemithorax

3. What accounts for the hyperlucent lung seen in Swyer-James syndrome?
   A. Combination of hypoperfusion and air trapping
   B. Air trapping
   C. Hypoperfusion
   D. Congenital absence of the pectoralis musculature in the chest wall

4. True or false?
   A. Bronchiolitis obliterans is a nonspecific pathologic finding that can occur after infection, after exposure to toxic fumes, as a complication after organ transplant, in adverse drug reactions, and for other reasons.

## CASE 115

### Swyer-James Syndrome

1. C

2. C

3. A

4. True

### Comment

Swyer-James syndrome (SJS) is an acquired unilateral pulmonary hypoplasia secondary to postinfectious bronchiolitis obliterans (also known as constrictive bronchiolitis) early in life (<8 years). Bronchiolitis obliterans is a nonspecific pathologic process related to concentric fibrosis of the submucosal and peribronchial tissues of the terminal and respiratory bronchioles, resulting in bronchial narrowing or obliteration. In addition to infectious causes, bronchiolitis obliterans can occur following lung transplantation, after toxic fume inhalation, as a drug reaction, in connective tissue disorders, and for other reasons. In SJS, postinfectious bronchiolitis obliterans early in life results in disturbance of normal lung development due to progressive peripheral air trapping and diminished pulmonary blood flow. The most common inciting organisms are believed to be adenovirus, respiratory syncytial virus, influenza A, and *Mycoplasma pneumoniae*. Imaging reflects the underlying pathogenesis, with asymmetric hyperlucent lung with a diminished number and caliber of vessels, as well as air trapping on expiration. The affected segment or lobe may show reduced volume related to hypoplasia. Although proximal interruption of the pulmonary artery may also present with a small oligemic hyperlucent lung, there will not be air trapping on expiration, and blood flow to the affected lung will be from the systemic circulation via bronchial, internal mammary, and intercostal collateral arteries.

### Reference

Damle NA, Mishra R, Wadhwa JK. Classical imaging triad in a very young child with Swyer-James syndrome. *Nucl Med Mol Imaging*. 2012;46(2):115-118.

### Cross-reference

Walters MM, Robertson RL. *Pediatric Radiology: The Requisites*. 4th ed. Philadelphia: Elsevier; 2017:39-40.

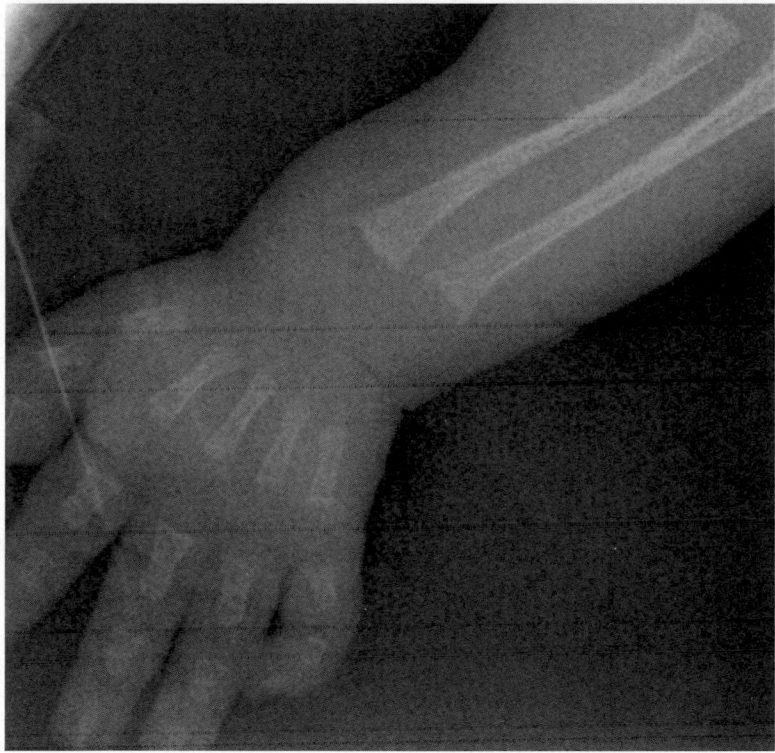

Fig. 116.1

**HISTORY:** 6-month-old male presenting with slow growth rate

1. Based on the imaging findings, which of the following should be included in the differential diagnosis? (Choose all that apply.)
   A. Hypophosphatemic rickets
   B. Vitamin D–deficiency rickets
   C. Leukemia
   D. Hypophosphatasia

2. What is the most common inheritance pattern of hypophosphatemic (vitamin D–resistant) rickets?
   A. Autosomal dominant
   B. Autosomal recessive
   C. X-linked dominant
   D. X-linked recessive

3. What is the underlying pathogenesis in hypophosphatemic rickets?
   A. Malabsorption of phosphate
   B. Decreased phosphate reabsorption from the proximal renal tubules and inhibition of 1-α-hydroxylation of 25-hydroxy vitamin D
   C. Defective hydrolysis of inorganic phosphate leading to extracellular accumulation of inorganic pyrophosphate, which inhibits formation of hydroxyapatite
   D. Defective formation of 25-hydroxy vitamin D in the liver

4. True or false?
   A. Vitamin D–deficiency rickets and hypophosphatemic (vitamin D–resistant) rickets can be differentiated based on their characteristic imaging findings.

## CASE 116

### Hypophosphatemic Rickets

1. A, B, D

2. C

3. B

4. False

### *Comment*

Bone consists mostly of mineral (hydroxyapatite) deposited on a matrix (osteoid) that is composed primarily of collagen. Rickets arises in the immature skeleton when there is failure to mineralize osteoid and cartilage at growth plates, resulting in metaphyseal cupping and splaying, physeal widening, bowing of long bones, and loss of dense zones of provisional calcification. The most common cause is vitamin D deficiency, related to decreased dietary uptake, malabsorption, inadequate exposure to sunlight, liver disease (decreased formation of 25-hydroxy vitamin D), or renal disease (decreased 1-α-hydroxylation of 25-hydroxy vitamin D). Vitamin D is necessary to promote maturation and mineralization of the osteoid matrix by osteoblasts. To mineralize the osteoid matrix, osteoblasts require adequate levels of calcium and phosphate (key components of hydroxyapatite). Thus, disorders of calcium and phosphate metabolism may also cause rickets. Hypophosphatemic rickets, also known as vitamin D–resistant rickets, is most commonly inherited in an X-linked dominant pattern and is caused by various impairments of renal tubular reabsorption of phosphate and inhibition of 1-α-hydroxylation of 25-hydroxy vitamin D in the proximal renal tubules. This results in decreased serum phosphate levels, normal serum calcium levels, and low-normal circulating levels of 1,25-dihydroxy vitamin D (the activated form of vitamin D). Treatment consists of activated vitamin D (calcitriol) and phosphate supplementation. Hypophosphatasia is a rare, potentially life-threatening disorder that may appear in a severe form in utero or in a milder form in childhood or even later in life. In this disorder, there is failure to hydrolyze inorganic phosphate, which accumulates extracellularly and inhibits formation of hydroxyapatite. Rickets due to vitamin D deficiency, hypophosphatasia, and hypophosphatemic rickets cannot be reliably differentiated by imaging alone.

### Reference

Pavone V, Testa G, Iachino SG, Evola FR, Avondo S, Sessa G. Hypophosphatemic rickets: etiology, clinical features and treatment. *Eur J Orthop Surg Traumatol*. 2015;25(2):221–226.

### Cross-reference

Walters MM, Robertson RL. *Pediatric Radiology: The Requisites*. 4th ed. Philadelphia: Elsevier; 2017:211–212.

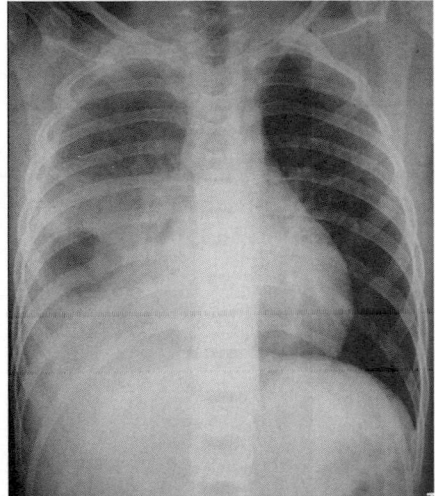

Fig. 117.1

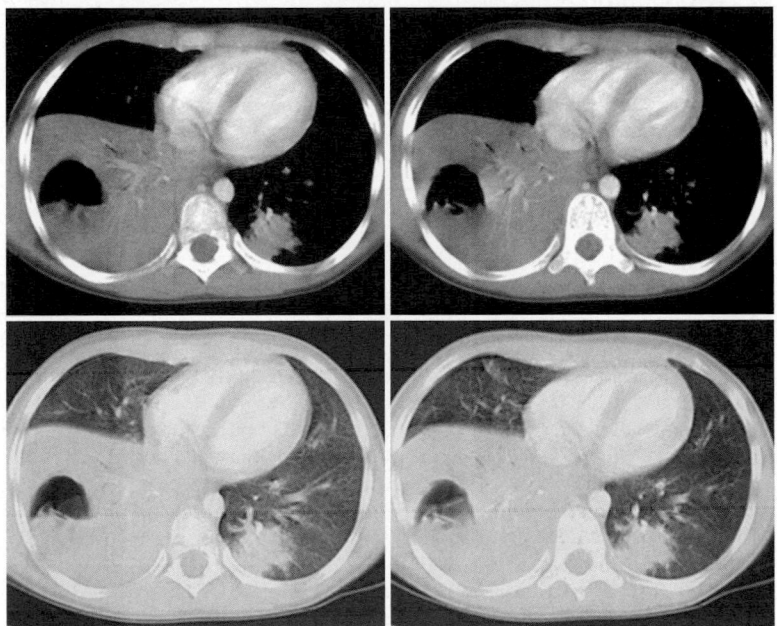

Fig. 117.2

**HISTORY:** Adolescent patient presenting with persistent cough

1. Based on the imaging findings, what is the most likely diagnosis?
   A. Pyogenic bacterial abscess
   B. Hydatid disease
   C. Tuberculous abscess
   D. Fungal infection

2. Which option is *not* a differential diagnostic consideration in the setting of an air crescent sign?
   A. Mycetoma
   B. Invasive aspergillosis
   C. Pyogenic abscess
   D. Hydatid disease

3. What is the causative organism in hydatid disease?
   A. *Taenia soltum*
   B. *Entamoeba histolytica*
   C. *Echinococcus granulosus*
   D. *Toxoplasma gondii*

4. Which option is *not* a component of the hydatid cyst?
   A. Endocyst
   B. Ectocyst
   C. Pericyst
   D. Epicyst

## CASE 117

### Pulmonary Hydatid Disease

1. B

2. C

3. C

4. D

### Comment

Cystic echinococcosis, also called hydatid disease, is caused by the tapeworm *Echinococcus granulosus*. In the normal life cycle of *Echinococcus* species, adult tapeworms inhabit the small intestine of carnivorous definite hosts, such as dogs or wolves, and the echinococcal cyst stage occurs in herbivorous intermediate hosts like sheep or horses. Humans may become an accidental intermediate host when they inadvertently ingest food or drink water contaminated with fecal material containing tapeworm eggs. Larval cysts may develop in every organ, most commonly in the liver and lungs. In the pediatric age group, the lungs are commonly involved and are often the only site of involvement. Pulmonary hydatid cysts may become very large (>10 cm), especially in young patients, due to the increased elasticity of their lung tissue. The larval cyst is surrounded by the pericyst, which is dense and fibrous, and represents the host reaction to the parasite. The exocyst is the outer laminated cyst membrane, an acellular portion of the parasite that permits passage of nutrients. The endocyst is the inner membrane and contains the germinal layer, which produces the larval scolices. On imaging, uncomplicated/unruptured pulmonary hydatid disease presents as a solitary (most common) or multiple spherical or ovoid masses with well-defined borders, typically located in the lower lobes. When they rupture, the cysts can take on a number of different appearances. When air dissects between the pericyst and the exocyst, an air crescent sign develops (this sign is also associated with mycetomas and angioinvasive aspergillosis with pulmonary infarction). When air dissects through to the endocyst, and fluid is partially expelled into the airways, an air-fluid level develops, and floating remnants of the endocyst give rise to the water lily sign. If the membranes collapse into the cyst fluid without an air-fluid level, the collapsed membranes within the fluid give rise to the serpent sign. If multiple membranes of the collapsed cyst are outlined by air, findings may mimic the appearance of onion peels, which is known as the onion peel or Cumbo sign.

### References

Kayhan S, Sahin U, Turut H, Yurdakul C. An unusual radiological presentation of a pulmonary hydatid cyst in a child. *J Clin Imaging Sci*. 2013;3:20.

Koul P, Koul A, Wahid A, Mir FA. CT in pulmonary hydatid disease. Unusual appearances. *Chest*. 2000;118(6):1645–1647.

### Cross-reference

Walters MM, Robertson RL. *Pediatric Radiology: The Requisites*. 4th ed. Philadelphia: Elsevier; 2017:125.

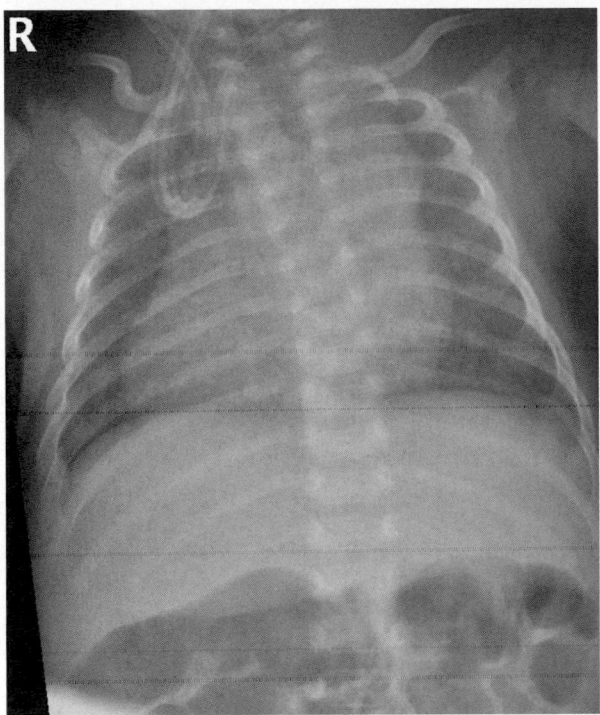

Fig. 118.1

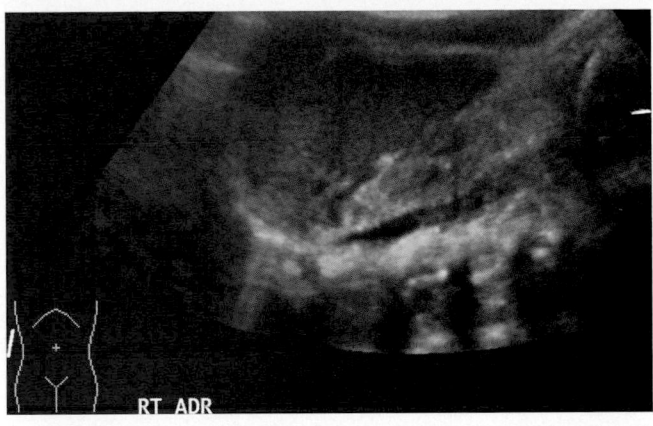

Fig. 118.2

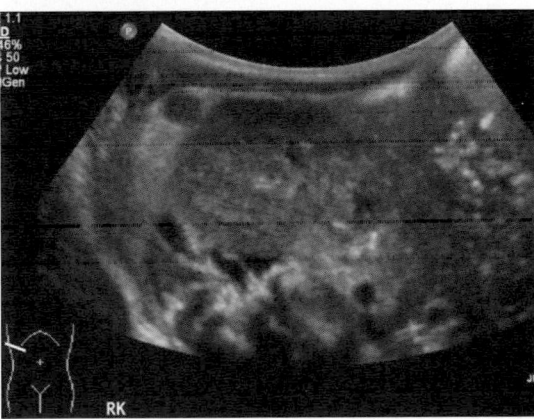

Fig. 118.3

**HISTORY:** 6-month-old male presenting with palpable mass in the left upper quadrant

1. What is the most likely diagnosis?
   A. Right atrial isomerism
   B. Left atrial isomerism
   C. Dextroversion of the heart
   D. Situs inversus totalis

2. Which of the following can be seen in heterotaxy syndromes?
   A. Cardiac malposition
   B. Transverse liver
   C. Right-sided stomach bubble with levocardia
   D. All of the above

3. Which of the following contributes most to the prognosis of heterotaxy patients?
   A. Associated cardiac anomalies
   B. Malrotation
   C. Preduodenal portal vein
   D. Absence of spleen

4. Which of the following provides the best clue to heterotaxy syndromes?
   A. Bronchial anatomy
   B. Position of the stomach
   C. Position of the cardiac apex
   D. Drainage pattern of the hepatic veins

## CASE 118

### Heterotaxy syndrome

1. B
2. D
3. A
4. A

### Comment

Heterotaxy syndromes represent a spectrum of anomalies, occur in 1 in 10,000, and represent 3% of all cardiac anomaly cases. In heterotaxy syndromes, there is a lack of normal abdominal lateralization. Historically, the syndrome was categorized on the basis of the splenic anatomy as asplenia or polysplenia. However, this was later recognized as being less than ideal because cardiac anatomy is a better discriminator between the two subsets of heterotaxy than is splenic anatomy. From a cardiac point of view, significant emphasis has been given to atrial morphology, and based on this, heterotaxy cases are defined in two major categories: left atrial isomerism (LAI) and right atrial isomerism (RAI). In patients with RAI, most frequently the spleen is absent, whereas a poorly functioning spleen is typically seen in LAI. RAI is typically associated with complex congenital cardiac malformations, such as complete unbalanced atrioventricular septal defects, an absence of the spleen, and intestinal malrotation. Left isomerism, in contrast, is more frequently associated with interruption of the inferior caval vein and multiple spleens, but less severe intracardiac lesions. Most patients with heterotaxy syndromes have cardiac anomalies that significantly contribute to their prognosis. In LAI, patients usually demonstrate bilateral left lung bronchial anatomy and hyparterial bronchi, whereas in RAI, right lung bronchial anatomy and eparterial bronchi are seen.

Plain radiography in this case shows a midline liver and dextrocardia. The ultrasound image demonstrates a relatively small but nearly normal-appearing spleen and a smaller round spleen under the hemidiaphragm. Based on the polysplenia, the patient is most likely to have left isomerism.

### Reference

Teele SA, Jacobs JP, Border WL, Chanani NK. Heterotaxy syndrome: proceedings from the 10th international PCICS meeting. *World J Pediatr Congenit Heart Surg.* 2015;6(4):616–629.

### Cross-reference

Walters MM, Robertson RL. *Pediatric Radiology: The Requisites.* 4th ed. Philadelphia: Elsevier; 2017:65–67.

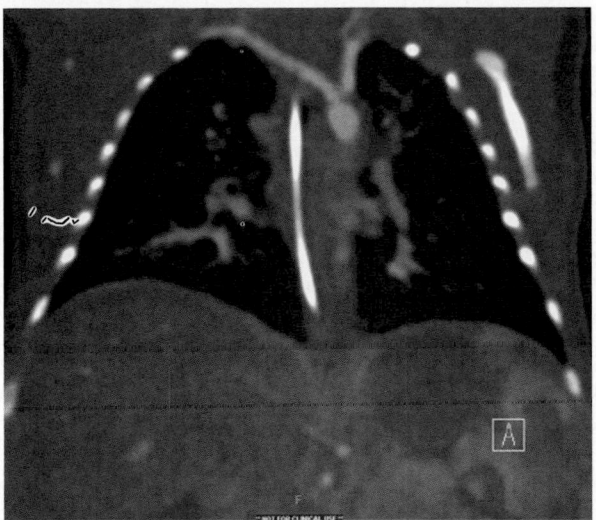

**Fig. 119.1**

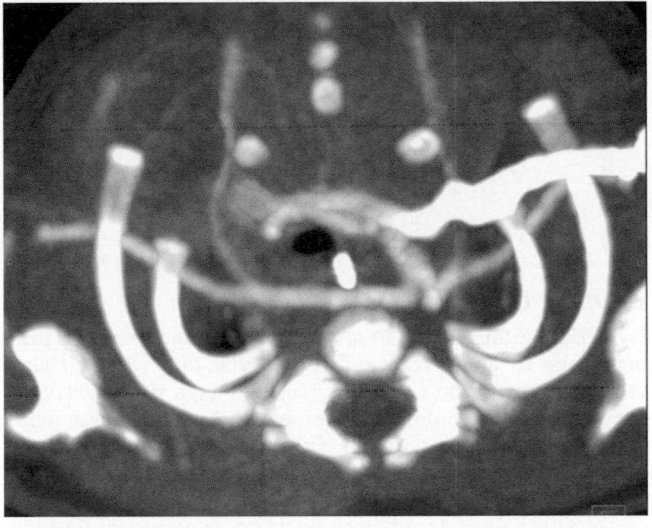

**Fig. 119.2**

**HISTORY:** Adolescent child with difficulties swallowing, occasional wheezing, and recurrent aspirations

1. Which signature pathologic imaging finding do you see?
   A. Right descending aorta
   B. Aortic coarctation
   C. Aberrant right subclavian artery
   D. Vascular ring

2. What is the exact location of the aberrant vessel in relation to the esophagus/trachea?
   A. Between the esophagus and trachea
   B. Posterior to the esophagus
   C. Anterior to the trachea
   D. Superior to the trachea

3. What is the clinical diagnosis/name associated with this finding?
   A. Dysphagia lusoria
   B. Dysphagia of Kommerell
   C. Stridor lusoria
   D. Stridor of Kommerell

4. Which statement is correct?
   A. A right aortic arch with an aberrant left subclavian artery is the most common aortic arch anomaly.
   B. A left aortic arch with an aberrant right subclavian artery is the most common aortic arch anomaly.
   C. A right aortic arch is rarely (<2%) associated with congenital heart disease.
   D. A left aortic arch is, in most instances (>85%), associated with congenital heart disease.

## CASE 119

### Dysphagia Lusoria

1. C
2. B
3. A
4. B

### Comment

Dysphagia lusoria refers to a symptomatic compression of the esophagus by an aberrant right subclavian artery (arteria lusoria) arising from the descending aorta, which runs dorsally to the esophagus. Children present with difficulties swallowing and/or recurrent episodes of aspiration. Simultaneous stridor is usually present only when a complete, tight vascular ring is present circumferentially compressing the trachea and esophagus. Vascular rings or slings result from an abnormal development of the initially paired aortic arch system.

The combination of a left aortic arch with an aberrant right subclavian artery is the most common anomaly of the aortic arch system and is usually asymptomatic. A right-sided aortic arch with an aberrant left subclavian artery (originating from the descending aorta) is much rarer (0.5% of asymptomatic patients). Associated cardiac anomalies are somewhat more frequent, especially when a right aortic arch is present. In addition, there is frequently an aberrant course of the phrenic nerve, which can be of importance for surgical repair. Normally, the right recurrent inferior laryngeal nerve passes below the right subclavian artery. If the normal right subclavian artery is absent, the recurrent nerve will move cranially.

Chest radiography can demonstrate a mild widening of the upper mediastinum but usually fails to identify the aberrant right subclavian artery. Upper gastrointestinal swallow studies may show an indentation of the posterior esophageal wall suggesting the aberrant right subclavian artery. In skilled hands, mediastinal ultrasound studies can show the anomalous relation between the esophagus and arteries; however, computed tomography angiography (CTA) and magnetic resonance angiography (MRA) are the best diagnostic modalities for identifying the aberrant vessels directly.

### Reference

De Araujo G, Junqueira Bizzi JW, Muller J, Cavazzola LT. "Dysphagia lusoria"—right subclavian retroesophageal artery causing intermittent esophageal compression and eventual dysphagia—a case report and literature review. *Int J Surg Case Rep*. 2015;10:32–34.

### Cross-reference

Walters MM, Robertson RL. *Pediatric Radiology: The Requisites*. 4th ed. Philadelphia: Elsevier; 2017:27.

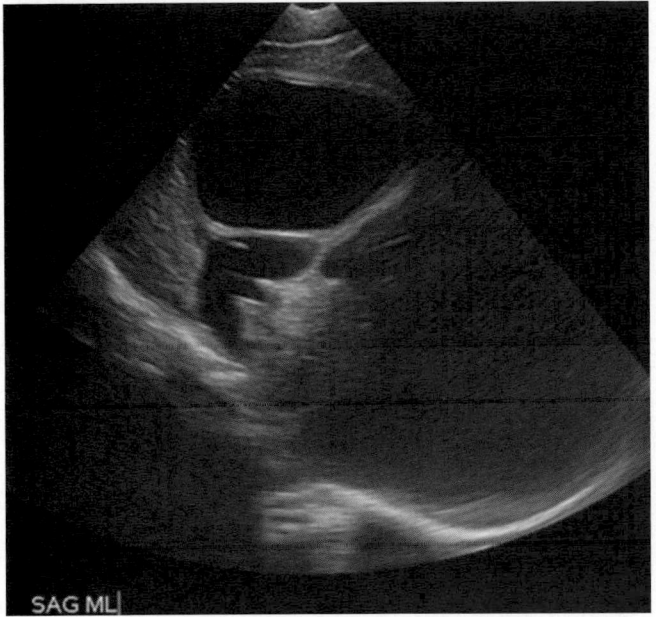

Fig. 120.1

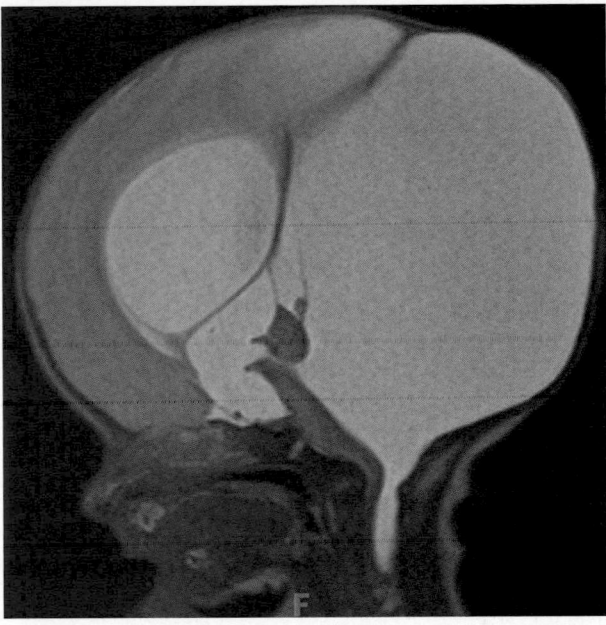

Fig.120.2

**HISTORY:** Sagittal cranial ultrasound and multiplanar ultrafast T2-weighted magnetic resonance (MR) images in a newborn child with marked macrocephaly

1. Which signature pathologic imaging finding do you see on the ultrasound (US) and magnetic resonance imaging (MRI)?
   A. Obstructed outflow tracts of the fourth ventricle with resultant dilated fourth ventricle
   B. Primary cystic dilation of the fourth ventricle with upward rotated hypoplastic vermis
   C. Large posterior fossa arachnoid cyst compressing the brain stem
   D. Occipital encephalocele with high-grade global ventriculomegaly

2. What is the most likely diagnosis?
   A. Chiari 2 malformation
   B. Joubert syndrome
   C. Dandy-Walker malformation
   D. Rhombencephalosynapsis

3. Dandy-Walker malformations may be associated with which of the following conditions?
   A. Polydactyly
   B. Cardiac anomalies
   C. Developmental delay
   D. All of the above

4. Which option would you *not* include in your differential diagnosis?
   A. Blake pouch cyst
   B. Mega cisterna magna
   C. Retrocerebellar arachnoid cyst
   D. Pontocerebellar hypoplasia

## CASE 120

### Dandy-Walker Malformation

1. B
2. C
3. D
4. D

### Comment

Dandy-Walker malformation (DWM) is characterized by hypoplasia of the cerebellar vermis and a cystic dilation of the fourth ventricle. DWM is a relatively common malformation with an estimated prevalence of about 1 in 11,000. The etiology of DWM remains poorly understood and is probably multifactorial and highly heterogeneous. In most DWM patients, a genetic etiology is present. DWM may occur in isolation or as part of a defined Mendelian disorder, including syndromes (e.g., posterior fossa malformations, hemangiomas, arterial anomalies, cardiac defects, eye abnormalities, sternal cleft and supraumbilical raphe (PHACES syndrome)) and various chromosomal anomalies such as trisomy 9, 13, and 18.

Most children are asymptomatic during the neonatal period and present with hydrocephalus and increased intracranial pressure (e.g., bulging of the anterior fontanel and upward gaze palsy). Cognitive functions are normal in at least 30% of patients.

Most cases are diagnosed on prenatal ultrasound (US) or fetal magnetic resonance imaging (MRI). Postnatally, transfontanellar ultrasound is the first-line imaging modality followed by MRI of the brain and upper spinal cord. Pre- and postnatal imaging findings are similar. The cerebellar vermis is hypoplastic or aplastic, and the residual superior vermis is typically elevated and rotated upward by the cystic dilated fourth ventricle. The posterior fossa is enlarged with various degrees of elevation of the torcular Herophili. The cerebellar hemispheres are usually displaced anterolaterally by the enlarged fourth ventricle, but their size and morphology is usually normal. The brain stem may be thin, mostly due to pontine hypoplasia. In about 30% to 50% of patients, DWM is associated with additional brain malformations such as agenesis or dysgenesis of the corpus callosum, occipital encephaloceles, and neuronal migrational abnormalities (e.g., subependymal heterotopia).

Alternative terms have been introduced to describe various forms of vermian hypoplasia that do not fulfill the diagnostic criteria of a true DWM, such as the Dandy-Walker variant, Dandy-Walker complex, or Dandy-Walker spectrum. This leads to lack of specificity and confusion and should be avoided.

### References

Bosemani T, Orman G, Boltshauser E, Tekes A, Huisman TA, Poretti A. Congenital abnormalities of the posterior fossa. *Radiographics*. 2015;35(1):200–220.

Poretti A, Meoded A, Rossi A, Raybaud C, Huisman TA. Diffusion tensor imaging and fiber tractography in brain malformations. *Pediatr Radiol*. 2013;43(1):28–54.

### Cross-reference

Walters MM, Robertson RL. *Pediatric Radiology: The Requisites*. 4th ed. Philadelphia: Elsevier; 2017:270–271.

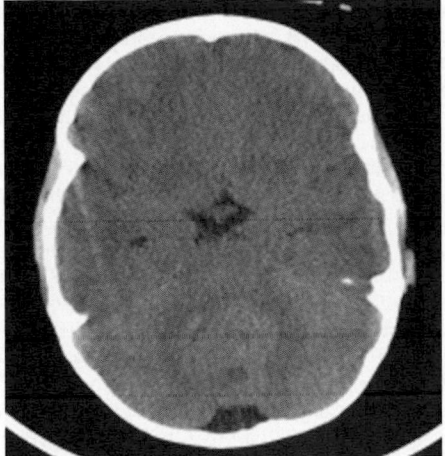

Fig. 121.1

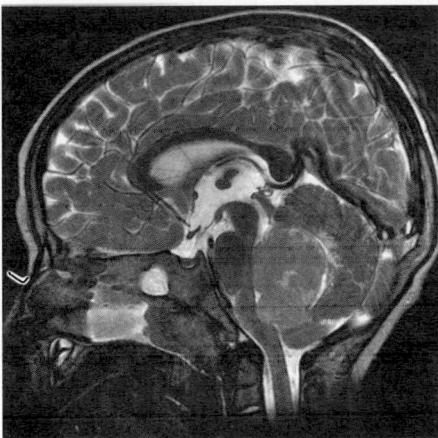

Fig. 121.2

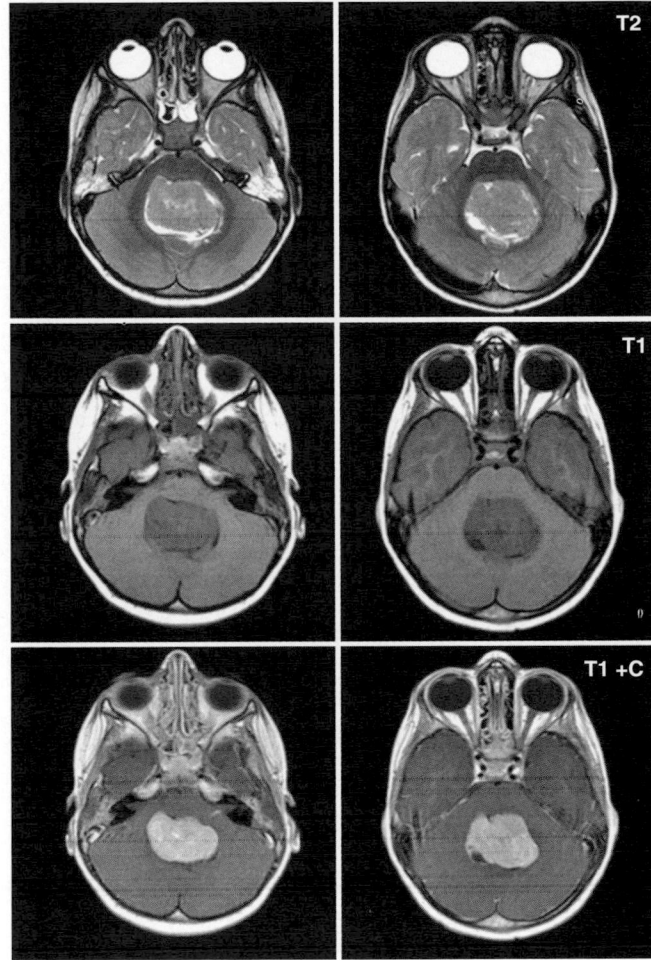

Fig. 121.3

**HISTORY:** Non–contrast-enhanced computed tomography (CT) and multiplanar magnetic resonance imaging (MRI) of a 6-year-old boy presenting with ataxia, gait disturbance, and intermittent headache with vomiting

1. Which signature pathologic imaging finding do you see?
   A. Focal mass lesion within the fourth ventricle
   B. Focal mass lesion dorsal to the fourth ventricle
   C. Focal mass lesion within the dorsal pons
   D. Focal mass lesion originating from the lower dorsal brain stem

2. Based upon the location, gender, and age, what is the most likely diagnosis?
   A. Medulloblastoma (MB)
   B. Ependymoma
   C. Pilocytic astrocytoma
   D. Diffuse intrinsic pontine glioma

3. What is the most frequent initial epicenter of this tumor?
   A. Vermis
   B. Cerebellar hemispheres
   C. Fourth ventricle
   D. Brain stem

4. Which statement is correct?
   A. Leptomeningeal dissemination rarely occurs in MB.
   B. MBs occur twice as often in girls than in boys.
   C. MBs have a peak incidence in the second decade of life.
   D. MBs are hyperdense because of the high cellularity.

## CASE 121

### Medulloblastoma

1. B

2. A

3. A

4. D

## *Comment*

Medulloblastoma (MB), the most frequent malignant brain tumor of childhood, is an invasive embryonal tumor of the cerebellum with an inherent tendency to metastasize via subarachnoid seeding. MBs occur bimodally with peak incidences between ages 3 and 4 and ages 8 and 9. About 10% to 15% of cases are diagnosed within the first year of life. MB is twice as common in boys as in girls.

Approximately 75% to 90% of MBs occur in the midline, mostly arising in the inferior vermis. Consequently, the epicenter of the tumor is typically located dorsally to the fourth ventricle in contrast to ependymomas, which usually arise from the roof of the fourth ventricle. With progression of the MB, the fourth ventricle may become invaded. Hemispheric locations account for 10% to 15% of the cases and are associated with an older age and desmoplastic histology. Dissemination along the craniospinal axis is found in about 11% to 43% of patients.

On non–contrast-enhanced computed tomography (CT), the typical feature of MB is a midline, well-defined, and homogeneous mass that appears hyperdense or isodense compared to the surrounding tissue due to the high cellularity. Peritumoral vasogenic edema is reported in 90% to 95% of children. Most MBs enhance diffusely and homogeneously, but patchy enhancement has been reported. Calcifications can be found in up to 20% of cases, and cysts or necrotic nonenhancing regions in about 50%.

On magnetic resonance imaging (MRI), the appearance of MBs is variable. MBs most often appear as a round, slightly lobulated, T1-isointense or T1-hypointense mass lesion located dorsal to the fourth ventricle. The T2 signal is heterogeneous, and the solid portion is often T2 hypointense to isointense compared to the gray matter. Contrast enhancement is usually present, but may be variable in degree, ranging from diffuse and homogeneous to focal and patchy. On diffusion-weighted imaging, the tumor typically has low apparent diffusion coefficient values.

### Reference

Huisman TA. Posterior fossa tumors in children. Differential diagnosis and advanced imaging techniques. *Neuroradiol J*. 2007;20(4): 449-460.

### Cross-reference

Walters MM, Robertson RL. *Pediatric Radiology: The Requisites*. 4th ed. Philadelphia: Elsevier; 2017:300-301.

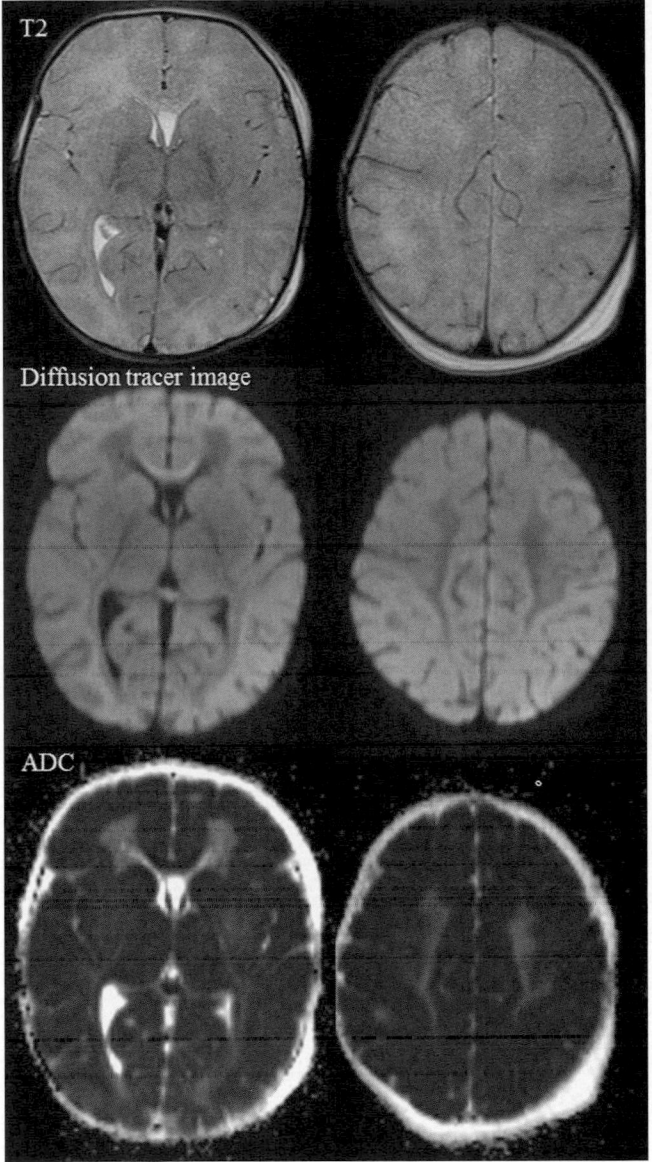

**Fig. 122.1**

See Supplemental Figures section for additional figures for this case.

**HISTORY:** 39 gestational week (GW) infant, born via emergent C-section due to placental abruption. No respiratory effort, flaccid, cyanotic. Appearance, pulse, grimace, activity, and respiration (Apgar) score 1/4/5, cord pH 6.53. Brain magnetic resonance imaging (MRI) at day of life 5

1. What is the best diagnosis?
   A. Herpes simplex encephalitis (HSE)
   B. Hypoxic-ischemic encephalopathy (HIE)
   C. Bilateral middle cerebral artery stroke
   D. Neonatal hypoglycemia (NHG)

2. Which of the following has been postulated in the etiology/pathologica mechanism of HIE?
   A. Infection
   B. Inflammation
   C. Failure of secondary energy metabolism and free radicals
   D. All of the above

3. Which statement about the neuroimaging findings of HIE is most accurate?
   A. Midbrain and brain stem injury is highly suggestive of severe insult such as acute complete placental abruption.
   B. Lack of a T2 dark signal in the posterior limb of the internal capsule (PLIC) in a 34-GW infant is indicative of moderate injury.
   C. Low resistive indices in the circle of Willis, increased echogenicity of the white matter, and slit-like ventricles are usually seen in head US in the acute phase of HIE.
   D. A and C

4. Which statement about HIE in newborns is true?
   A. The pattern of injury may depend on the maturity of the brain.
   B. The pattern of injury may depend on the severity of the insult.
   C. The pattern of injury may depend on the duration of the insult.
   D. The pattern of injury may depend on superimposed infection and metabolic derangement.
   E. All of the above.

## CASE 122

### Hypoxic-Ischemic Encephalopathy

1. B
2. D
3. D
4. E

### Comment

Hypoxic-ischemic encephalopathy (HIE) may be a result of prenatal, perinatal, and postnatal insult to the brain, generally attributed to cerebral hypoperfusion. The pattern of injury can be affected by the maturity of the brain (term vs. preterm), severity of the insult (severe, moderate, mild), duration of the injury (brief, intermittent, prolonged), and other superimposed diseases such as infection, thrombosis, hemorrhage, or metabolic derangements. Diagnostic criteria for HIE are profound metabolic or mixed acidemia ($pH < 7$) in an umbilical artery blood sample; appearance, pulse, grimace, activity, and respiration (Apgar) score of 0 to 3 for more than 5 minutes; neonatal neurologic sequelae (seizures, coma, hypotonia); and multiple organ involvement (kidney, lungs, liver, heart, intestines). As the previously mentioned criteria imply, this is a clinical diagnosis; however, neuroimaging is critical in confirming the suspected diagnosis, determining prognosis, and family counseling.

Despite neuroprotective treatments such as cooling (head only or whole body), HIE is still the leading cause of disability and death in neonates. Three major patterns of injury can be observed, although none of which is exclusive of each other: deep gray matter (thalamus and basal ganglia), periventricular white matter, or peripheral (cortex and/or subcortical white matter). The case shown here is an example of severe injury secondary to placental abruption. Magnetic resonance imaging (MRI) shows diffuse increased T2 signal of the cortex, white matter, basal ganglia, and thalami, with associated restricted diffusion. Findings are typically bilateral and symmetric in HIE unless there is additional superimposed thrombosis, hemorrhage, and infectious disease.

Periventricular injury is commonly seen in preterms, whereas watershed injury is typically seen in term infants. Lack of a dark T2 signal in the posterior limb of the internal capsule (PLIC) is an important prognosticator; however, it is important to keep in mind that the PLIC is myelinated in term infants, but not in preterm infants.

### Reference

Johnston MV, Fatemi A, Wilson MA, Northington F. Treatment advances in neonatal neuroprotection and neurointesive care. *Lancet Neurol.* 2011;10(4):372–382.

### Cross-reference

Walters MM, Robertson RL. *Pediatric Radiology: The Requisites.* 4th ed. Philadelphia: Elsevier; 2017:306–307.

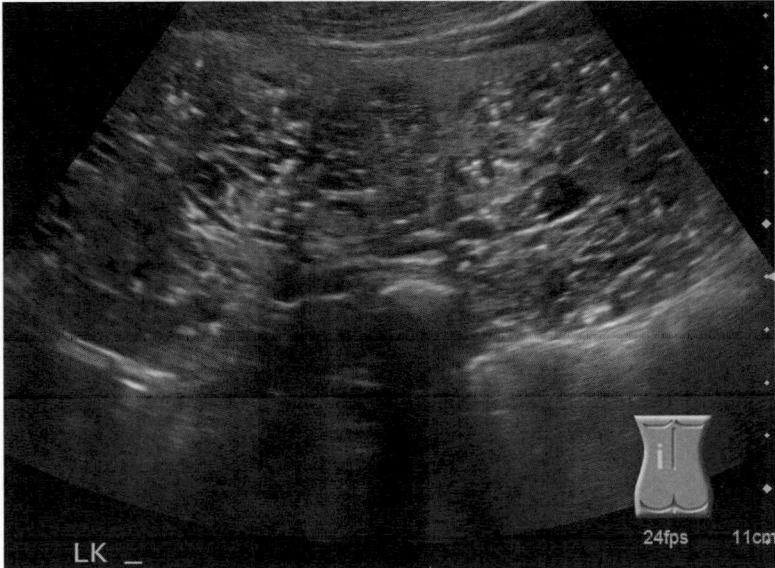

**Fig. 123.1**

**HISTORY:** Infant presenting with renal insufficiency.

1. What is your diagnosis?
   A. Autosomal recessive polycystic kidney disease (ARPCKD)
   B. Meckel-Gruber syndrome
   C. Tuberous sclerosis
   D. Autosomal dominant polycystic kidney disease (ADPCKD)

2. Which of the following is suggestive of ARPCKD in a fetus?
   A. Oligohydramnios
   B. Enlarged kidneys >2 standard deviations (SD) at 24 gestational weeks (GWs)
   C. Lack of urine in the bladder
   D. All of the above

3. True or false?
   A. Associated with musculoskeletal abnormalities
   B. Associated with hepatic fibrosis

4. Which statement is accurate regarding the imaging findings?
   A. The reniform shape of the kidneys is preserved despite enlargement.
   B. Punctate calcification can be seen over time, which correlates with worsening renal function.
   C. There are enlarged hyperechoic kidneys with or without discernible cysts.
   D. All of the above.

## CASE 123

### Autosomal Recessive Polycystic Kidney Disease

1. A

2. D

3. A) True, B) True

4. D

### Comment

Autosomal recessive polycystic kidney disease (ARPCKD) is the most common ciliopathy in the pediatric population, and renal manifestations are the most common presentation. ARPCKD maps to chromosome 6, and the involved gene is PKHD1 (polycystic kidney and hepatic disease 1). Dilation in collecting ducts and ectatic convoluted tubules are the hallmark of pathology in ARPCKD. This results in increased volume of the medulla, leading to renal enlargement. An increase in reflective interfaces from dilated tubules creates increased echogenicity on ultrasound. Discernible cysts may not be appreciable on imaging. Oligohydramnios is an important feature in prenatal imaging. Kidney size may be within normal limits until 20 gestational weeks, and there is no gender predilection. More severe disease presents in infancy, and milder forms can present in childhood. Approximately 75% of survivors develop hypertension, and 30% to 50% require ventilator support. The treatment is symptomatic, and renal replacement therapy is required via dialysis or transplant.

### Reference

Chung EM, Conran RM, Schroeder JW, Rohena-Quinquilla IR, Rooks VJ. From the radiologic pathology archives: pediatric polycystic kidney disease and other ciliopathies: radiologic-pathologic correlation. *Radiographics*. 2014;34(1):155–178.

### Cross-reference

Walters MM, Robertson RL. *Pediatric Radiology: The Requisites*. 4th ed. Philadelphia: Elsevier. 2017:166–167.

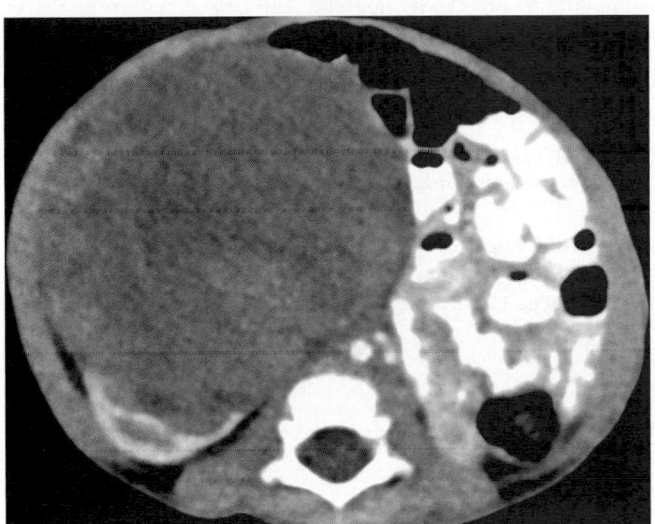

Fig. 124.1

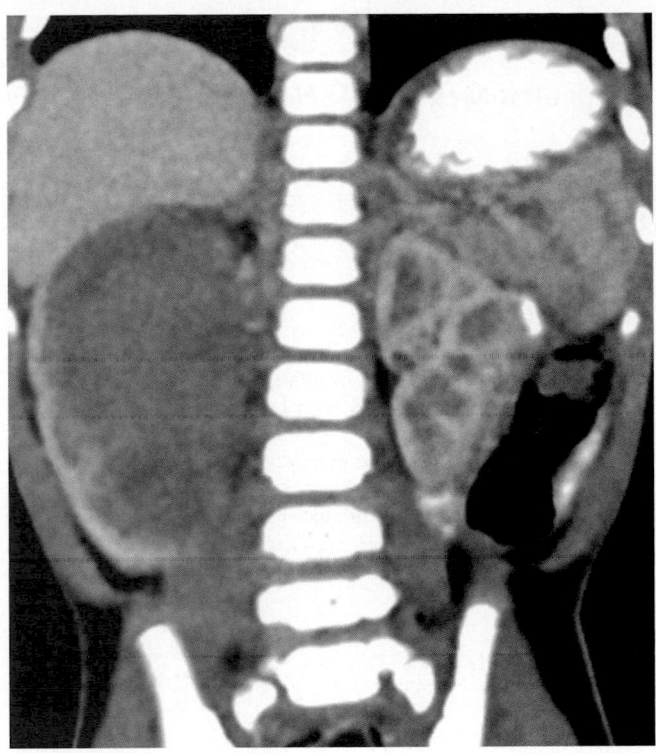

Fig. 124.2

**HISTORY:** 5-month-old infant presenting with a palpable abdominal mass

1. Which of the following would you include in your differential diagnosis? (Choose all that apply.)
   A. Wilms tumor
   B. Multicystic dysplastic kidney (MCDK)
   C. Congenital mesoblastic nephroma (CMN)
   D. Multilocular cystic renal tumor (MCRT)

2. What is the best preoperative predictor that a renal mass is due to CMN rather than Wilms tumor?
   A. Size of the mass
   B. Age of the patient
   C. Presence of cystic/necrotic change
   D. Presence of intratumoral hemorrhage

3. What is the 5-year event-free survival rate in patients with CMN?
   A. 12%
   B. 42%
   C. 73%
   D. 94%

4. Which statement about CMN is *not* correct?
   A. The three different subtypes are classic, cellular, and mixed.
   B. Most are diagnosed before 6 months of age.
   C. CMN cannot be reliably differentiated from Wilms tumor on imaging alone.
   D. CMN can commonly affect both kidneys.

## CASE 124

### Congenital Mesoblastic Nephroma

1. A, C
2. B
3. D
4. D

### Comment

Congenital mesoblastic nephroma (CMN) is the most common renal tumor in neonates and in infants under 1 year of age and represents 3% of all pediatric renal neoplasms. Most of these tumors are diagnosed before 6 months of age, and most are unilateral. The best preoperative predictor that a renal mass is due to CMN rather than Wilms tumor is the patient's age, because Wilms tumor is rare under the age of 6 months. There are three variants of CMN: the classic subtype, the more aggressive cellular subtype, and the mixed type, which displays characteristics of both the classic and cellular subtypes. The classic subtype typically presents at a younger age (<3 months) and is more circumscribed and solid in appearance on imaging. The cellular subtype commonly presents slightly later (3 to 6 months) and is more cystic, more heterogeneous, and larger on imaging compared to the classic subtype. The risk of recurrence after resection is higher with cellular CMN than with classic CMN. However, both are treated with radical nephrectomy, and complete excision with negative margins is curative in most cases.

### Reference

Sheth MM, Cai G, Goodman TR. AIRP best cases in radiologic-pathologic correlation: congenital mesoblastic nephroma. *Radiographics*. 2012;32(1):99–103.

### Cross-reference

Walters MM, Robertson RL. *Pediatric Radiology: The Requisites*. 4th ed. Philadelphia: Elsevier. 2017:160.

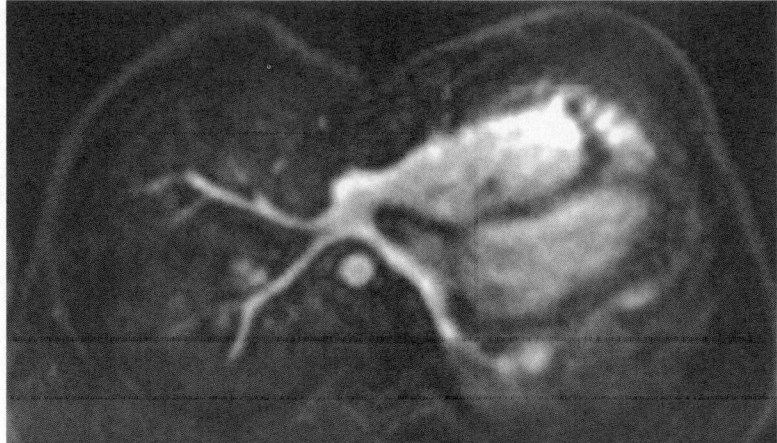

Fig. 125.1

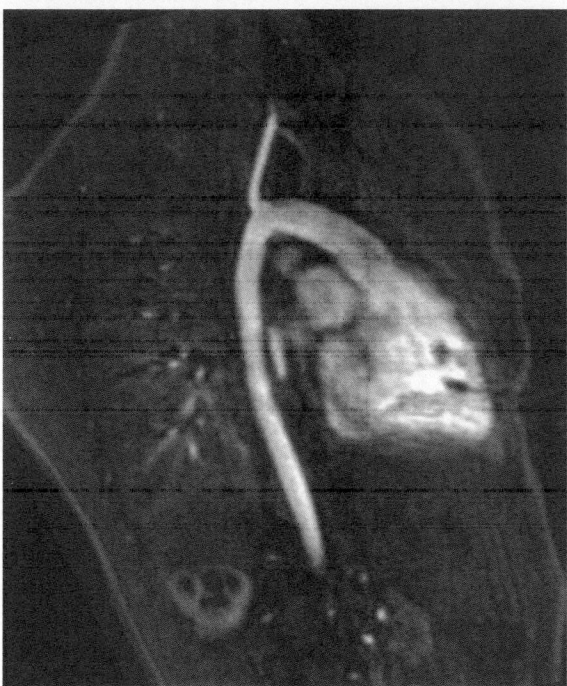

Fig. 125.2

See Supplemental Figures section for additional figures for this case.

**HISTORY:** 14-year-old status post cardiac surgery as an infant for cyanosis

1. Based on the clinical history and imaging findings, which of the following is the most likely diagnosis?
   A. L-transposition of the great arteries
   B. D-transposition of the great arteries
   C. Epstein anomaly
   D. Tetralogy of Fallot

2. Which option correctly describes the Jatene procedure?
   A. Rerouting of venous flow in the atria with a pericardial baffle
   B. Arterial switch with transposition of the coronary arteries
   C. Rerouting of venous flow in the atria with reorientation of the atrial septum
   D. Rerouting of a subclavian artery branch to the pulmonary artery

3. Which statement about D-transposition is *not* correct?
   A. It includes atrioventricular discordance and ventriculoarterial discordance.
   B. Surgical interventions include the Jatene, Mustard, and Senning procedures.
   C. It is lethal without admixture of the left and right circulations.
   D. It presents with cyanosis and often with increased pulmonary vasculature.

4. True or false?
   A. Patients with L-transposition of the great arteries ("congenitally corrected transposition") typically have good prognosis and normal life expectancy.

## CASE 125

### D-Transposition of the Great Arteries

1. B

2. B

3. A

4. False

### Comment

D-transposition of the great arteries is characterized by atrio-ventricular concordance and ventriculoarterial discordance. In other words the right and left atrium appropriately connect to the right and left ventricle, respectively (atrioventricular concordance), but the ventricles then connect to the inappropriate respective great artery (ventriculoarterial discordance). This results in complete separation between the systemic and pulmonary circulations, which is why D-transposition of the great arteries is lethal without admixture between the two systems, for example, via patent foramen ovale, ventricular septal defect (VSD), atrial septal defect, or patent ductus arteriosus. The aorta arises from the right ventricle, and its origin is located anterior and to the right of the origin of the pulmonary artery arising from the left ventricle. This anteroposterior relationship of the great vessels gives rise to the classic "egg on a string appearance" of the heart and mediastinum on plain chest radiograph. The Jatene procedure consists of an arterial switch with concomitant transposition of the coronary arteries to the neoaorta and has largely replaced the previous atrial switch procedures (Mustard and Senning; the patient in this case is status post Senning procedure as an infant—notice how the pulmonary veins are routed to the right atrium). L-transposition of the great arteries, also known as "congenitally corrected transposition," is characterized by atrioventricular discordance and ventriculoarterial discordance. Although there is no separation between the systemic and pulmonary circulations, these patients commonly have other anomalies, including VSD, left ventricular outflow tract obstruction, Ebstein anomaly, and tricuspid atresia, so the prognosis remains guarded despite corrective surgery.

### Reference

Files MD, Arya B. Preoperative physiology, imaging, and management of transposition of the great arteries. *Semin Cardiothorac Vasc Anesth*. 2015;19(3):210–222.

### Cross-reference

Walters MM, Robertson RL. *Pediatric Radiology: The Requisites*. 4th ed. Philadelphia: Elsevier. 2017:75–76.

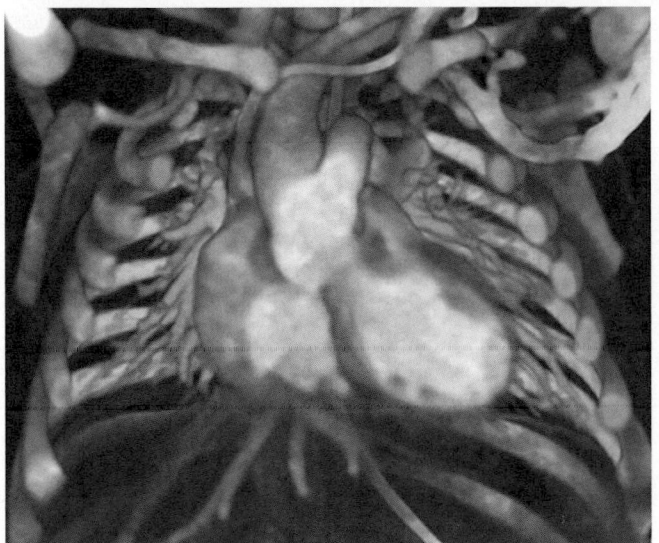

Fig. 126.1

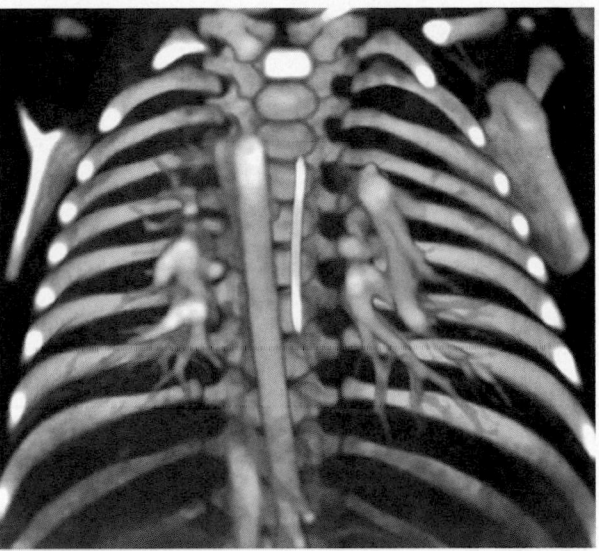

Fig. 126.2

See Supplemental Figures section for additional figures for this case.

**HISTORY:** 2-week-old infant presenting with increasing cyanosis and progressive heart failure

1. What should be included in the differential diagnosis for an infant presenting with increased pulmonary vascularity and cyanosis? (Choose all that apply.)
   A. D-transposition of the great arteries
   B. Tetralogy of Fallot
   C. Truncus arteriosus
   D. Total anomalous pulmonary venous return

2. What is the most likely diagnosis in this patient?
   A. D-transposition of the great arteries
   B. Tetralogy of Fallot
   C. Truncus arteriosus
   D. Total anomalous pulmonary venous return

3. Which statement about truncus arteriosus is *not* true?
   A. Cyanosis is due to flow admixture associated with a ventricular septal defect (VSD) and truncus.
   B. There may be a main pulmonary artery arising from the trunk, but the right and left pulmonary arteries may also arise directly from the trunk.
   C. Surgical repair consists of creating a conduit from a subclavian artery to a pulmonary artery branch (Blalock-Taussig [BT] shunt).
   D. Truncus arteriosus is the heart lesion most commonly associated with a right aortic arch.

4. Which other cyanotic heart disease is frequently associated with a right aortic arch?
   A. D-transposition of the great arteries
   B. Tetralogy of Fallot
   C. Ebstein anomaly
   D. Total anomalous pulmonary venous return

## CASE 126

### Truncus Arteriosus

1. A, C, D
2. C
3. C
4. B

### Comment

Truncus arteriosus is a cyanotic admixture lesion with a high ventricular septal defect (VSD) and a common arterial trunk providing outflow for both ventricles. Cyanosis is due to flow admixture within the VSD and the truncus. The main pulmonary artery may arise from the trunk, but in some patients, the right and left pulmonary arteries arise separately from the trunk. Truncus arteriosus is the heart lesion most commonly associated with a right aortic arch. Surgery consists of closure of the VSD and creation of a conduit from the right ventricle to the pulmonary arteries. Postoperative complications include conduit stenosis or regurgitation and truncal stenosis or regurgitation.

### Reference

Hong SH, Kim YM, Lee CK, Lee CH, Kim SH, Lee SY. 3D MDCT angiography for the preoperative assessment of truncus arteriosus. *Clin Imaging*. 2015;39(6):938-944.

### Cross-reference

Walters MM, Robertson RL. *Pediatric Radiology: The Requisites.* 4th ed. Philadelphia: Elsevier; 2017:77-78.

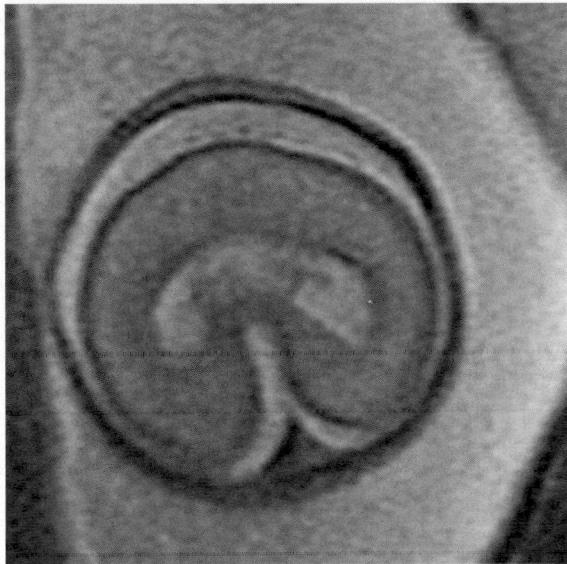

Fig. 127.1

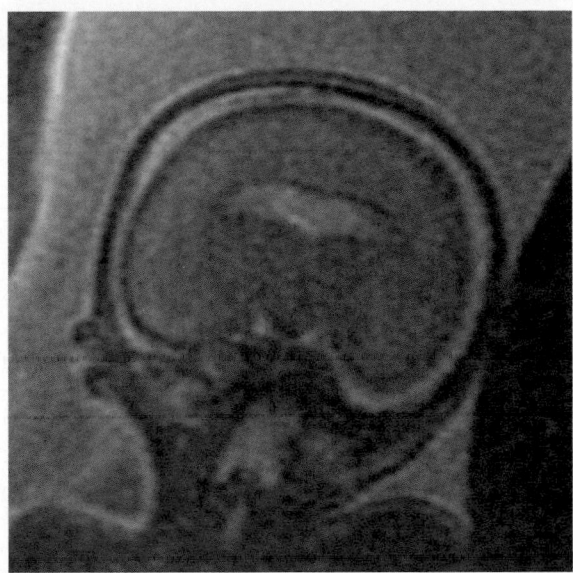

Fig. 127.2

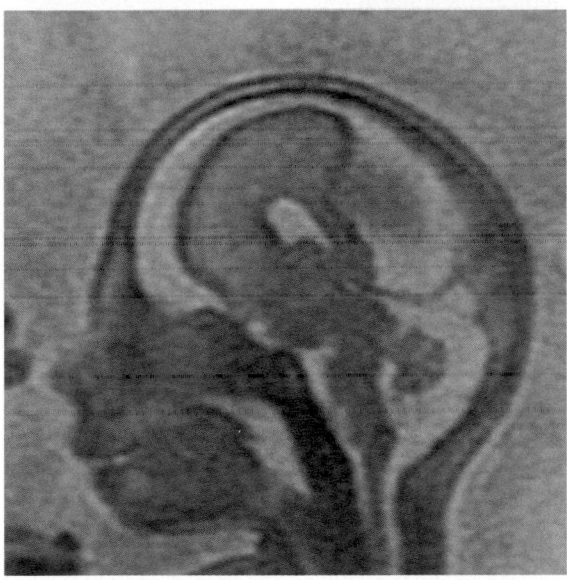

Fig. 127.3

**HISTORY:** Fetal magnetic resonance imaging (MRI) of a child within the first trimester of gestation

1. Which signature pathologic imaging finding do you see on the fetal MRI?
   A. Fused frontal lobes with a monoventricle
   B. Z-shaped brain stem
   C. Cystic dilation of the fourth ventricle
   D. Skull base meningoencephalocele

2. This abnormality belongs to which group?
   A. Ciliopathies
   B. Tubulinopathies
   C. Cleavage disorders
   D. Neural tube closure defects

3. What is the most likely diagnosis?
   A. Septooptic dysplasia
   B. Lobar holoprosencephaly (HPE)
   C. Semilobar HPE
   D. Alobar HPE

4. Which statement is incorrect?
   A. Children with lobar HPE do better than those with alobar HPE.
   B. The thalami are typically fused in alobar HPE.
   C. The metopic suture is typically wide open.
   D. Midline craniofacial defects may include midfacial hypoplasia and cyclopia.

## CASE 127

### Alobar Holoprosencephaly

1. A
2. C
3. D
4. C

## Comment

Holoprosencephaly (HPE) is a complex human brain malformation due to incomplete cleavage of the telencephalon and absent or poor development of the midline structures. The etiology of HPE is very heterogeneous and includes environmental and multiple chromosomal and genetic causes. Children with HPE present with a variety of neurologic and developmental deficits including epileptic seizures, spasticity movement disorders, cognitive impairment, and endocrinopathies. Furthermore, midline craniofacial defects like midfacial hypoplasia, cyclopia, and fused/absent metopic suture (the face predicts the brain) may occur. The severity of clinical deficits appears to be related to the degree of structural brain abnormalities in HPE.

Prenatal ultrasound and fetal MRI typically recognize the characteristic anomalous features; however, postnatal MRI is necessary for correct classification of the malformation. HPE is traditionally classified into three grades of increasing severity based on the major neuroanatomical findings: (1) In lobar HPE, the cerebral hemispheres are rather well developed and separated (including thalamic nuclei), and there is rudimentary formation of the frontal horns of the lateral ventricles and nonseparation of only the most rostral/ventral parts of the striatum and neocortex with absence of the corpus callosum in the affected region. (2) In semilobar HPE, there is lack of separation of the anterior part of the hemispheres and incomplete separation of the deep gray matter nuclei, but separation of the posterior and inferior parts of the hemispheres resulting in the presence of the posterior horns and trigones of the lateral ventricles and of the splenium of the corpus callosum. (3) In alobar HPE, the most severe form, there is a complete or nearly complete lack of separation of the cerebral hemispheres; fused basal ganglia, thalami, and hypothalamic nuclei; a single midline forebrain ventricle (monoventricle) that often communicates with a dorsal cyst; and a complete absence of the interhemispheric fissure, falx cerebri, and corpus callosum.

### Reference

Poretti A, Meoded A, Rossi A, Huisman TA. Diffusion tensor imaging and fiber tractography in brain malformations. *Pediatr Radiol.* 2013;43:28–54.

### Cross-reference

Walters MM, Robertson RL. *Pediatric Radiology: The Requisites.* 4th ed. Philadelphia: Elsevier. 2017:265–266.

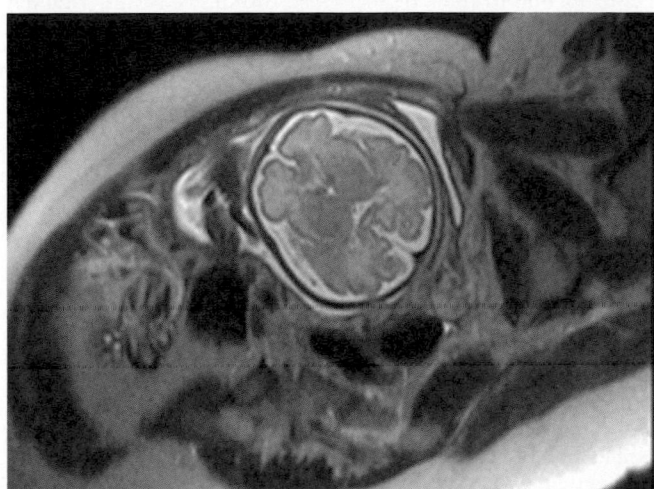

Fig. 128.1

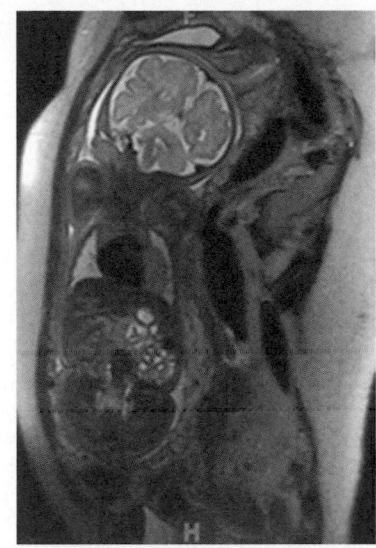

Fig. 128.2

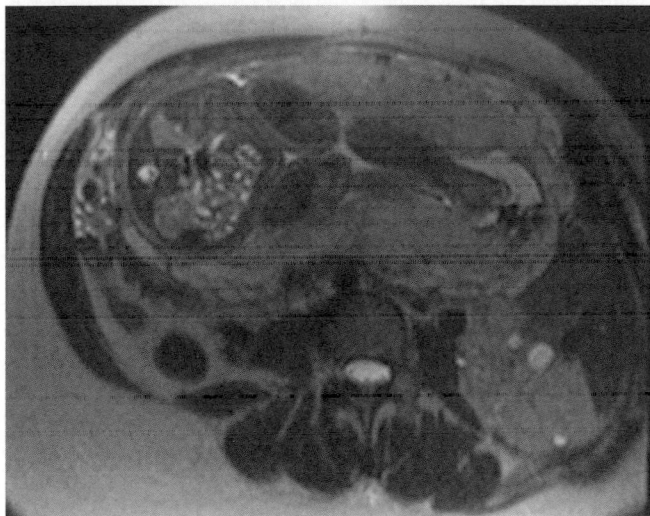

Fig. 128.3

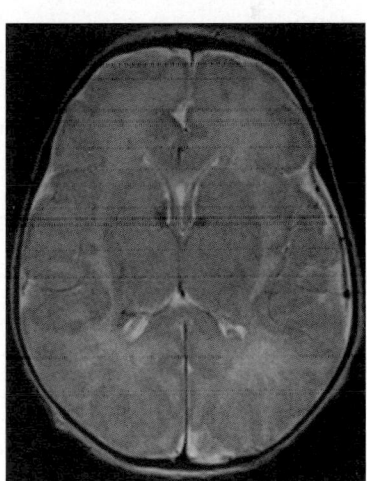

Fig. 128.4

**HISTORY:** Fetal magnetic resonance imaging (MRI) in the second trimester of gestation after prenatal ultrasound showed a suspicious lesion at the foramen of Monro.

1. Which signature pathologic imaging finding do you see within the fetal brain?
   A. Bilateral T2-hypointense lesions at the foramen of Monro
   B. Global hypomyelination of the cerebral white matter
   C. Corpus callosum agenesis
   D. Vein of Galen aneurysmal malformation

2. Which additional fetal imaging finding do you see within the fetal chest or abdomen?
   A. Cardiomegaly
   B. Renal agenesis
   C. Cardiac mass lesion, e.g., a rhabdomyoma
   D. Pulmonary sequestration

3. Which findings do you see in the mother?
   A. Ovarian carcinoma with excessive ascites
   B. Lumbar myelomeningocele
   C. Wide open, insufficient cervical canal
   D. Multiple cysts within the kidneys

4. What is the final diagnosis based upon the fetal and postnatal imaging findings?
   A. Tuberous sclerosis complex (TSC)
   B. Sturge-Weber-Dimitri syndrome
   C. Von Hippel-Lindau syndrome
   D. Neurofibromatosis type 1

## CASE 128

### Tuberous Sclerosis

1. A

2. C

3. D

4. A

### Comment

Tuberous sclerosis complex (TSC), also known as Bourneville-Pringle disease, is a neurocutaneous disorder with simultaneous involvement of the skin and multiple organs (heart, kidneys, lungs, eyes) in addition to the central nervous system. The skin lesions include hypomelanotic macules, subcutaneous shagreen patches, ungual or periungual fibromas, and facial angiofibromas. Angiomyolipomas and cysts are seen in the kidneys, rhabdomyomas occur in the heart, and lymphangiomyomatosis may affect the lungs.

Neuroimaging is essential to identify the multitude of central nervous system lesions that may include cortical tubers, subependymal nodules, radial glial bands, and giant cell astrocytomas. The cortical tubers and subependymal nodules are seen in nearly all patients and may calcify with age. The radial glial bands are also seen in nearly all TSC patients; they represent islets or bands of arrested disordered neurons intermixed with glial cells. Giant cell astrocytomas are seen in about 15%

of patients and may be complicated by supratentorial hydrocephalus due to their typical close proximity to the foramen of Monro.

All TSC lesions are easily diagnosed on magnetic resonance imaging (MRI). The cortical tubers change their relative signal intensities with progressing white matter myelination and typically enlarge the affected gyrus. The hyperintense signal on T2-weighted and fluid-attenuated inversion recovery (FLAIR) MR images give the appearance of "empty gyri." Calcifications may appear on follow-up. The subependymal nodules are typically located along the lateral ventricles and may show calcifications. The white matter radial glial bands are best seen on FLAIR images as hyperintense ill-defined bands that extend from the ventricles toward the overlying cortex. Subependymal nodules at the level of the foramen of Monro, when larger than 1 cm in diameter, are concerning for subependymal giant cell astrocytomas. The subependymal giant cell astrocytomas are T2-hyperintense, highly vascularized tumors with avid contrast enhancement and prominent tumor vessels. Cerebellar lesions are seen in about one-third of children.

### Reference

Huisman TA. Neurocutaneous syndromes with cerebellar involvement. In: Boltshauser E, Schmahmann J, eds. *Cerebellar Disorders in Children. Clinics in Developmental Medicine No 191–192.* London: Mac Keith Press; 2012;29:291–302.

### Cross-reference

Walters MM, Robertson RL. *Pediatric Radiology: The Requisites.* 4th ed. Philadelphia: Elsevier. 2017:281–283.

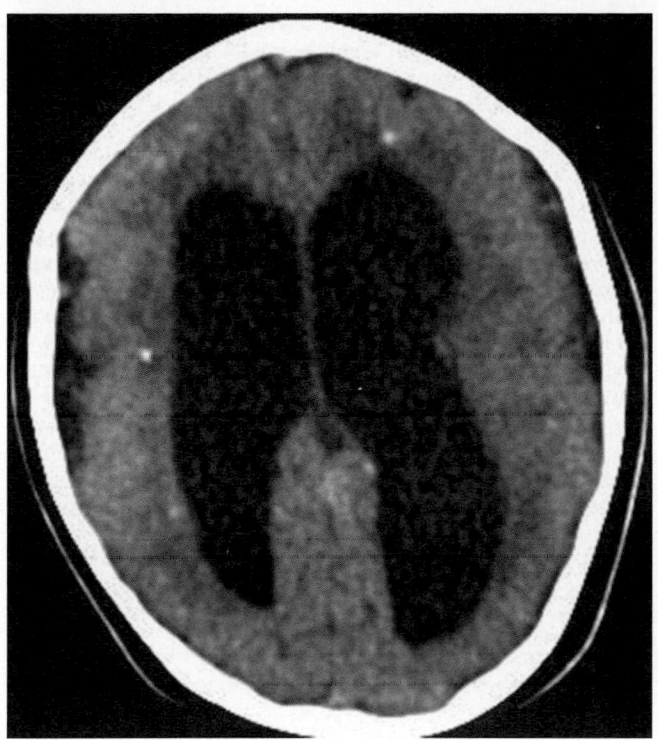

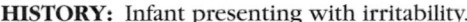

**Fig. 129.1**

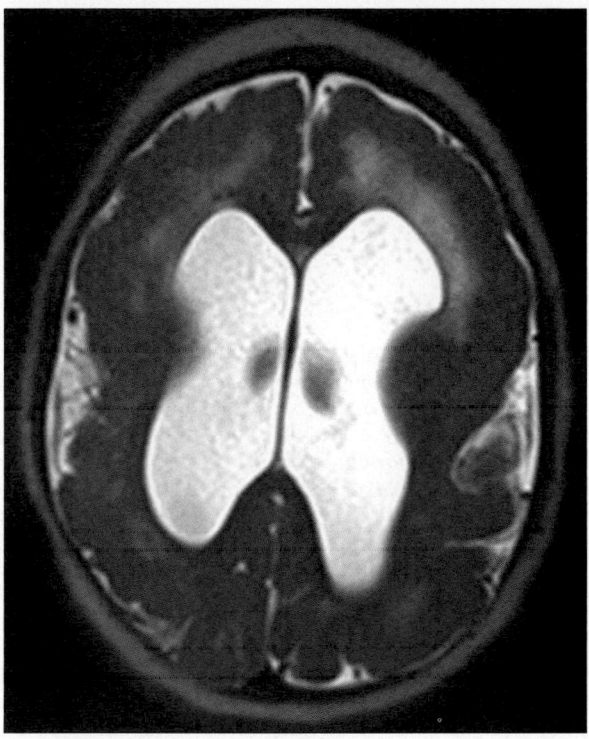

**Fig. 129.2**

**HISTORY:** Infant presenting with irritability.

1. Which of the following is the most common TORCH (toxoplasmosis, other [e.g. human immunodeficiency virus (HIV), lymphocytic choriomeningitis (LCM), syphilis, zika virus, varicella zoster], rubella, cytomegalovirus [CMV], and herpes) infection?
   A. CMV
   B. Herpes simplex type 1
   C. Human immunodeficiency virus (HIV)
   D. Rubella

2. Which of the following are seen in the case shown?
   A. Microcephaly
   B. Neuronal migrational disorder
   C. Myelination defect
   D. All of the above

3. Which head ultrasound (US) finding is accurate for TORCH infections?
   A. The periventricular/parenchymal calcifications typically have acoustic shadowing.
   B. Mineralizing vasculopathy indicates poor prognosis.
   C. Cerebellar hypoplasia is present.
   D. All of the above.

4. True or false?
   A. Active inflammatory lesions may have elevated *myo*-inositol (mI).
   B. Most TORCH infections will result in neuronal loss and ↓ NAA (*N*-acetylaspartate).

## CASE 129

### TORCH, Cytomegalovirus

1. A

2. D

3. C

4. A) True, B) True

## Comment

TORCH is the acronym for congenital infection of the central nervous system, which includes the following pathogens: *Toxoplasma gondii*, rubella virus, cytomegalovirus (CMV), herpes simplex virus 2 (HSV-2), human immunodeficiency virus (HIV), and *Treponema pallidum* (syphilis). Toxoplasmosis, CMV, HIV, and rubella all cause parenchymal calcifications, which are more extensive with CMV than with toxoplasmosis. The neuroimaging findings are variable depending on the timing and severity of injury. Microcephaly, intracranial calcifications, pachygyria/agyria, neuronal migrational anomalies, white matter abnormalities/delayed myelination, and cysts can be seen. It is important to remember that intracranial calcifications are not specific for congenital infections, and that ischemic/metabolic diseases may result in dystrophic calcifications as well. Linear branching hyperechogenicities can be seen in the basal ganglia with transfontanellar head ultrasound (US) and represent mineralizing vasculopathy, which can be seen in TORCH, trisomies, prenatal drug exposure, congenital heart disease and a variety of anoxic/toxic injuries, and as a normal variant (far more commonly). Therefore, mineralizing vasculopathy is a nonspecific finding, and unless additional abnormalities are seen in the brain, TORCH should not be strongly considered. Head US can be the first line of imaging for screening. It is important to note that calcifications in the brain do not result in acoustic shadowing. Toxoplasmosis is 10 times less common than CMV. The principal central nervous system (CNS) findings are chorioretinitis, hydrocephalus, and seizures. Unlike CMV, malformations of cortical development are uncommon. Toxoplasmosis calcifies the most frequently of the congenital infections (71% of the time in one series), but remember that the incidence of CMV is much higher. With treatment of congenital toxoplasmosis, 75% of cases show diminution or resolution of the intracranial calcifications by 1 year of age. The status of the calcifications often mirrors neurologic function. Rubella and HSV cause lobar destruction/encephalomalacia. HSV is often hemorrhagic, and syphilis causes basilar meningitis. Magnetic resonance imaging (MRI) is the modality of choice for full characterization of the lesions, and protocols should include susceptibility weighted imaging (SWI) or T2* gradient echo (GRE) sequences, which are sensitive for $Ca^{++}$ or hemorrhagic foci.

### Reference

Bale Jr JF. Congenital infections. *Neurol Clin*. 2002;20(4):1039–1060, vii.

### Cross-reference

Walters MM, Robertson RL. *Pediatric Radiology: The Requisites*. 4th ed. Philadelphia: Elsevier. 2017:291–293.

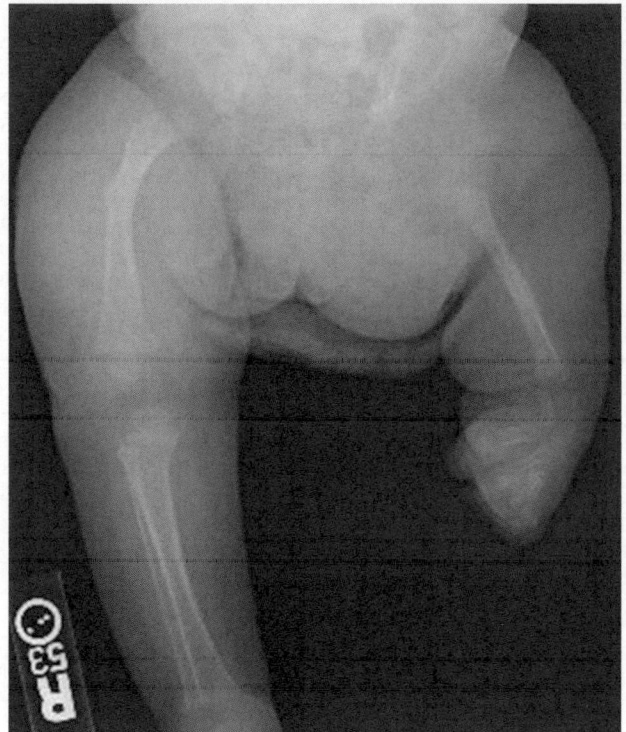

Fig. 130.1

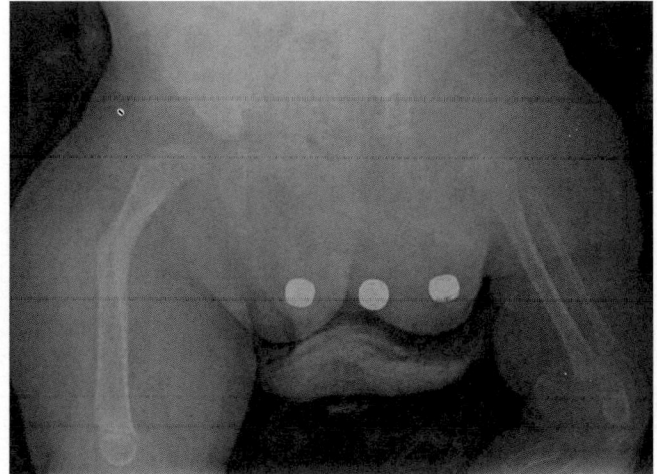

Fig. 130.2

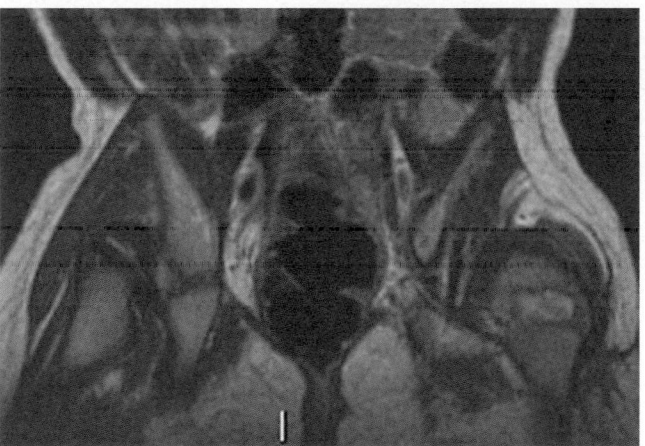

Fig. 130.3

1. What is the most likely diagnosis?
   A. Proximal femoral deficiency
   B. Proximal femoral deficiency with terminal fibular and tibial hemimelia
   C. Femoral deficiency and tibial hemimelia
   D. Femoral deficiency and fibular hemimelia

2. Which statement is true?
   A. Associated congenital defects in the lower extremities are rare in this entity.
   B. Associated congenital defects in the lower extremities are found in more than 50% of patients, with contralateral tibial deficiency being the most common.
   C. Associated congenital defects in the lower extremities are found in more than 50% of patients, with ipsilateral fibular deficiency being the most common.
   D. Associated congenital anomalies are seen in approximately one-third of patients, with renal anomalies being the most common.

3. Regarding the preferred imaging modality for diagnosis, which statement is accurate?
   A. Plain radiography of the lower extremities and pelvis is the choice for initial workup.
   B. Magnetic resonance imaging (MRI) is not necessary because the congenital anomaly itself and leg length discrepancy can be evaluated on radiographs.
   C. MRI is useful, especially in the young immature skeleton, because cartilaginous/nonossified structures are not seen in radiographs.
   D. None of the above.

4. True or false:
   A. Fibular shortening and foot abnormalities are highly associated; more severe limb shortening is associated with a greater amount of metatarsal agenesis.
   B. Tibial hemimelia is at least as common as fibular hemimelia.

## CASE 130

### Femoral Deficiency and Fibular Hemimelia

1. D

2. C

3. C

4. A) True, B) False

## Comment

Proximal focal femoral deficiency (PFFD) and fibular hemimelia (FH) are the most common causes of congenital lower extremity shortening. PFFD is characterized by variable degrees of shortening or absence of the femoral head, with associated dysplasia of the acetabulum and femoral shaft. It ranges from mild shortening to severe deficiency of the femoral head, acetabulum, and femoral shaft, as presented in this case (complete deficiency of the femur). Several factors, such as mutations or teratogens, can cause impairment of mesenchymal condensation and decelerate, or even abort, the onset of chondrification. This can partially explain the phylogenetic loss of certain skeletal structures, as in PFFD and FH. The classification of congenital skeletal limb deficiencies by Frantz and O'Rahilly has been used for evaluation since its publication in 1961. Conventional radiograph of the affected extremity in the frontal plane is the first line of imaging and is often sufficient for initial diagnosis. Magnetic resonance imaging (MRI) allows more complete characterization of the anatomical abnormalities, especially in skeletally immature patients, for early diagnosis and surgical planning. Radiographs cannot demonstrate fibrous or fibrocartilaginous connections between the femoral head and the femoral shaft, and the associated delay in the ossification of the femoral head. MRI examination should include evaluation of the size and configuration of the acetabulum and femoral head, femoroacetabular joint, femoral physis, subtrochanteric pseudarthrosis, and surrounding muscle atrophy.

Anteroposterior (AP) radiography of bilateral lower extremities nicely depicts the leg length discrepancy in this child. Angular deformity of the contralateral femur was appreciated on the radiographs in this case. MRI clearly contributes with identification of the right hip dislocation and presence of small right proximal femoral epiphysis, and confirmation of complete absence of the left femur, absence of the left acetabulum, and visualization of the proximal left tibial epiphysis creating pseudarthrosis with the ileum. Associated congenital anomalies are present in more than 50% of cases, with fibular hemimelia being the most common in up to 80%, as shown in this case.

### Reference

Bedoya MA, Chauvin NA, Jaramillo D, Davidson R, Horn BD, Ho-Fung V. Common patterns of congenital lower extremity shortening: diagnosis, classification, and follow-up. *Radiographics*. 2015;35(4): 1191–1207.

### Cross-reference

Walters MM, Robertson RL. *Pediatric Radiology: The Requisites*. 4th ed. Philadelphia: Elsevier. 2017:206–208.

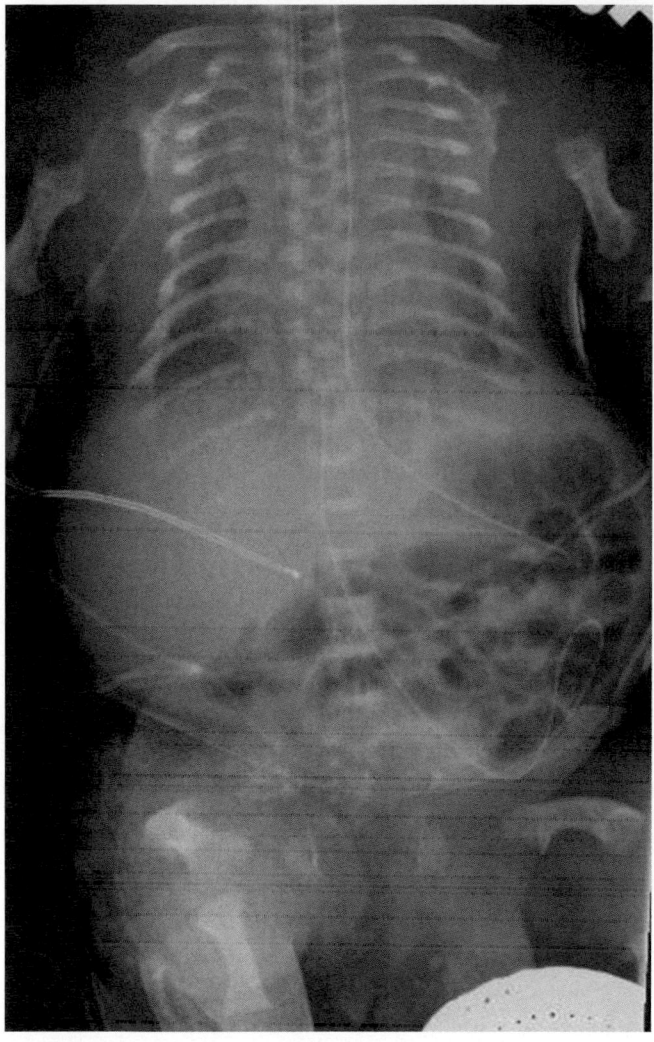

Fig. 131.1

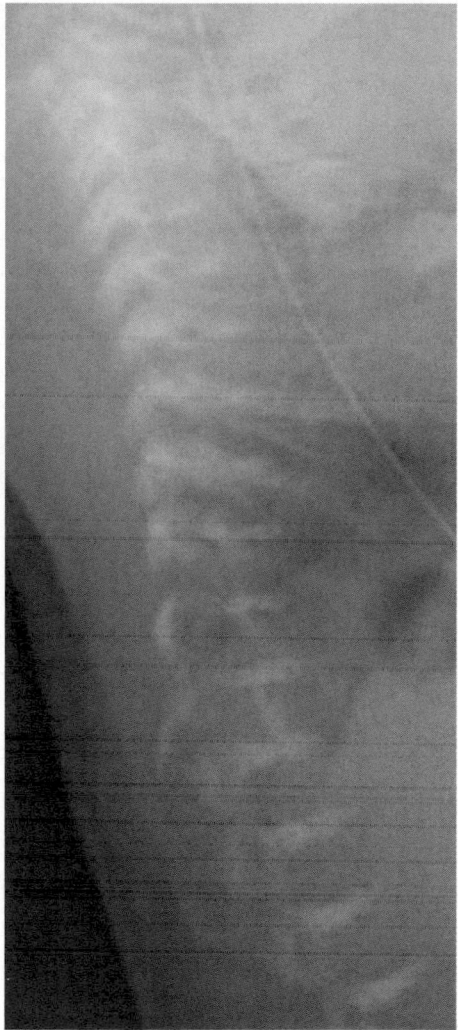

Fig. 131.2

**HISTORY:** Newborn presenting with rhizomelic limb shortening and respiratory insufficiency

1. Based on the images provided, which of the following is the best diagnosis?
   A. Jeune syndrome
   B. Thanatophoric dysplasia
   C. Morquio syndrome
   D. Osteogenesis imperfecta type II

2. Which of the following is the most common lethal skeletal dysplasia?
   A. Jeune syndrome
   B. Thanatophoric dysplasia
   C. Morquio syndrome
   D. Osteogenesis imperfecta type II

3. Which option is *not* a characteristic imaging finding in thanatophoric dysplasia?
   A. Small thorax with short horizontal ribs
   B. Platyspondyly
   C. Multiple fractures with hypertrophic callus formation
   D. Short, curved femurs

4. True or false?
   A. Thanatophoric dysplasia is uniformly fatal within hours to days.

## CASE 131

### Thanatophoric Dysplasia

1. B
2. B
3. C
4. True

## Comment

Thanatophoric dysplasia is the most common type of lethal skeletal dysplasia, occurring in about 1 out of 20,000 to 50,000 live births. It is uniformly fatal within hours to days due to respiratory insufficiency. Characteristic imaging findings include platyspondyly, a small thorax with short horizontal ribs, trident acetabulum, and rhizomelia with short, curved ("telephone receiver") femurs. Unlike osteogenesis imperfecta, multiple fractures are not characteristic. Jeune syndrome can also present with a small chest, but the spine is typically normal. Morquio syndrome is a member of the mucopolysaccharidosis group, which presents with findings of anteriorly beaked vertebral bodies, gibbus deformity of the spine, and thick "canoe-paddle" ribs (together referred to as dysostosis multiplex).

### Reference

Miller E, Blaser S, Shannon P, Widjaja E. Brain and bone abnormalities of thanatophoric dwarfism. *Am J Roentgenol*. 2009;192(1):48–51.

### Cross-reference

Walters MM, Robertson RL. *Pediatric Radiology: The Requisites*. 4th ed. Philadelphia: Elsevier. 2017:203–204.

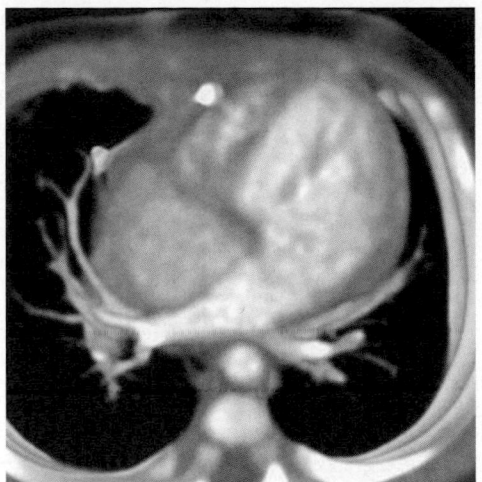

Fig. 132.1

See Supplemental Figures section for additional figures for this case.

**HISTORY:** Neonate presenting with congenital heart disease

1. Based on the imaging findings, which of the following would you include in your differential diagnosis?
   A. Ebstein anomaly
   B. Pulmonary atresia
   C. Tricuspid atresia
   D. Tetralogy of Fallot

2. What is the usual clinical presentation of tricuspid atresia?
   A. Incidental heart murmur
   B. Heart failure with poor feeding and failure to thrive
   C. Cyanosis
   D. Decreased blood pressure in the lower extremities

3. Which of the following associated congenital cardiac defects is obligatory for survival in the neonatal period in patients with tricuspid atresia?
   A. Patent ductus arteriosus
   B. Ventricular septal defect
   C. Atrial septal defect
   D. D-transposition of the great arteries

4. Which statement about tricuspid atresia is *not* correct?
   A. It is associated with D-transposition of the great arteries in 12% to 25% of cases.
   B. There is no established associated genetic predisposition.
   C. Prostaglandins are contraindicated in the immediate neonatal period to allow for closure of the ductus arteriosus.
   D. Cardiac size depends in part on the size of the ventricular septal defect (VSD).

## CASE 132

### Tricuspid Atresia

1. C

2. C

3. C

4. C

### Comment

Tricuspid atresia is the third most common cyanotic heart lesion. An atrial septal defect (ASD) is obligatory for survival, and if flow through the ASD is restrictive, the patient may need an emergent atrial septostomy. A patent ventricular septal defect (VSD) and/or patent ductus arteriosus (PDA) are required for pulmonary arterial flow, and prostaglandins are typically given to keep the ductus arteriosus open after birth. It is associated with D-transposition of the great arteries (in up to 25% of cases). Extracardiac anomalies occur in 20% of cases. It is typically diagnosed in utero, and 50% present with cyanosis in the first 24 hours. Surgery is staged, beginning with a modified Blalock-Taussig shunt with systemic artery-to-pulmonary artery (PA) anastomosis, followed by a bidirectional Glenn shunt (superior vena cava [SVC]-to-PA anastomosis) at 3 to 6 months, and finally completed with modified Fontan with inferior vena cava (IVC)-to-PA conduit at 2 to 3 years of age.

### Reference

Helbing WA, Ouhlous M. Cardiac magnetic resonance imaging in children. *Pediatr Radiol*. 2015;45(1):20–26.

### Cross-reference

Walters MM, Robertson RL. *Pediatric Radiology: The Requisites*. 4th ed. Philadelphia: Elsevier. 2017:81–82.

# Supplemental Figures

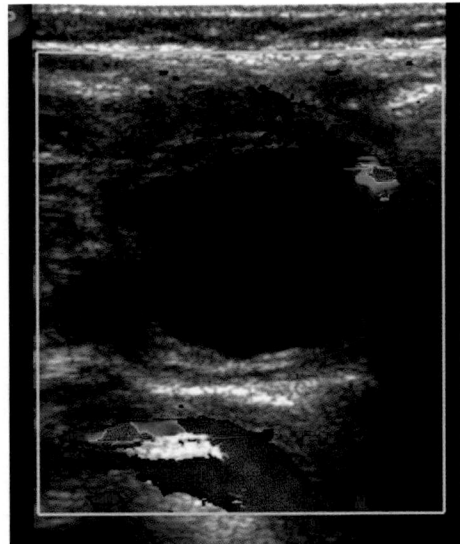

Fig. 26.3

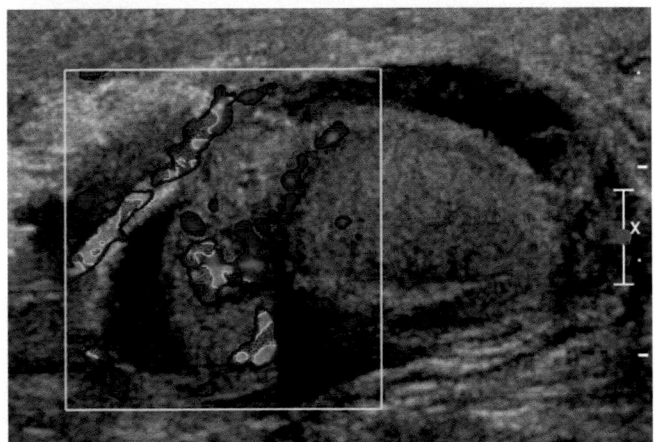

Fig. 40.2

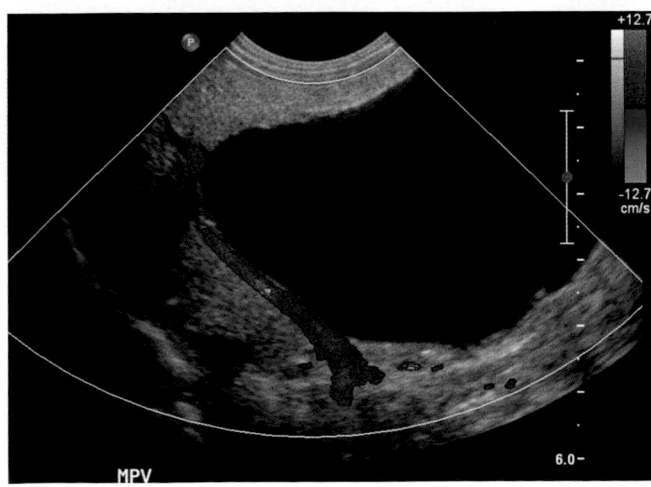

Fig. 71.4

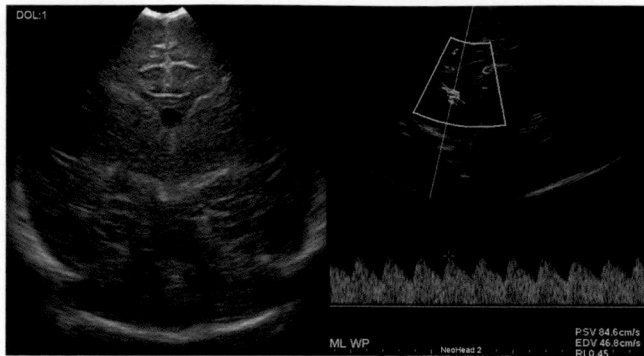

Fig. 122.2

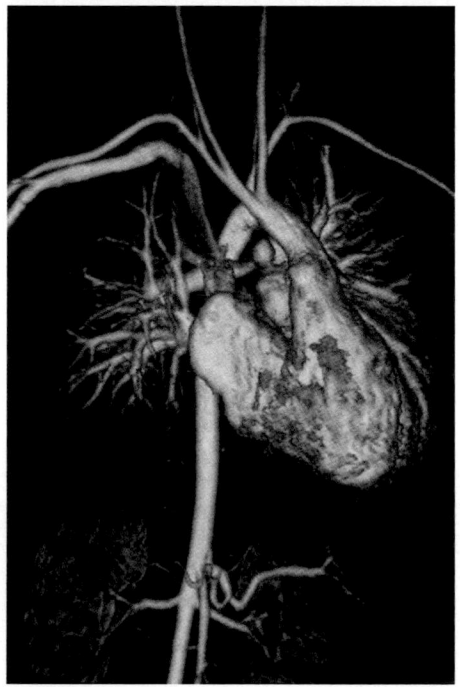

Fig. 125.3

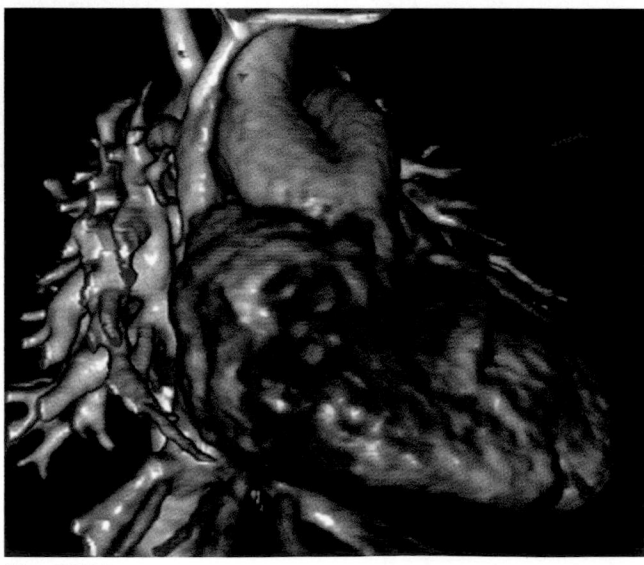

Fig. 126.3

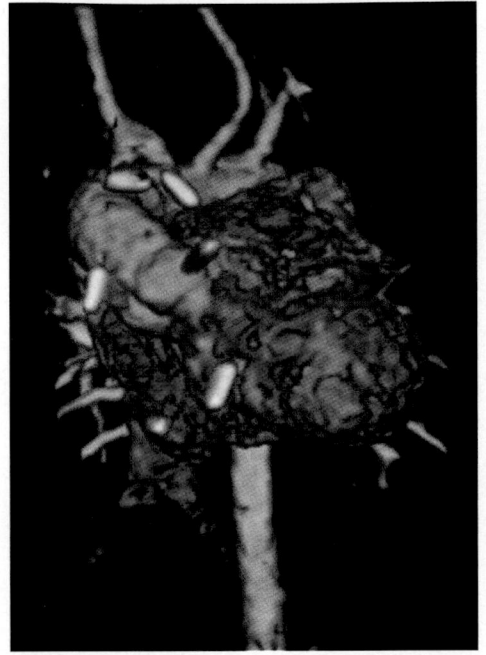

Fig. 132.2

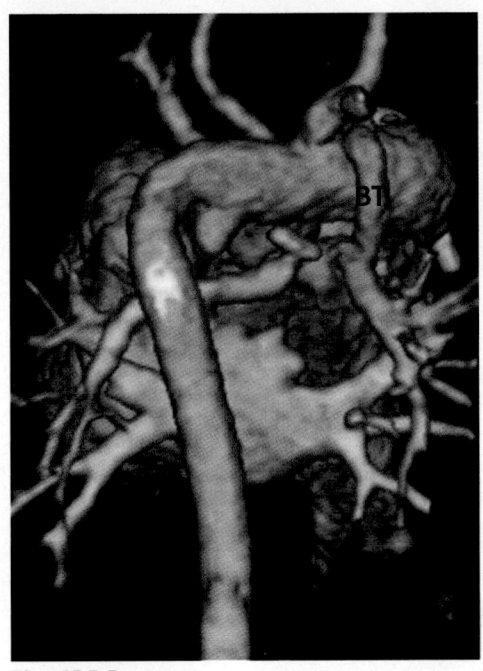

Fig. 132.3

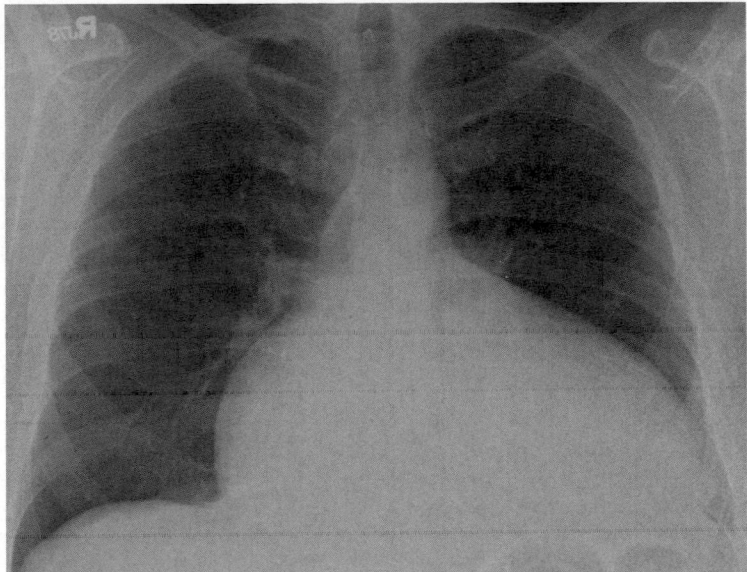

Fig. 133.1

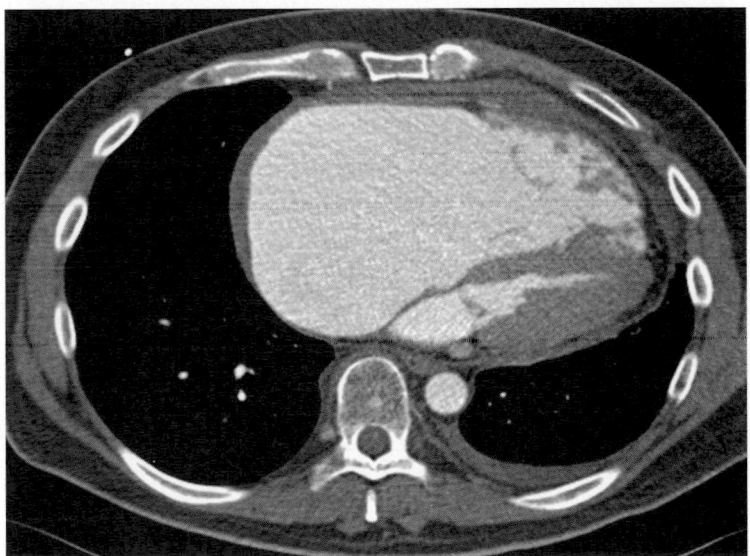

Fig. 133.2

**HISTORY:** Young adult male presenting with history of congenital cardiac anomaly

1. Based on the imaging findings, which of the following is the best diagnosis?
   A. Ebstein anomaly
   B. Pulmonary atresia with ventricular septal defect
   C. Pulmonary atresia with intact ventricular septum
   D. Tricuspid atresia
   E. Tetralogy of Fallot

2. Which option is *not* a potential therapeutic approach in the management of Ebstein anomaly?
   A. Right heart bypass with Glenn and Fontan shunts
   B. Tricuspid valve repair with valvuloplasty or prosthetic valve replacement
   C. Supportive management
   D. Systemic-to-PA (pulmonary artery) conduit with modified Blalock-Taussig shunt

3. Which statement about Ebstein anomaly is *not* true?
   A. It is the second most common cyanotic congenital heart defect.
   B. Presentation is variable, ranging from asymptomatic to profoundly cyanotic.
   C. Functional obstruction and massive tricuspid regurgitation leads to right atrial enlargement and the classic "box-shaped" heart appearance on plain film.
   D. It occurs with higher frequency in infants of mothers who take lithium during early pregnancy.

4. True or false?
   A. The prognosis in Ebstein is highly variable and is most dependent on the presence of cyanosis and the degree to which tricuspid regurgitation is hemodynamically significant.

## CASE 133

### Ebstein Anomaly

1. A

2. D

3. A

4. True

## Comment

Ebstein anomaly is a rare congenital cyanotic heart disease caused by downward displacement of septal and posterior leaflets of the tricuspid valve into the right ventricle ("atrialization of the right ventricle"). Presentation is variable, ranging from asymptomatic to profound cyanosis, depending on the hemodynamic significance of tricuspid atresia. Imaging classically shows massive right-sided cardiomegaly (box-shaped heart), although heart size may be normal early on, with enlargement over time. Pulmonary flow is typically decreased. In the setting of functional obstruction and regurgitation at the tricuspid valve, deoxygenated blood is shunted from the right atrium into the left atrium through a patent foramen ovale, resulting in cyanosis. Treatment in neonates is supportive, including treatment with nitric oxide to lower pulmonary vascular resistance. Definitive repair is with tricuspid valve bioprosthesis and/or reconstruction (valvuloplasty). Systemic-to-pulmonary arterial shunting (Blalock-Taussig shunt) is ineffective in these patients.

### Reference

Malik SB, Kwan D, Shah AB, Hsy JY. The right atrium: gateway to the heart—anatomic and pathologic imaging findings. *Radiographics*. 2015;35(1):14-31.

### Cross-reference

Walters MM, Robertson RL. *Pediatric Radiology: The Requisites*. 4th ed. Philadelphia: Elsevier. 2017:82.

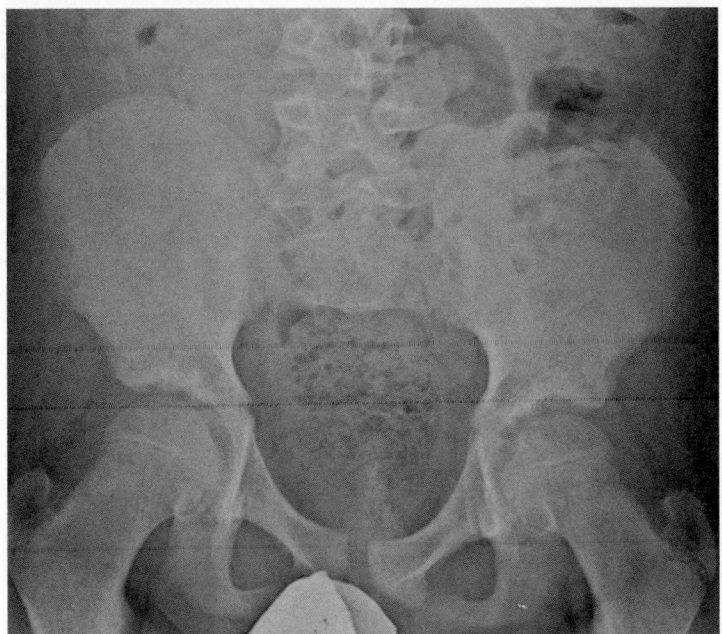

Fig. 134.1

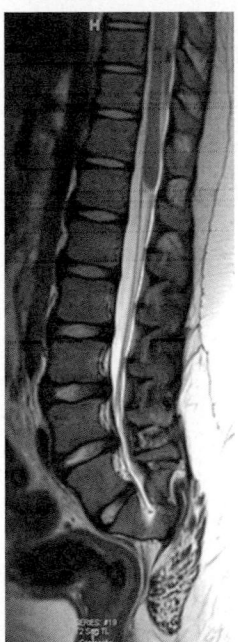

Fig. 134.2

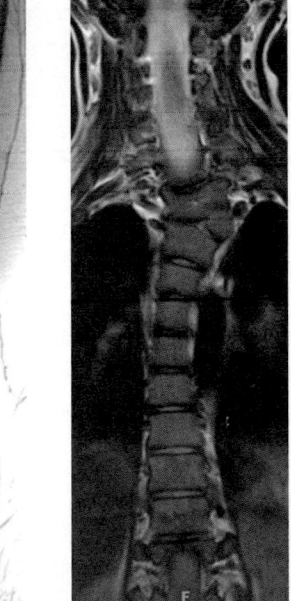

Fig. 134.3

**HISTORY:** Plain radiography and matching T2-weighted magnetic resonance imaging (MRI) of the pelvis and lumbar spine in a boy with hypoplastic lower extremities and coprostasis

1. Which signature pathologic imaging finding do you see on the plain radiograph?
   A. Bilateral coxa valga
   B. Bladder exstrophy
   C. Sacral agenesis
   D. Spina bifida occulta

2. What is the additional key finding noted on MRI to make the final diagnosis?
   A. Low positioned spinal cord
   B. Segmented spinal cord
   C. Club- or wedge-shaped inferior border of the spinal cord
   D. Widened terminal ventricle

3. What is the most likely diagnosis?
   A. Sacrococcygeal teratoma
   B. Caudal regression syndrome
   C. Diastematomyelia
   D. Myelomeningocele

4. Which additional findings are often found in association with the diagnosed entity?
   A. Vertebral segmentation anomalies
   B. Motility disorder of the bowel with coprostasis
   C. Hypoplastic lower extremities
   D. All of the above

## CASE 134

### Caudal Regression Syndrome

1. C
2. C
3. B
4. D

## Comment

Caudal regression syndrome is a severe disorder of the lower vertebral column with partial absence of the caudal spinal cord and matching vertebral osseous elements. Caudal regression syndrome is frequently associated with various urogenital tract malformations, pulmonary hypoplasia (due to renal insufficiency), imperforate anus, and lower limb abnormalities. In addition, caudal regression syndrome may be seen as part of the omphalocele, exstrophy, imperforate anus, spinal defects (OEIS) association.

Ultrasound and magnetic resonance imaging (MRI) are diagnostic. Imaging findings are characteristic with lack of the most distal segments of the spinal cord and matching musculoskeletal elements. Typically, the spinal cord abruptly terminates with a club- or wedge-shaped inferior border. The conus medullaris and terminal ventricle are lacking as well as the terminal filum. The overlying skin is intact but the lower extremities may be severely hypo- or dysplastic. In the most severe forms, the lower extremities may be fused (sirenomelia). The sacrum and coccyx are typically absent. Depending on the level of affection, additional lumbar or thoracic vertebral bodies may be lacking. The malformation can be categorized into two types depending on the location and shape of the conus medullaris: high and abrupt (type I) or low and tethered (type II). The hips are frequently dislocated and the musculature highly hypoplastic. Additional segmentation/formation anomalies of the thoracic or cervical vertebral bodies may be seen. The brain is typically normally developed.

Caudal regression syndrome is believed to result from a deficient secondary neurulation that involves the caudal cell mass.

### Reference

Huisman TA, Rossi A, Tortori-Donati P. MR imaging of neonatal spinal dysgraphia: what to consider? *Magn Reson Imaging Clin North Am.* 2012;20:45–61.

### Cross-reference

Walters MM, Robertson RL. *Pediatric Radiology: The Requisites.* 4th ed. Philadelphia: Elsevier. 2017:328.

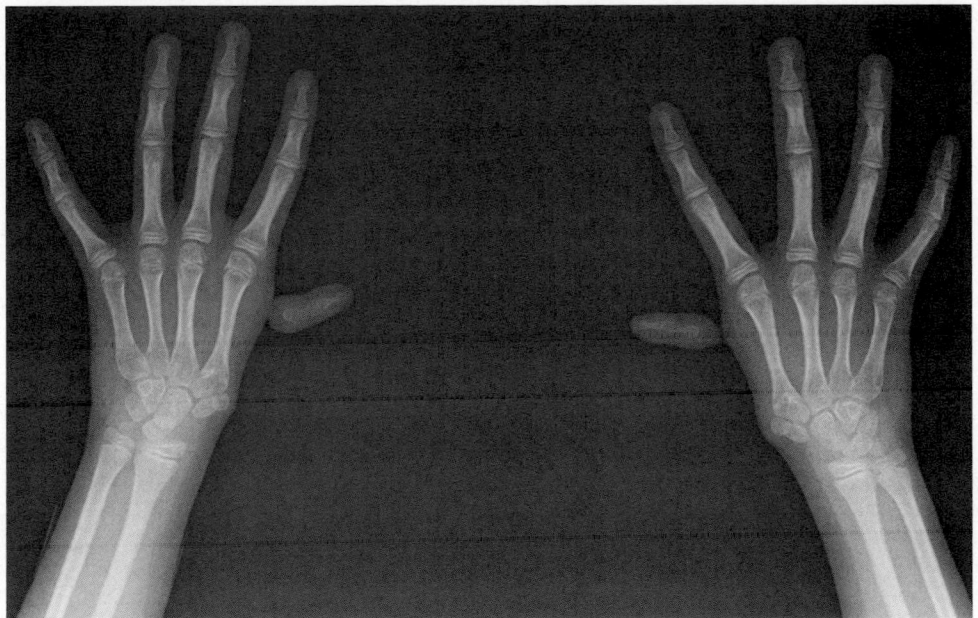

Fig. 135.1

**HISTORY:** Infant born with congenital defects

1. Given the imaging findings, which of the following would you include in your differential diagnosis? (Choose all that apply.)
   A. Thrombocytopenia absent radius (TAR) syndrome
   B. Holt-Oram syndrome
   C. VACTERL association
   D. Fanconi anemia

2. Which additional congenital anomalies could you expect to see in a patient with Holt-Oram syndrome?
   A. Polycystic kidneys
   B. Aqueductal stenosis
   C. Atrial septal defect (ASD)
   D. Biliary atresia

3. Which additional congenital anomalies could you expect to see in a patient with VACTERL association? (Choose all that apply.)
   A. Vertebral anomalies
   B. Alimentary tract/gastrointestinal (GI) anomalies
   C. Cardiac anomalies
   D. Thymic anomalies
   E. Eye anomalies
   F. Renal anomalies
   G. Laryngeal anomalies

4. Which statement about radial ray malformations is *not* true?
   A. TAR syndrome may present with an absent thumb.
   B. Holt-Oram syndrome may present with a triphalangeal thumb.
   C. Fanconi anemia may present with pancytopenia.
   D. Diagnosis is typically in utero during anatomical screening at 16 to 18 weeks' gestation.

## CASE 135

### Radial Ray Malformation

1. A, B, C, D

2. C

3. A, C, F

4. A

## Comment

Radial ray malformations comprise a spectrum of anomalies characterized by the absence or hypoplasia of the radius, the radial carpal bones, or the thumb. These are typically detected during a routine anatomical survey in utero at 16 to 18 weeks' gestational age and are associated with various syndromes, including Holt-Oram syndrome, thrombocytopenia absent radius (TAR) syndrome, VACTERL (vertebral defects, anal atresia, cardiac defects, tracheoesophageal fistula, renal anomalies, and limb abnormalities) association, and Fanconi anemia. Holt-Oram syndrome has associated cardiac defects, including atrial septal defect (ASD) and ventricular septal defect (VSD), and presents with variable degrees of radial deficiency, often asymmetric, and may include a triphalangeal thumb. Patients with TAR syndrome have radial ray anomalies, but always have both thumbs present and have associated thrombocytopenia. Patients with Fanconi anemia have associated pancytopenia, and radial ray defect in about 50% of cases, including thumb abnormalities (as seen in the patient in this case). Characteristic anomalies in patients with VACTERL association include vertebral, anorectal, cardiac, tracheoesophageal fistula with or without esophageal atresia, renal, and limb (including radial ray).

### Reference

Kennelly MM, Moran P. A clinical algorithm of prenatal diagnosis of radial ray defects with two and three dimensional ultrasound. *Prenat Diagn.* 2007;27(8):730-737.

### Cross-reference

Walters MM, Robertson RL. *Pediatric Radiology: The Requisites.* 4th ed. Philadelphia: Elsevier. 2017:208.

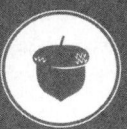

# Non-Interpretive Skills

1. During annual review, the chair of the radiology department notes that the number of head computed tomography (CT) scans ordered from the pediatric emergency room has significantly increased compared to prior years. Which of the following quality improvement tools could be used to evaluate all contributing causes of the overordering of head CTs?
   A. Cause-and-effect diagram ("Fishbone diagram")
   B. Six Sigma
   C. Peer review program
   D. Morbidity and mortality conference

2. A radiologist observes that reporting times are too long for radiographs performed in the pediatric emergency room. Which quality improvement tool could be used to visualize the contributing factors in order of significance?
   A. Pareto chart
   B. Control diagram
   C. Dashboard
   D. Check sheet

3. A pediatric radiologist aims to reduce patient wait time for outpatient ultrasound exams using Lean Six Sigma methodology. Which of the following is part of the Lean process?
   A. Involve staff members at all levels of the department.
   B. Allow for variations within different examination rooms to offer flexibility in the process.
   C. Limit the use of visual clues to avoid distractions.
   D. Focus only on adding value regardless of waste.

4. A pediatric radiologist at a tertiary care hospital is planning a quality improvement project to reduce the unnecessary chest radiographs ordered in the pediatric intensive care unit (PICU). Which of the following describes a methodology that emphasizes the ongoing nature of quality improvement?
   A. Benchmarking
   B. Plan-do-study-act (PDSA)
   C. Strengths-weaknesses-opportunities-threats (SWOT) analysis
   D. Root cause analysis

5. The chief of pediatric interventional radiology is asked to analyze and reduce the error rate in interventional radiology procedures. Which methodology can be used prospectively to prevent errors?
   A. Root cause analysis
   B. Strengths-weaknesses-opportunities-threats (SWOT) analysis
   C. Failure modes and effects analysis (FMEA)
   D. Six Sigma

6. What is the most appropriate study to perform in an 18-month-old child with suspected nonaccidental trauma without focal neurologic symptoms?
   A. Tc-99m bone scan
   B. Radiographic skeletal survey
   C. Head computed tomography (CT) with intravenous contrast
   D. Brain magnetic resonance imaging (MRI) without contrast.

7. A 13-year-old male presents with a history of right-sided partial seizures. What is the most appropriate imaging study to perform?
   A. Computed tomography (CT) of the head with and without contrast
   B. Positron emission tomography with computed tomography (PET/CT) of the brain
   C. Single-photon emission computed tomography (SPECT) of the brain
   D. Magnetic resonance imaging (MRI) scan of the head without contrast

8. Which of the following is a component of the Image Gently Pledge?
   A. To accept suggestions only from radiologists, but not from technologists or other members of the care team.
   B. To always perform a right lower quadrant ultrasound for suspected appendicitis prior to ordering an abdominal computed tomography (CT) scan.
   C. To review recommended protocols and implement changes when necessary.
   D. To promote Image Gently to parents and the community at large.

9. An 8-year-old male has a history of hives after intravenous contrast administration in the past. He now requires a computed tomography (CT) scan of the abdomen and pelvis with contrast. What is the most appropriate next step in this case?
   A. Perform the exam without premedication.
   B. Premedicate with prednisone 0.5–0.7 mg/kg PO (up to 50 mg) at 13, 7, and 2 hours prior to contrast administration and diphenhydramine 1.25 mg/kg PO (up to 50 mg) 1 hour prior to contrast administration.
   C. Premedicate with solumedrol 0.5 mg/kg IV 4 hours prior to contrast administration.
   D. Premedicate with diphenhydramine 1.25 mg/kg PO (up to 50 mg) only.

10. A 10-year-old girl presents with her mother for a magnetic resonance imaging (MRI) scan of the abdomen. In which MRI zone does patient screening typically takes place?
    A. Zone 1
    B. Zone 2
    C. Zone 3
    D. Zone 4

## Question 1

Answer: A

### Comment

A cause-and-effect diagram is a useful quality improvement tool for identifying multiple contributing factors of a particular problem. The causes can be separated by category, which aids in visualization and understanding of all possible elements. Other analysis tools for quality improvement include Pareto charts, flow charts, and control charts. Six Sigma is a technique to improve processes. Peer review is a method to evaluate radiologist performance. A morbidity and mortality conference is used to evaluate an adverse outcome.

### References

Kruskal JB, Eisenberg R, Sosna J, Yam CS, Kruskal JD, Boiselle PM. Quality improvement in radiology: basic principles and tools required to achieve success. *Radiographics.* 2011;31(6):1499–1509.

Kruskal JH, Anderson S, Yam CS, Sosna J. Strategies for establishing a comprehensive quality and performance improvement program in a radiology department. *Radiographics.* 2011;29(2):315–329.

## Question 2

Answer: A

### Comment

A Pareto chart is a bar graph that ranks the significance of causes that contribute to a problem from highest to lowest value. This allows identification of the most important factors to focus on when making improvements. A control diagram allows visualization of data over time. A dashboard is a visualization of benchmarks that allows real-time review of data. A checksheet is a structured form that can be used to collect data.

### References

Katzman GL, Paushter DM. Building a culture of continuous quality improvement in an academic radiology department. *J Am Coll Radiol.* 2016;13(4):453–460.

Kruskal JB, Eisenberg R, Sosna J, Yam CS, Kruskal JD, Boiselle PM. Quality Improvement in radiology: basic principles and tools required to achieve success. *Radiographics.* 2011;31(6):1499–1509.

## Question 3

Answer: B

### Comment

The Lean practice is a system created by Toyota with the goals of improving quality and eliminating waste. Lean principles include: respecting and involving staff at all levels of the organization, assessing the current state of the workplace, eliminating waste, standardizing work and processes, and using visual clues.

### References

Katzman GL, Paushter DM. Building a culture of continuous quality improvement in an academic radiology department. *J Am Coll Radiol.* 2016;13(4):453–460.

Kruskal JB, Reedy A, Pascal L, Rosen MP, Boiselle PM. Quality initiatives: lean approach to improving performance and efficiency in a radiology department. *Radiographics.* 2012;32(2):573–587.

## Question 4

Answer: B

### Comment

The plan-do-study-act (PDSA) cycle is a widely used methodology for quality improvement that consists of planning a change to implement, doing the implementation, studying the results of the change, and acting on the results by starting another cycle. Benchmarking refers to comparing measurable metrics to acceptable levels. A strengths-weaknesses-opportunities-threats (SWOT) analysis may be used to identify possible quality improvement projects. A root cause analysis is a method used to evaluate the causes of an adverse outcome.

### References

Bruno MA, Nagy P. Fundamentals of quality and safety in diagnostic radiology. *J Am Coll Radiol.* 2014;11:1115–1120.

Tamm EP, Szklaruk J, Puthooran L, Stone D, Stevens BL, Modaro C. Quality initiatives: planning, setting up, and carrying out radiology process improvement projects. *Radiographics.* 2012;32:1529–1542.

## Question 5

Answer: C

### Comment

Failure modes and effects analysis (FMEA) describes a prospective method used to evaluate a process in an attempt to determine what might go wrong, to reduce the risk that such events might happen. A root cause analysis, on the other hand, is a retrospective method used to evaluate what *did* go wrong after an adverse event has occurred.

### References

Abujudeh HH, Kaewlai R. Radiology failure mode and effect analysis: what is it? *Radiology.* 2009;252(2):544–550.

Bruno MA, Nagy P. Fundamentals of quality and safety in diagnostic radiology. *J Am Coll Radiol.* 2014;11:1115–1120.

## Question 6

Answer: B

### Comment

According to the American College of Radiology (ACR) Appropriateness Criteria, a radiographic skeletal survey is the most appropriate imaging study in the evaluation of suspected child abuse in children younger than 24 months. A Tc-99m bone scan may be used if the skeletal survey is negative and clinical concern for nonaccidental trauma remains high. A head computed tomography (CT) or brain magnetic resonance imaging (MRI) scan is usually appropriate if the child presents with neurologic signs and symptoms.

### Reference

Meyer JS, Coley BD, Karmazyn B. ACR appropriateness criteria® suspected physical abuse-child. *J Am Coll Radiol.* <https://acsearch.acr.org/docs/69443/Narrative/>; Accessed July 2016.

## Question 7

Answer: D

### Comment

According to the American College of Radiology (ACR) Appropriateness Criteria, the most appropriate imaging study for this patient is a magnetic resonance imaging (MRI) scan of the head without contrast. Abnormal imaging findings are much more likely to be found in patients with partial seizures as opposed to those presenting with generalized seizures. MRI is more sensitive than computed tomography (CT) in these cases. Nuclear medicine imaging with positron emission tomography (PET) or single-photon emission computed tomography (SPECT) of the brain may be useful in patients with recurrent seizures in whom MRI was normal.

### References

Dory CE, Coley BD, Karmazyn B. ACR appropriateness criteria® seizures-child. *J Am Coll Radiol*. <https://acsearch.acr.org/docs/69441/Narrative/>;Accessed July 2016.

Garvey MA, Gaillard WD, Rusin JA, et al. Emergency brain computed tomography in children with seizures: who is most likely to benefit? *J Pediatr*. 1998;133(5):664-669.

Sharma S, Riviello JJ, Harper MB, Baskin MN. The role of emergent neuroimaging in children with new onset afebrile seizures. *Pediatrics*. 2003;111(1):1-5.

## Question 8

Answer: C

### Comment

The Image Gently campaign was created in 2007 by a coalition of major healthcare associations. The goal of the campaign is to improve safe and effective imaging of children. A major goal of the Image Gently Pledge is to raise awareness of opportunities to reduce radiation dose in pediatric imaging.

### References

Goske MJ, Applegate KE, Boylan J, et al. The Image Gently campaign: working together to change practice. *Am J Roentgenol*. 2008;190:273-274.

Image Gently. <http://www.imagegently.org/>;Accessed July 2016.

## Question 9

Answer: B

### Comment

Although there have been no controlled, prospective studies evaluating the efficacy of premedication for intravenous contrast allergies, the American College of Radiology (ACR) recommends premedication for pediatric patients that is similar to that recommended for adult patients. Allergic reactions to iodinated contrast may still occur after premedication, and therefore, close monitoring of premedicated patients is still recommended.

### References

*ACR Committee on Drugs and Contrast Media*. ACR manual on contrast media, version 10.1. Reston, VA. <http://www.acr.org/quality-safety/resources/contrast-manual/>; 2015.

Dillman JR, Strouse PJ, Ellis JH, Cohan RH, Jan SC. Incidence and severity of acute allergic-like reactions to i.v. nonionic iodinated contrast material in children. *AJR Am J Roentgenol*. 2007;188(6):1643-1647.

## Question 10

Answer: B

### Comment

A magnetic resonance (MR) facility is divided into four zones to facilitate site restrictions. Zone 1 is accessible to the general public. Zone 2 is the zone between the accessible areas and controlled areas, and is where patient screening typically takes place. Zone 3 is where the control room is typically located and Zone 4 is the MRI scanner room.

### Reference

Kanal EK, Barkovich AJ, Bell C, et al. ACR guidance document on MR safe practices: 2013. *J Magn Reson Imaging*. 2013;37:501-530.

# Radiation

1.  If a pregnant patient undergoes a computed tomography (CT) scan of the chest, what is the main source of radiation exposure to the fetus?
    A. Primary x-ray radiation
    B. Leakage radiation
    C. Internal scatter radiation
    D. Natural background radiation

2.  What is the effect on the radiation dose of lowering the tube voltage in pediatric computed tomography (CT) when all other scan parameters remain unchanged?
    A. Decreases
    B. Increases
    C. No change
    D. Initially increases then decreases

3.  How does radiation dose in computed tomography (CT) vary with tube current (in milliamperes [mA])?
    A. Linearly
    B. Inversely
    C. Exponentially
    D. Logarithmically

4.  Which parameter, when changed, results in a directly proportional change in patient dose?
    A. Tube current (in milliamperes [mA])
    B. Tube voltage (in kilovolts [kV])
    C. Pitch
    D. Slice thickness

5.  Which quantity represents the total energy deposited in a standard phantom?
    A. Effective dose
    B. Dose length product (DLP)
    C. Computed tomography dose index volume (CTDIvol)
    D. Size-specific dose estimate

## Question 1

Answer: C

### Comment

Because the fetus is not in the primary path of exposure during a chest computed tomography (CT) scan, the main source of exposure to the fetus is internal scatter radiation. Internal scatter radiation diminishes with distance from the primary source of exposure.

### Reference

Tremblay E, Therasse E, Naggara IT, Trop I. Guidelines for use of medical imaging during pregnancy and lactation. *Radiographics*. 2012;32:897–911.

## Question 2

Answer: A

### Comment

Tube voltage is one of the primary factors that impacts radiation dose and image quality. It is established that lower tube voltage is advantageous in lowering the radiation dose in pediatric computed tomography (CT). Because the patients are small in pediatric CT, lowering the tube voltage from 120 kV to 100 kV reduces the radiation dose by nearly 30%. Hence, adjusting the tube voltage based on patient size is recommended.

### References

Mahesh M. *MDCT Physics: The Basics—Technology, Image Quality and Radiation Dose*. Philadelphia, PA: Lippincott Williams and Wilkins; 2009.

Mayo-Smith WW, Hara AK, Mahesh M, Sahani DV, Pavlicek W. How I do it: managing radiation dose in CT. *Radiology*. 2014;273(3):657–672.

## Question 3

Answer: A

### Comment

Tube current is one of the primary factors that impacts radiation dose and image quality. Tube current can be considered as the indicator of "quantity" in x-ray imaging. The relationship between tube current and patient dose is linear. Hence, doubling tube current would double the patient dose and vice versa.

### References

Bushberg JT, Seibert JA, Leidholdt EM, Boone JM. *The Essential Physics of Medical Imaging*. Philadelphia, PA; London: Wolters Kluwer Health/Lippincott Williams & Wilkins; 2012.

Singh S, Kalra MK, Thrall JH, Mahesh M. CT radiation dose reduction by modifying primary factors. *J Am Coll Radiol*. 2011;8(5):369–372.

## Question 4

Answer: A

### Comment

Tube current is one of the primary factors that impacts radiation dose and image quality. Tube current can be considered as the indicator of "quantity" in x-ray imaging. The relationship between tube current and patient dose is linear. Hence, doubling tube current would double the patient dose and vice versa.

### References

Durand DJ, Mahesh M. Understanding CT dose display. *J Am Coll Radiol*. 2012;9(9):669–671.

Bushberg JT, Seibert JA, Leidholdt EM, Boone JM. *The Essential Physics of Medical Imaging*. Philadelphia, PA; London: Wolters Kluwer Health/Lippincott Williams & Wilkins; 2012

## Question 5

Answer: B

### Comment

The two main radiation dose descriptors are $CTDI_{vol}$ and dose length product (DLP). $CTDI_{vol}$ is an index that provides radiation dose output of a scanner measured at the center of a tissue-equivalent phantom. DLP is a product of $CTDI_{vol}$ and scan length. Therefore, DLP represents the total energy deposited in a standard phantom.

### Reference

Durand DJ, Mahesh M. Understanding CT dose display. *J Am Coll Radiol*. 2012;9(9):669–671.

Mayo-Smith WW, Hara AK, Mahesh M, Sahani DV, Pavlicek W. How I do it: managing radiation dose in CT. *Radiology*. 2014;273(3):657–672.

## Cardiovascular

## Chest

## GI

## GU

## Head & Neck

## MSK

## Neuro

## Radiation

## Various

# A

Group B streptococcal pneumonia, surfactant deficiency disease *vs.*, 19-20

Growth disturbance, in Salter-Harris fractures, 36

## H

Haemophilus influenzae
  as causative agents in round pneumonia, 67-68
  type B, epiglottitis due to, 41-42
Hand- Schuller-Christian, Langerhans cell histiocytosis and, 140
Head and neck, vascular anomalies in, 185-186
Heart failure, in infants with symptomatic coarctation, 123-124
Hemangioendothelioma, Kaposiform, 215-216, 215f
Hemangioma, infantile hepatic, 203-204, 203f
Hematomas, testicular germ cell tumor and, 162
Hemihypertrophy, 159-160
Hemihypertrophy syndrome, perilobar nephrogenic rests and, 229-230
Hemorrhage
  adrenal, neonatal, 127-128, 127f
  germinal matrix, 85-86, 85f
  pulmonary, acute complications of surfactant deficiency disease, 19-20
  rim of, invasive aspergillosis and, 129-130
Hepatic cirrhosis, biliary obstruction and, 145-146
Hepatic fibrosis, ARPCKD associated with, 251-252
Hepatoblastoma, 149-150, 149f
  clinical presentation of, 149-150
  treatment of, 149-150
Hernia
  congenital diaphragmatic, 55-56, 55f
  congenital inguinal, 75-76, 75f
Herniation
  in omphalocele, 212
  solid organ, incidence of, 75-76
Heterotaxy syndromes, 241-242
Hirschsprung disease, 51-52, 51f
Hodgkin lymphoma, 121-122, 121f
  staging options for, 121-122
  type IV, 121-122
Holoprosencephaly, 260
Holt-Oram syndrome
  atrial septal defect and, 275-276
  radial ray malformations and, 275-276
  triphalangeal thumb and, 275-276
Horseshoe kidney, 79-80
H-type malformation, 22
Human papilloma virus (HPV), papillomatosis and, 138
Hurler syndrome, 187-188
Hyaline membrane disease, 19-20
Hydatid cyst, component of, 239-240
Hydatid disease, 239-240, 239f
Hydrocele, testicular torsion and, 82
Hydrometrocolpos, 97-100, 99f
Hydronephrosis, marked, in ureteropelvic junction obstruction, 43-44
Hydroxyapatite, 238
Hyperdensity, medulloblastoma, 247-248
Hyperechoic kidneys, enlarged, 251-252
Hyperechoic masses, in meconium ileus, 28
Hyperinflation, in bronchiolitis, 33-34
Hyperlucent lung, in Swyer-James syndrome, 235-236
Hyperosmotic enema, for meconium ileus, 28
Hypertrophic pyloric stenosis, 93-94
Hypophosphatasia, hypophosphatemic rickets and, 237-238
Hypophosphatemic rickets, 237-238, 237f
Hypoplastic left heart, 101-102
Hypoplastic left heart syndrome, 101-102, 101f
Hypothyroidism
  infantile hepatic hemangioma and, 203-204
  slipped capital femoral epiphysis and, 47-48
Hypoxic-ischemic encephalopathy (HIE), 249-250, 249f
  neuroimaging findings of, 249-250
  in newborns, 249-250

## I

Idiopathic intussusception, 54
Ileocecal syndrome, 73-74

Ileum
  distal
    homogeneous enhancement and thickening of bowel wall, in Crohn disease, 169-170
    neonatal obstruction of, 27-28
  terminal, in Crohn disease, 169-170
  thickened wall of terminal, 5-6
Iliac osteotomy, OEIS and, 231-232
Image-defined risk factors (IDRFs), 16
Image-guided pressure reduction, for intussusception, 54
Immune system disorder, chronic granulomatous disease, 205-206, 205f
Infantile hemangioma, 151-152, 151f
  clinical presentation of, 151-152
  hepatic, 203-204, 203f
Infants
  alpha angle in, 11-12
  preterm, ventilation support for, 17-18
  screening of, for DDH, 11-12
Infection, in hypoxic-ischemic encephalopathy, 249-250
Inferior herniation, of bowel loops, 75-76
Inflammation, in hypoxic-ischemic encephalopathy, 249-250
Inguinal hernia, 222
  congenital, 75-76, 75f
Inlet/inflow ventricular septal defect, endocardial cushion defect and, 189-190
International Neuroblastoma Risk Group Staging System (INRGSS), 16
International Reflux Study Committee, grading system, 25-26
International Society for the Study of Vascular Anomalies (ISSVA), for vascular tumors and vascular malformation classification, 151-152
Interpediculate distance, reduced, in achondroplasia, 3-4
Intestinal malrotation, 63-64, 63f, 214
  midgut volvulus and, 141-142
  omphalocele, incidence of, 63-64
Intraabdominal injuries, in children, 61-62
Intralobar nephrogenic rests, 229-230
Intralobar sequestration, 30
Intraperitoneal tumor seeding, 23-24
Intrascrotal appendages, torsion of, 82
Intrauterine vascular obstruction, jejunal atresia due to, 59-60
Intravesical ureteroceles, 117-118
Intrinsic obstruction of airway, by foreign body, 77-78
Intussusception, 53-54, 53f
Ipsilateral fibular deficiency, 265-266
Irritability, idiopathic intussusception and, 53-54

## J

Jatene procedure, 255-256
Jaundice, neonatal, 7
Jejunal atresia, 59-60, 59f
Jejunoileal atresia, 60
Joint spaces, Langerhans cell histiocytosis and, 139-140

## K

Kaposiform hemangioendothelioma, 215-216, 215f
Kasabach-Merritt phenomenon, 215-216
Kasai procedure, biliary atresia and, 7-8
Kidneys
  autosomal recessive polycystic disease, 251-252, 251f
  clear cell sarcoma of, 159-160
  duplicated, segmentation of, multicystic dysplastic kidney and, 65-66
  horseshoe, 79-80
  hyperechoic, enlarged, 251-252
  left, hydrometrocolpos and, 99-100
  multicystic dysplastic, 65-66, 65f
    multilocular cystic renal tumor and, 227-228
  multiple cysts in, 261-262
  pelvic, in Mayer-Rokitansky-Küster-Hauser syndrome, 226
  reniform shape of, 251-252
Klippel-Trenaunay syndrome, lymphatic malformation and, 185-186

## L

Labor, prolonged, TTN in, 125-126
Langerhans cell histiocytosis, 139-140, 139f
Large bowel, wall of, air in, 37-38